T0263697

Vascular Disease

Editor

LEONARDO C. CLAVIJO

CARDIOLOGY CLINICS

www.cardiology.theclinics.com

Consulting Editors
ROSARIO FREEMAN
JORDAN M. PRUTKIN
DAVID M. SHAVELLE
AUDREY H. WU

February 2015 • Volume 33 • Number 1

ELSEVIER

1600 John F. Kennedy Boulevard • Suite 1800 • Philadelphia, Pennsylvania, 19103-2899

http://www.theclinics.com

CARDIOLOGY CLINICS Volume 33, Number 1
February 2015 ISSN 0733-8651, ISBN-13: 978-0-323-35436-3

Editor: Adrianne Brigido
Developmental Editor: Susan Showalter

© **2015 Elsevier Inc. All rights reserved.**

This periodical and the individual contributions contained in it are protected under copyright by Elsevier, and the following terms and conditions apply to their use:

Photocopying
Single photocopies of single articles may be made for personal use as allowed by national copyright laws. Permission of the Publisher and payment of a fee is required for all other photocopying, including multiple or systematic copying, copying for advertising or promotional purposes, resale, and all forms of document delivery. Special rates are available for educational institutions that wish to make photocopies for non-profit educational classroom use. For information on how to seek permission visit www.elsevier.com/permissions or call: (+44) 1865 843830 (UK)/(+1) 215 239 3804 (USA).

Derivative Works
Subscribers may reproduce tables of contents or prepare lists of articles including abstracts for internal circulation within their institutions. Permission of the Publisher is required for resale or distribution outside the institution. Permission of the Publisher is required for all other derivative works, including compilations and translations (please consult www.elsevier.com/permissions).

Electronic Storage or Usage
Permission of the Publisher is required to store or use electronically any material contained in this periodical, including any article or part of an article (please consult www.elsevier.com/permissions). Except as outlined above, no part of this publication may be reproduced, stored in a retrieval system or transmitted in any form or by any means, electronic, mechanical, photocopying, recording or otherwise, without prior written permission of the Publisher.

Notice
No responsibility is assumed by the Publisher for any injury and/or damage to persons or property as a matter of products liability, negligence or otherwise, or from any use or operation of any methods, products, instructions or ideas contained in the material herein. Because of rapid advances in the medical sciences, in particular, independent verification of diagnoses and drug dosages should be made.

Although all advertising material is expected to conform to ethical (medical) standards, inclusion in this publication does not constitute a guarantee or endorsement of the quality or value of such product or of the claims made of it by its manufacturer.

Cardiology Clinics (ISSN 0733-8651) is published quarterly by Elsevier Inc., 360 Park Avenue South, New York, NY 10010-1710. Months of issue are February, May, August, and November. Business and Editorial Offices: 1600 John F. Kennedy Blvd., Ste. 1800, Philadelphia, PA 19103-2899. Customer Service Office: 3251 Riverport Lane, Maryland Heights, MO 63043. Periodicals postage paid at New York, NY and additional mailing offices. Subscription prices are $320.00 per year for US individuals, $530.00 per year for US institutions, $155.00 per year for US students and residents, $390.00 per year for Canadian individuals, $665.00 per year for Canadian institutions, $455.00 per year for international individuals, $665.00 per year for international institutions and $220.00 per year for Canadian and international students/residents. To receive student/resident rate, orders must be accompanied by name of affiliated institution, data of term, and the *signature* of program/residency coordinator on institution letterhead. Orders will be billed at individual rate until proof of status is received. Foreign air speed delivery is included in all *Clinics* subscription prices. All prices are subject to change without notice. **POSTMASTER:** Send address changes to *Cardiology Clinics*, Elsevier Health Sciences Division, Subscription Customer Service, 3251 Riverport Lane, Maryland Heights, MO 63043. **Customer Service: 1-800-654-2452 (U.S. and Canada); 314-447-8871 (outside U.S. and Canada). Fax: 314-447-8029. E-mail: journalscustomerservice-usa@ elsevier.com (for print support); journalsonlinesupport-usa@elsevier.com (for online support).**

Reprints. For copies of 100 or more, of articles in this publication, please contact the Commercial Reprints Department, Elsevier Inc., 360 Park Avenue South, New York, NY 10010-1710. Tel.: 212-633-3874; Fax: 212-633-3820; E-mail: reprints@elsevier.com.

Cardiology Clinics is also published in Spanish by McGraw-Hill Interamericana Editores S. A., P.O. Box 5-237, 06500, Mexico D. F., Mexico; in Portuguese by Reichmann and Alfonso Editores Rio de Janeiro, Brazil; and in Greek by Dimitrios P. Lagos, 8 Pondon Street, GR115-28 Ilissia, Greece.

Cardiology Clinics is covered in *MEDLINE/PubMed (Index Medicus), Excerpta Medica, The Cumulative Index to Nursing and Allied Health Literature* (CINAHL).

Contributors

EDITORIAL BOARD

ROSARIO FREEMAN, MD, MS, FACC
Associate Professor of Medicine; Director, Coronary Care Unit; Director, Echocardiography Laboratory, University of Washington Medical Center, Seattle, Washington

JORDAN M. PRUTKIN, MD, MHS, FHRS
Assistant Professor of Medicine, Division of Cardiology/Electrophysiology, University of Washington Medical Center, Seattle, Washington

DAVID M. SHAVELLE, MD, FACC, FSCAI
Associate Professor, Keck School of Medicine; Director, General Cardiovascular Fellowship Program; Director, Cardiac Catheterization Laboratory, Los Angeles County + USC Medical Center; Division of Cardiovascular Medicine, University of Southern California, Los Angeles, California

AUDREY H. WU, MD
Assistant Professor, Internal Medicine, University of Michigan, Ann Arbor, Michigan

EDITOR

LEONARDO C. CLAVIJO, MD, PhD
Director, Interventional Cardiology Fellowship Program; Director, Vascular Medicine and Peripheral Interventions, Division of Cardiovascular Medicine, University of Southern California, Los Angeles, California

AUTHORS

KUSH AGRAWAL, MD
Fellow, Cardiovascular and Endovascular Intervention, Cardiovascular Medicine, Boston Medical Center, Boston, Massachusetts

LEONARDO C. CLAVIJO, MD, PhD
Director, Interventional Cardiology Fellowship Program; Director, Vascular Medicine and Peripheral Interventions, Division of Cardiovascular Medicine, University of Southern California, Los Angeles, California

ROBERT S. DIETER, MD, RVT
Associate Professor of Medicine, Loyola University Medical Center, Stritch School of Medicine, Maywood, Illinois

ROBERT T. EBERHARDT, MD
Director of Vascular Medical Services, Boston Medical Center; Associate Professor of Medicine, Boston University School of Medicine, Boston, Massachusetts

SARAH ELSAYED, MD
Fellow in Cardiology, Vascular Medicine Graduated Fellow, Division of Cardiovascular Medicine, University of Southern California, Los Angeles, California

GIOVANNI ESPOSITO, MD, PhD
Division of Cardiology, Department of Advanced Biomedical Sciences, University of Napoli "Federico II", Napoli, Italy

ANNA FRANZONE, MD
Division of Cardiology, Department of Advanced Biomedical Sciences, University of Napoli "Federico II", Napoli, Italy

TAKI GALANIS, MD
Assistant Professor of Medicine, Department of Surgery, Jefferson Vascular Center, Thomas Jefferson University Hospitals, Philadelphia, Pennsylvania

PARVEEN K. GARG, MD, MPH
Division of Cardiology, Keck School of Medicine, University of Southern California, Los Angeles, California

HOSSEIN GHOFRANI, MD
Nephrology Fellow, Division of Nephrology, Department of Medicine, Keck School of Medicine, University of Southern California, Los Angeles, California

NESTOR R. GONZALEZ, MD
Associate Professor, Departments of Neurosurgery and Radiology, University of California, Los Angeles, Los Angeles, California

ASIF JAFFERANI, MD
Loyola University Medical Center, Maywood, Illinois

MICHELLE P. LIN, MD, MPH
Department of Neurology, University of Southern California, Los Angeles, California

GENO J. MERLI, MD
Professor of Medicine, Department of Surgery, Jefferson Vascular Center, Thomas Jefferson University Hospitals, Philadelphia, Pennsylvania

MITRA K. NADIM, MD
Associate Professor of Clinical Medicine, Division of Nephrology, Department of Medicine, Keck School of Medicine, University of Southern California, Los Angeles, California

YINN CHER OOI, MD
Senior Resident, Department of Neurosurgery, University of California, Los Angeles, Los Angeles, California

AMBROSE PANICO, DO
Loyola University Medical Center, Maywood, Illinois

NERSES SANOSSIAN, MD
Director, Department of Neurology, Roxanna Todd Hodges Comprehensive Stroke Clinic, University of Southern California, Los Angeles, California

FALAK SHAH, MD
Loyola University Medical Center, Maywood, Illinois

EUGENIO STABILE, MD, PhD
Division of Cardiology, Department of Advanced Biomedical Sciences, University of Napoli "Federico II", Napoli, Italy

JOSE DAVID TAFUR-SOTO, MD
Cardiology Fellow, Department of Cardiology, Ochsner Clinic Foundation, New Orleans, Louisiana

BRUNO TRIMARCO, MD
Division of Cardiology, Department of Advanced Biomedical Sciences, University of Napoli "Federico II", Napoli, Italy

FRED A. WEAVER, MD, MMM
Chief, Division of Vascular Surgery & Endovascular Therapy; Professor, Department of Surgery, Keck School of Medicine, University of Southern California, Los Angeles, California

CHRISTOPHER J. WHITE, MD, FSCAI, FACC, FAHA, FESC
Professor and Chairman of Medicine, Ochsner Clinical School, University of Queensland; AMD for Medical Specialties and System Chair for Cardiovascular Diseases; Medical Director, John Ochsner Heart & Vascular Institute, Ochsner Medical Center; Department of Cardiology, Ochsner Clinic Foundation, New Orleans, Louisiana

Contents

Stroke is the third leading cause of death in developed nations. Up to 88% of strokes are ischemic in nature. Extracranial carotid artery atherosclerotic disease is the third leading cause of ischemic stroke in the general population and the second most common nontraumatic cause among adults younger than 45 years. This article provides comprehensive, evidence-based recommendations for the management of extracranial atherosclerotic disease, including imaging for screening and diagnosis, medical management, and interventional management.

Critical limb ischemia (CLI), the most advanced form of peripheral artery disease (PAD), carries grave implications with regard to morbidity and mortality. Within 1 year of CLI diagnosis, 40% to 50% of diabetics will experience an amputation, and 20% to 25% will die. Management is optimally directed at increasing blood flow to the affected extremity to relieve rest pain, heal ischemic ulcerations, avoid limb loss, and prevent cardiovascular events. This management is achieved by guideline-directed medical therapy and risk factor modification, whereas the mainstay of therapy remains revascularization by endovascular or surgical means for patients who are deemed potential candidates.

Venous thromboembolism (VTE) is a potentially fatal condition and includes deep vein thrombosis and pulmonary embolism. The novel oral anticoagulants, which include the direct thrombin and factor Xa inhibitors, have been shown to be safe and effective for the treatment of VTE. Additional interventions include thrombolysis and the use of inferior vena cava filters. The purpose of this article is to provide a contemporary review of the treatment of VTE.

Atherosclerotic renal artery stenosis (RAS) is the single largest cause of secondary hypertension; it is associated with progressive renal insufficiency and causes cardiovascular complications such as refractory heart failure and flash pulmonary edema. Medical therapy, including risk factor modification, renin-angiotensin-aldosterone system antagonists, lipid-lowering agents, and antiplatelet therapy, is advised in all patients. Patients with uncontrolled renovascular hypertension despite optimal medical therapy, ischemic nephropathy, and cardiac destabilization syndromes who have severe RAS are likely to benefit from renal artery revascularization.

Screening for RAS can be done with Doppler ultrasonography, CT angiography, and magnetic resonance angiography.

agents for the treatment of symptomatic PAD, such as cilostazol, statins, and angiotensin-converting enzyme inhibitors, are highlighted.

Vascular surgery is associated with a higher incidence of perioperative cardiovascular morbidity and mortality compared with other noncardiac surgeries. Patients undergoing vascular surgery represent a higher-risk population, usually because of the presence of generalized arterial disease and multiple comorbidities. The overwhelming perioperative cardiac event is myocardial infarction. This article offers a tailored approach to preoperative cardiovascular management for patients undergoing vascular surgery. The use and limitations of well-established guidelines and clinical risk indices for patients undergoing noncardiac surgery are described as it pertains to vascular surgery in particular. Furthermore, the role and benefit of noninvasive stress testing, coronary revascularization, and medical therapy before vascular surgery are discussed.

This article reviews current knowledge and applications of drug-eluting devices in the treatment of peripheral arterial disease. The authors briefly report on the performance of plain old balloon angioplasty and bare metal stents in femoro-popliteal and below-the-knee lesions. This article explains the rationale behind the development of drug-eluting devices and describes the main technical features of currently available drug-eluting stents and drug-coated balloons. Dedicated sections discuss the results of trials investigating the potential benefits of these devices used in femoro-popliteal and infra-popliteal arterial vascular beds. Finally, ongoing studies and potential novel applications of drug-eluting technologies in other vascular beds are mentioned.

CARDIOLOGY CLINICS

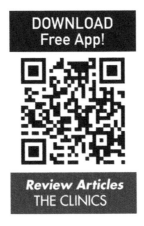

DOWNLOAD
Free App!

Review Articles
THE CLINICS

NOW AVAILABLE FOR YOUR iPhone and iPad

Preface
Vascular Disease

 CrossMark

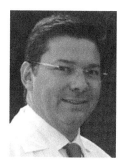

Leonardo C. Clavijo, MD, PhD
Editor

Vascular medicine–related diseases are the most common cause of death and disability in the United States; they affect more than 30 million people and account for more than $100 billion of health care expenditure every year. Vascular medicine is a relatively new specialty and encompasses multiple disciplines, including vascular surgery, interventional radiology, cardiology, rheumatology, hematology, and neurology. As cardiologists, we are looked upon as experts in cardiovascular disease and are often the first health care contact for patients with vascular disease. This means that we are therefore required to codify an initial diagnostic evaluation and to then formulate a treatment plan.

The practice of medicine is experiencing profound change as we are currently at a juncture among informatics, increased computational power that allows for high-resolution imaging and processing, bioscience, and genetics, all the while being challenged by increasing health care costs and regulatory restrictions.

Vascular medicine is at the forefront of these changes, having benefited from advancements in vascular biology, pharmacology, imaging, and endovascular technology.

The vascular practitioner's challenge is to administer excellent care while keeping in mind cost effectiveness and the safety and efficacy of new treatments.

This issue of *Cardiology Clinics* focuses on the general aspects of vascular medicine: peripheral arterial disease (medical treatment, critical limb ischemia, and applied drug-eluting technologies), cerebrovascular disease (carotid disease and stroke interventions), venous thromboembolic disease, resistant hypertension, and renal artery stenosis. We asked experts from various specialties to provide balanced state-of-the-art reviews of common vascular medical problems encountered by the cardiovascular practitioner.

It is my hope that this issue of *Cardiology Clinics* will help the reader effectively manage patients with vascular disease and ultimately provide a foundation for continued learning.

Leonardo C. Clavijo, MD, PhD
Interventional Cardiology Fellowship Program
Vascular Medicine and Peripheral Interventions
Division of Cardiovascular Medicine
University of Southern California
Los Angeles, CA 90033, USA

E-mail address:
lclavijo@usc.edu

0733-8651/15/$ – see front matter © 2015 Elsevier Inc. All rights reserved.

Management of Extracranial Carotid Artery Disease

Yinn Cher Ooi, MD[a], Nestor R. Gonzalez, MD[a,b],*

KEYWORDS

- Carotid disease • Carotid stenosis • Atherosclerotic disease • Stroke • Carotid endarterectomy
- Carotid angioplasty and stenting • Antiplatelet therapy

KEY POINTS

- Asymptomatic patients without risk factors should not be screened for carotid atherosclerotic disease.
- Carotid ultrasonography should be the initial screening tool for symptomatic patients.
- Medical management, including antiplatelet therapy, is indicated in all symptomatic patients with carotid atherosclerotic disease, independent of degree of stenosis.
- In general, carotid revascularization is indicated in symptomatic patients with nonocclusive moderate to severe stenosis (>50%) and asymptomatic patients with severe stenosis (>70%).
- When revascularization is indicated, patient anatomy, risk factors, and plaque factors should be considered in the decision for carotid endarterectomy versus angioplasty and stenting.

INTRODUCTION
Epidemiology

When considered as an independent diagnosis separate from other cardiovascular diseases, stroke is the third leading cause of death in developed nations and a leading cause of long-term disability.[1] Approximately 87% of all strokes are ischemic, 10% are hemorrhagic, and 3% are subarachnoid hemorrhages.[2–10]

Based on the Framingham Heart Study and Cardiovascular Health Study populations, the prevalence of greater than 50% carotid stenosis is approximately 9% in men and 6% to 7% in women.[11,12] Carotid stenosis or occlusion as a cause of stroke has been more difficult to determine from population studies. Approximately 7% to 18% of all first strokes were associated with carotid stenosis.[13,14] The risk for recurrent strokes among survivors is 1% to 15% within a year after the initial stroke, and 25% by 5 years.[8]

Extracranial atherosclerotic disease accounts for up to 15% to 20% of all ischemic strokes.[15,16] Whereas intracranial atherosclerotic disease has been shown to be consistently more common among Blacks, Hispanics, and Asians in comparison with Whites,[15,17] the racial differences for extracranial atherosclerotic disease are less apparent. The Northern Manhattan Stroke study reported equal incidence of extracranial atherosclerotic disease among patients of all races presenting with an acute ischemic stroke.[15] However, a smaller study reported that Whites were

Research reported in this publication was supported by the National Institute of Neurological Disorders and Stroke of the National Institutes of Health (award number K23NS079477-01A1). The content is solely the responsibility of the authors and does not necessarily represent the official views of the National Institutes of Health.
[a] Department of Neurosurgery, University of California, Los Angeles, 300 Stein Plaza, Suite 562, Los Angeles, CA 90095-69, USA; [b] Department of Radiology, University of California, Los Angeles, 300 Stein Plaza, Suite 562, Los Angeles, CA 90095-69, USA
* Corresponding author. Department of Neurosurgery, University of California, Los Angeles, 300 Stein Plaza, Suite 562, Los Angeles, CA 90095-69.
E-mail address: NGonzalez@mednet.ucla.edu

Cardiol Clin 33 (2015) 1–35
http://dx.doi.org/10.1016/j.ccl.2014.09.001
0733-8651/15/$ – see front matter © 2015 Elsevier Inc. All rights reserved.

more likely than Blacks to have extracranial carotid artery lesions (33% vs 15%, $P = .001$).[16] Male gender appears to be an independent predictor for intracranial atherosclerotic disease, whereas no gender differences were reported for extracranial disease.[16]

Natural History

Stroke associated with extracranial carotid atherosclerotic disease could occur via several mechanisms[18]:

- Atheroembolism of cholesterol crystals or other debris
- Artery to artery embolism of thrombus
- Structural disintegration of the wall (dissection)
- Acute thrombotic occlusion
- Reduced cerebral perfusion with plaque growth

In symptomatic patients, there is a clear correlation between the degree of stenosis and the risk of stroke.[19] In the North America Symptomatic Carotid Endarterectomy Trial (NASCET), the stroke rate after 18 months of medical therapy without revascularization was 19% in patients with 70% to 79% stenosis, 28% in patients with 80% to 89% stenosis, and 33% in patients with 90% to 99% stenosis.[19]

This correlation is less apparent in asymptomatic patients. In the Asymptomatic Carotid Atherosclerosis Study (ACAS) and the Asymptomatic Carotid Surgery Trial (ACST), asymptomatic patients with 60% to 80% stenosis had higher strokes rates compared with those with more severe stenosis.[20,21] The presence of a carotid bruit also does not appear to be a reliable predictor of stroke risk in asymptomatic patients. Despite the Framingham Heart Study population showing that asymptomatic patients with carotid bruit had a 2.6-fold increased incidence of strokes in comparison with those without carotid bruit, less than half of these stroke events involved the ipsilateral cerebral hemisphere.[3]

Although the degree of carotid stenosis remains the main determinant of disease severity, additional imaging markers of plaque vulnerability are also important in determining the risk for transient ischemic attack (TIA) and strokes.[22–24] Imaging markers for plaque vulnerability on ultrasonography (US) include[22,23]:

- Ulceration
- Echolucency
- Intraplaque hemorrhage
- High lipid content

Thin or ruptured fibrous caps, intraplaque hemorrhage and large lipid-rich or necrotic plaque cores, and overall plaque thickness seen on MRI have also been associated with subsequent ischemic events.[25]

The utility of biomarkers and imaging makers for inflammation in predicting plaque vulnerability and the risk for stroke has also been investigated. Carotid plaques from patients with ipsilateral stroke demonstrated infiltration of the fibrous cap by inflammatory cells.[26,27] ^{18}F-Fluorodeoxyglucose measured by PET is believed to reflect inflammation.[28,29] Macrophage activity quantified by PET has been observed in experimental models. In addition, biomarkers such as C-reactive protein and different matrix metalloproteinases are currently being studied for their predictive value of plaque instability.[30–32] However, the reliability of these markers remains uncertain.

EVALUATION OF CAROTID ATHEROSCLEROTIC DISEASE
Carotid Ultrasonography

When performed by well-trained, experienced technologists, carotid US is accurate and relatively inexpensive.[33–38] Carotid US is also noninvasive, and does not require a venipuncture or exposure to contrast material or radiation. As such, carotid US is recommended for the initial evaluation of symptomatic and asymptomatic patients with suspicion for carotid atherosclerotic disease.[39]

Carotid US should be performed in asymptomatic patients with 2 or more of the following risk factors:

- Hypertension
- Hyperlipidemia
- Family history of atherosclerosis or ischemic stroke before 60 years of age
- Tobacco smoking

US remains an appropriate screening tool for high-risk, asymptomatic patients irrespective of auscultation findings, because the sensitivity and positive predictive value of a carotid bruit for a hemodynamically significant carotid stenosis are relatively low.

Carotid US is not recommended, however, for routine screening of asymptomatic patients without risk factors for atherosclerotic disease, owing to the lack of data from health economic studies to support mass screening of the general population.[40,41]

Carotid US should also be performed annually to assess the progression or regression of disease and response to therapeutic measures in patients with greater than 50% stenosis. Once stability has been established or a patient's candidacy for further intervention has changed, longer intervals may be appropriate.[39]

Carotid US does not directly measure the luminal diameter of the artery or stenotic section. Instead, it relies on blood flow velocity as an indicator for the degree of stenosis. Several schemes have been developed for assessment of carotid stenosis.[42–44] Measuring the internal carotid artery (ICA) peak systolic velocity and the ratio of ICA peak systolic velocity over the ipsilateral common carotid artery velocity correlate best with angiographic stenosis. Potential pitfalls of velocity-based estimation of stenosis are the higher velocities in women than in men, and elevated velocities in the presence of a contralateral occlusion.[45,46] Subtotal arterial occlusion may also sometimes be mistaken for total occlusion, a crucial differentiation in determining management strategies. Other factors that may further reduce the accuracy of carotid US include highly operator-dependent reliability, obesity, high carotid bifurcation, severe arterial tortuosity, extensive calcifications, and presence of a carotid stent.[33–35,39,47]

Despite varying results between imaging centers and operators, the overall sensitivity and specificity for detection of occlusion or stenosis greater than 70% have been reported to be 85% to 90% when compared with catheter angiography.[48–50]

Computed Tomography Angiography and Magnetic Resonance Angiography

Both magnetic resonance angiography (MRA) and computed tomography angiography (CTA) are able to generate high-resolution images of the cervical arteries.[51–57] In comparison with catheter angiography, MRA has a sensitivity range of 97% to 100% and a specificity range of 82% to 96%,[58–62] whereas CTA has 100% sensitivity and 63% specificity (95% confidence interval [CI] 25%–88%).[63] Both are indicated in symptomatic patients when carotid US cannot be obtained, yield equivocal results, or show complete occlusion.[39] In patients with high pretest probability for disease, MRA and CTA may be used as the initial test. MRA and CTA of the intracranial vessels should be done when an extracranial source cannot be identified in symptomatic patients or in patients with risk factors for intracranial atherosclerotic disease. MRA and CTA are helpful in determining the exact severity of stenosis and anatomic details that will influence treatment decisions.

MRA has the benefit of its relative insensitivity to arterial calcification. Contrast-enhanced MRA allows for more detailed evaluation of the cervical arteries, especially in lesions with a slow blood flow, in comparison with noncontrast studies.[58–61,64,65] However, if contrast is contraindicated, non–contrast-enhanced MRA may be used.[51]

Potential pitfalls for MRA include a tendency to overestimate the degree of stenosis, and an inability to discriminate between total occlusion and subtotal occlusion. This effect is reduced with the use of contrast-enhanced MRA. Additional barriers of MRA include patients who are claustrophobic, extreme obesity, or incompatible implanted devices, such as pacemakers or defibrillators. For these patients, CTA is a good alternative.[39]

Unlike both MRA and carotid US, CTA provides direct imaging of the arterial lumen, making it suitable for evaluation of stenosis. It is an accurate test to determine severity of stenosis, and is also highly accurate for the detection or exclusion of complete occlusions.[55] However, CTA exposes patients to radiation, and the relatively high volume of iodinated contrast needed for the study precludes patients with impaired renal function. The presence of heavily calcified plaques may affect the accuracy of CTA in determining the degree of stenosis.[66] In addition, foreign metal objects, such as dental implants and surgical clips in the neck, can generate artifacts, which may obscure the targeted vessels.

Catheter Angiography

Although noninvasive imaging can provide the information needed in guiding the choice of medical, endovascular, or surgical treatment in most cases,[39] catheter angiography remains the gold standard for diagnosing and grading of carotid atherosclerotic disease.

Owing to its inherent cost and risk for complications, such as ischemic strokes, catheter angiography should be reserved for patients in whom noninvasive imaging is contraindicated, inconclusive, or yields discordant results. The risks of catheter angiography include allergic reactions to contrast, kidney dysfunction resulting from contrast toxicity, femoral artery injuries, infections or hematomas of the puncture site, strokes, or death, typically at a rate lower than 1 in 1000 for the most serious complications and less than 5% for the minor events in specialized centers with high volumes.[67,68]

Catheter angiography is useful in patients with renal insufficiency. Selective angiography of a single suspected vascular territory could provide definitive imaging with limited exposure to contrast material, and is unlikely to exacerbate renal insufficiency.[39]

Several methods to measure stenosis have been described, producing marked variability in measurements of vessels with the same degree of actual anatomic narrowing. Measurement methods based on the NASCET have been used in most modern clinical trials, taking into account the luminal diameter at the section with highest degree of stenosis (A), and the luminal diameter of a normal section just distal to the stenosis (B).[20]

$$\% \text{ Stenosis} = (B - A)/B \times 100$$

MEDICAL MANAGEMENT

Pharmacologic therapy for patients with carotid atherosclerotic disease consists mainly of antiplatelet therapy and medical management of the risk factors for atherosclerotic disease.

Antithrombotic Therapy

The use of antiplatelet agents has been shown to reduce the risk of stroke in patients with TIA or a previous stroke.[40,69–71] Single-agent antiplatelet therapies are recommended for all symptomatic patients, independent of whether they are candidates for revascularization. Aspirin 75 to 325 mg daily should be the first line of therapy. Clopidogrel 75 mg daily or ticlopidine 250 mg daily are reasonable alternatives when aspirin is contraindicated by factors other than active hemorrhage.[39,69,70,72]

Several randomized, controlled, double-blinded studies have shown that dual-antiplatelet combination therapy is not superior to single agents. The Clopidogrel for High Atherothrombotic Risk and Ischemic Stabilization, Management, and Avoidance (CHARISMA) trial and Management of Atherothrombosis with Clopidogrel in High-Risk Patients (MATCH) both showed that combination therapy of aspirin plus clopidogrel did not reduce stroke risk significantly compared with either drug alone.[73,74] The Second European Stroke Prevention Study (ESPS-2), which included 6602 patients, showed that the combination of aspirin and extended-release dipyridamole was superior to aspirin alone in patients with prior TIA or stroke.[75] However, a much larger study, with more than 20,000 patients, The Prevention Regimen for Effectively Avoiding Second Strokes (PROFESS) trial, showed that combination therapy of aspirin and extended-release dipyridamole was not superior to clopidogrel alone in recurrent stroke prevention.[76] Furthermore, there was an increased risk for major hemorrhagic events, including intracranial hemorrhage, in the combination therapy group.[76] Despite clopidogrel monotherapy showing equal efficacy and lower hemorrhage risk than aspirin plus extended-release dipyridamole, and equal efficacy with aspirin plus clopidogrel, the variations in response to clopidogrel attributable to genetic factors and drug interactions makes it crucial for individualized treatment selection for optimum stroke prevention.

Variability in response to clopidogrel is a result of both clinical and genetic factors. Conversion of clopidogrel to its active form by the cytochrome P450 system depends highly on CYP enzyme, which has significant genetic variability. CYP2C19*2 is the most common genetic variant associated with impaired response to clopidogrel.[39] However, other genetic polymorphisms may also contribute to poor response. Aspirin resistance has also been described, and was more frequent in patients taking low-dose aspirin (81 mg daily) and the enteric-coated preparations.[77] Clopidogrel or aspirin resistance resulting from the inability of these agents to inhibit platelet function is a potential cause of failure in stroke prevention. However, whether variations in response to antiplatelet therapy are associated with greater stroke risk and whether treatment of resistance improves outcomes have not been established. There is also a lack of consensus regarding which platelet function test should be used to determine such resistance.[39]

The efficacy of antiplatelet therapy in stroke prevention for asymptomatic patients is less apparent.[40,69,70,78] In the randomized, double-blinded Asymptomatic Cervical Bruit Study, the annual rate of ischemic events and death from any cause in patients with greater than 50% carotid stenosis was 11.0% in the aspirin group compared with 12.3% in the placebo group during a 2-year follow-up. However, the sample size of 372 patients may have been insufficient to detect a clinically meaningful difference.[79]

Anticoagulation with warfarin, along with its potential risk for increased hemorrhagic complications, has not been shown to be superior to antiplatelet agents. Antiplatelet therapy is recommended over anticoagulation for both symptomatic and asymptomatic patients in whom antithrombotic therapy is indicated.[39] The Warfarin-Aspirin Recurrent Stroke Study (WARSS), a randomized, double-blinded trial with 2206 patients, compared warfarin to aspirin for stroke prevention or recurrent ischemic stroke in patients with a recent stroke.[80] No significant benefit of warfarin over aspirin was found after 2 years. Parental anticoagulation with unfractionated heparin or low molecular weight heparin is also not recommended for patients with extracranial carotid atherosclerosis with acute ischemic stroke or TIA.[81–83] In patients who have other indications for anticoagulation, such as a mechanical prosthetic valve or atrial fibrillation, a vitamin K antagonist such as warfarin may be preferred to antiplatelet therapy. The target international normalized ratio should be 2.0 to 3.0.[84]

Treatment of Hypertension

Antihypertensive therapy has shown to reduce the risk of stroke, with a 33% reduction in stroke risk for every 10-mm Hg decrease in systolic blood pressure up to 115/75 mm Hg.[85,86] Antihypertensive therapy also reduces the risk for recurrent strokes by 24%.[87] These effects appear to be consistent between Whites and Blacks across a wide age range[88] and between sexes, regions, and stroke subtypes.[85] As such, antihypertensive treatment is recommended for all patients with concurrent hypertension and asymptomatic extracranial carotid atherosclerotic disease, with a target blood pressure lower than 140/90 mm Hg.[85–87,89,90] The protective value of antihypertensive therapy also seems to extend to patients without concurrent hypertension, as demonstrated by the Heart Outcomes Protection Evaluation (HOPE) trial.[91]

The exact benefits of antihypertensive treatment in symptomatic patients with severe carotid stenosis remain unclear because of concerns for reduction in cerebral perfusion and exacerbation of cerebral ischemia. Patients with severe carotid stenosis may have impaired cerebrovascular reactivity caused by chronic hypoperfusion, thereby increasing the risk for ipsilateral ischemic events.[92] Antihypertensive treatment is likely indicated in patients with hypertension and symptomatic extracranial atherosclerosis after the hyperacute period.[39] However, a specific blood pressure goal has yet to be established.

Treatment of Hyperlipidemia

According to the 2011 American Heart Association guidelines on the management of extracranial carotid and vertebral artery disease, statins are recommended for all patients with extracranial carotid stenosis to reduce low-density lipoprotein (LDL) levels to less than 100 mg/dL.[39,70,89,93] A target LDL level of 70 mg/dL is reasonable in patients who have sustained an ischemic stroke. Niacin and bile acid sequestrants are reasonable alternatives in patients who do not tolerate statins,[94–96] and can also be used in combination with a statin if treatment with a statin does not achieve target LDL levels.[94,95,97,98]

Epidemiologic studies have consistently shown a positive association between cholesterol levels and carotid artery atherosclerosis.[99–101] Lipid-lowering therapy with statins has been shown to reduce the risk of ischemic stroke in patients with atherosclerosis.[102,103] A meta-analysis of 26 trials involving approximately 90,000 patients showed that statins reduced the risk for all stroke by 21% (odds ratio [OR] 0.79, 95% CI 0.73–0.85), with a 15.6% reduction in stroke risk for every 10% decrease in serum LDL levels (95% CI 6.7–23.6).[103] Stroke Prevention by Aggressive Reduction in Cholesterol Levels (SPARCL), a randomized, prospective trial, showed that 80 mg daily of atorvastatin reduced the absolute risk for stroke at 5 years by 2.2%, the relative risk (RR) of all stroke by 16%, and the RR of ischemic stroke by 22%.[93] Statins also reduce the progression and induce regression of carotid atherosclerosis.[104] A meta-analysis of 9 randomized trials showed that statins reduced stroke risk by 15.6% and intima-media thickness (IMT) by 0.73% per year for every 10% reduction in LDL levels.[103] In the Atorvastatin versus Simvastatin on Atherosclerosis Progression (ASAP) trial involving patients with familial hypercholesterolemia, 80 mg daily of atorvastatin decreased carotid IMT after 2 years of treatment, but carotid IMT increased in patients randomized to simvastatin 40 mg daily.[105] Atorvastatin's effects on IMT were further supported by the Arterial Biology for Investigation of the Treatment Effects of Reducing Cholesterol (ARBITER) trial, which showed that carotid IMT regressed after 12 months of treatment with atorvastatin 80 mg daily, but remained unchanged with pravastatin 40 mg daily.[106] The Measuring Effects of Intima-Media Thickness: An Evaluation of Rosuvastatin (METEOR) trial showed that in patients with elevated LDL levels and a low Framingham risk score, rosuvastatin reduced the progression of carotid IMT over 2 years when compared with placebo.[107]

The effects of nonstatin lipid-modifying therapies on reduction of stroke risk are less apparent.[39] Niacin only showed a small benefit in reduction of risk of death caused by cerebrovascular disease in patients participating in the Coronary Drug Project.[108] Fenofibrate did not reduce stroke rates in patients with diabetes mellitus in the Fenofibrate Intervention and Event Lowering in Diabetes (FIELD) study.[109] Gemfibrozil reduced the risk of total strokes and ischemic strokes in patients with coronary artery disease and low high-density lipoprotein (HDL) levels in the Veteran Affairs HDL Intervention trial.[110]

The ARBITER-2 and Effect of Combination Ezetimibe and High-Dose versus Simvastatin Alone on the Atherosclerosis Process in Patients with Heterozygous Familial Hypercholesterolemia (ENHANCE) studies showed that the addition of extended-release niacin and ezetimibe, respectively, to statin therapy did not affect progression of carotid IMT more than statin therapy alone.[106,111] The Cholesterol Lowering Atherosclerosis (CLAS) trial, however, showed that combination therapy of niacin and colestipol reduced the progression of carotid IMT.[112]

Management of Diabetes Mellitus

Elevated fasting and postchallenge glucose levels were associated with an increased risk of stroke.[113] The risk of ischemic stroke in diabetic patients is increased 2- to 5-fold compared with nondiabetic patients.[114–116] The Cardiovascular Health Study showed that diabetes was associated with carotid IMT and severity of carotid stenosis.[12] Both the Atherosclerosis Risk in Communities (ARIC) study and Insulin Resistance Atherosclerosis Study and Epidemiology of Diabetes Interventions and Complications (EDIC) showed that diabetes was associated with progression of carotid IMT.[116–122] Several randomized, controlled, double-blinded studies have shown that the use of pioglitazone leads to substantial regression of carotid IMT.[123,124] The effect of pioglitazone appears to be independent of improved glycemic control.[123]

Smoking Cessation

Cigarette smoking increases the RR for ischemic stroke by 25% to 50%.[125–131] This risk decreases substantially within 5 years among those who quit smoking.[126,128] The Framingham Heart Study showed that the degree of extracranial carotid stenosis correlated with the quantity of cigarettes smoked over time.[132] These findings were corroborated by the Cardiovascular Health Study, in which the severity of carotid stenosis was greater among current smokers than in former smokers, and there was a significant association between pack-years of tobacco exposure with the severity of carotid stenosis.[133] The ARIC study revealed that current and past cigarette smoking was associated with a 50% and 25% increase, respectively, in risk of progression of IMT over a 3-year period when compared with nonsmokers.[130] Smoking cessation counseling and interventions should be offered to patients with extracranial carotid atherosclerosis to reduce the risk for disease progression and stroke.[125–128,134]

Obesity and Physical Inactivity

Abdominal adiposity has a strong positive association with the risk for stroke or TIA.[135] Adjusted OR for the waist-to-hip ratio showed successive increases in stroke/TIA risk for every successive tertile. There was also significant association with waist circumference and waist-to-stature ratio with the risk of stroke/TIA.

Physical inactivity is a significant modifiable risk factor for stroke, with 25% prevalence, 30%

attributable risk, and an RR of 2.7.[40,136] However, the risk reduction associated with intervention remains unclear. Several observational studies and meta-analyses have suggested a lower risk for stroke among individuals engaging in regular moderate to high levels of physical activity.[137] However, it is unclear whether exercise alone has a significant risk reduction for stroke in the absence of effects on other risk factors, such as reduction in obesity and improvement in glycemic control and serum lipid levels.

INTERVENTIONAL MANAGEMENT

Atherosclerotic disease of the extracranial carotid arteries carries significant morbidity and mortality risk despite maximal medical therapy. NASCET demonstrated a stroke rate of 19% to 33% after 18 months of medical therapy without intervention among symptomatic patients, depending on the degree of stenosis.[19] Interventional management, consisting mainly of carotid endarterectomy (CEA) and carotid angioplasty and stenting (CAS), has been shown to decrease the stroke rate among these patients.[8,19,138–146]

In general, intervention when indicated should be done within 6 months of original presentation.[8,19,147,148] However, intervention within 2 weeks of the index event is reasonable for patients with no contraindications for early revascularization.[149]

The indications for intervention are discussed in detail in the following sections. The general contraindications for interventions include:

- Severe, disabling stroke (modified Rankin Scale [mRS] score ≤3)
- Chronic total carotid artery occlusion
- Carotid stenosis less than 50%
- Extreme high risk for periprocedural complications

Carotid revascularization is not recommended for patients with near-complete occlusion or stenosis less than 50% because the risk for stroke is low in these patients.[19] Revascularization has also not been shown to have any benefit in these patients.[19] Moreover, carotid revascularization is also not recommended for patients with cerebral infarction causing severe disability that precludes preservation of useful function.

Carotid Endarterectomy

Carotid endarterectomy in symptomatic patients

CEA has been shown to significantly reduce the risk for ipsilateral stroke beyond the 30-day perioperative period in symptomatic patients. However, the inherent risk for periprocedural complications, such as stroke and myocardial infarction (MI), must be considered in the overall assessment of safety and efficacy.

Patients with a nondisabling ischemic stroke (mRS >3) or TIA and greater than 70% stenosis of the ipsilateral ICA by noninvasive imaging, or greater than 50% stenosis by catheter angiography, should undergo CEA.[8,147]

In NASCET, a randomized trial comparing stroke risk in symptomatic patients receiving CEA and medical management with medical management alone, patients were stratified according to severity of stenosis.[19] The trial for the high-grade stenosis group (70%–99%) was stopped after 18 months after randomizing 328 patients, because a significant benefit for CEA was evident. There was 17% absolute reduction in stroke risk with CEA at 2 years.[19] At the end of NASCET, the investigators also reported a benefit for CEA in patients with 50% to 69% stenosis. The rate of ipsilateral stroke including perioperative events was 15.7% at 5 years, compared with 22% in the medical management only group. The rate of operative mortality or perioperative stroke at 30 days was 6.7%. CEA had no benefit in patients with carotid stenosis less than 50%.

The European Carotid Surgery Trial (ECST), which randomized 2518 patients over a 10-year period, showed similar results to those of NASCET in symptomatic patients with 70% to 99% stenosis, showing a highly significant benefit for CEA, but did not show any benefit in patients with milder stenosis.[150,151] The lack of benefit of CEA in symptomatic patients with 50% to 69% stenosis based on ECST was attributed to the difference in angiographic measurement of stenosis.

The Veterans Affairs Cooperative Study (VACS) was stopped before completion, after only randomizing 109 symptomatic patients with a mean follow-up of 11.9 months, because of the significant benefit of CEA over medical therapy alone. The primary end point of death, stroke, or TIA occurred in 7.7% of CEA patients, compared with 19.4% of patients receiving medical therapy alone.[152]

A meta-analysis of these 3 trials showed that CEA was most effective in patients with greater than 70% stenosis without complete or near occlusion.[150] Benefits of CEA in patients with 50% to 69% stenosis were only modest, but increased with time. Surgery offered little to no long-term benefits in patients with complete or near occlusion. When the combined outcome of perioperative stroke or death and fatal or disabling ipsilateral ischemic stroke was considered, the clinical benefits of CEA were only evident in patients with 80% to 99% stenosis.

Carotid endarterectomy in asymptomatic patients

The benefits of CEA for reduction of stroke risk in asymptomatic patients are less profound than in symptomatic patients. CEA is reasonable in asymptomatic patients who have greater than 70% ICA stenosis if the risk of perioperative MI, stroke, and death is low.[138,153–156] Whereas CEA in symptomatic patients showed an increased benefit of surgery with increased degree of stenosis, CEA in asymptomatic patients did not show a similar trend. Equal benefits were seen in all patients within the 60% to 99% stenosis range.[156]

The VACS group conducted the first major trial of CEA in asymptomatic patients.[153] A total of 444 patients with 50% or greater stenosis were randomized over a 54-month period into either the CEA group or the medical therapy group. The 30-day mortality rate among patients undergoing CEA was 1.9% and the incidence of stroke was 2.4%. The study showed a statistically significant reduction in TIA, stroke, and death 5 years post-CEA, with a 10% overall rate of adverse events in the surgical group compared with 20% in the group given medical therapy alone. However, the inclusion of TIA in the primary composite end point remains controversial, given that the study was underpowered to detect a difference in a composite end point of death and stroke without TIA.[153,157,158]

ACAS also sought to determine whether the addition of CEA to medical management reduced the incidence of cerebral infarction in asymptomatic patients, but excluded TIA in its primary end point.[138] The trial was stopped before completion after randomizing 1662 patients, owing to the apparent advantage of CEA among patients with greater than 60% carotid stenosis. After a mean follow-up of 2.7 years, the projected 5-year risk for ipsilateral stroke and any perioperative stroke or death was estimated as 5.1% for surgical patients and 11.0% for patients treated medically. The aggregate risk reduction was 53% (95% CI 22%–72%).

These findings were further corroborated by the ACST, which randomized 3120 asymptomatic patients with greater than 60% stenosis to immediate CEA versus delayed surgery with initial medical management.[21] The 30-day stroke risk was 3.1% in both groups, but the 5-year rates were 6.4% in the early surgery group compared with 11.8% in the group initially managed medically.[139]

The benefits of CEA for asymptomatic patients are even less apparent in women, because of the higher operative risk and lower stroke risk without intervention among asymptomatic women compared with men.[156] Such benefits remain unclear despite a meta-analysis combining the data from both ACST and ACAS.[156]

Interpretation of carotid endarterectomy trials

The interpretation of CEA trials for both symptomatic and asymptomatic patients should be done in the context of the evolution of medical therapy for atherosclerotic disease. Although pharmacotherapy was included in most trials, guidelines and strategies for medical management have changed over the years. Best medical therapy during the period of older trials such as NASCET was scant by modern standards. In NASCET, only approximately 70% of patients were placed on antihypertensive drugs and an even smaller proportion were given lipid-lowering agents.[8] Medical therapy was not described in ACAS. The ACST investigators reported a change in medical therapy over the 10-year trial period.[139] Toward the end of the trial in 2003, 70% of patients were on lipid-lowering agents and 81% were on antihypertensive drugs. However, the outcomes for CEA were only reported for the first 5 years of the trial, ending in 1998, during which such medical therapy was considerably less frequent. In addition, 60% of patients had systolic blood pressure (SBP) greater than 160 mm Hg while 33% had total serum cholesterol greater than 250 mg/dL.

Concurrently surgical outcomes of CEA have improved over time, with advances in training, increased hospital and surgeon volumes, and improved perioperative medical management.[159–162]

Therefore, with advances in both medical management and operative/perioperative management and outcomes over time, which has led to a decline in rates of adverse events, the comparative outcomes of CEA over medical therapy must be interpreted with caution.

Demographic and clinical considerations

Advanced age does not preclude CEA in appropriately selected patients. Despite several reports showing a higher risk for complications among older patients,[163,164] patients 75 years and older with few cardiovascular risk factors have been shown to have comparable risk for perioperative stroke and death in comparison with younger patients.[165] However, in ACST no benefit from CEA was observed in patients 80 years of age and older.[21] In NASCET, the greatest benefit of CEA was observed in older patients up to 80 years of age.[19] Patients older than 80 years were excluded from NASCET (before 1991) and ACAS.[19,138]

Women undergoing CEA have a higher risk than men for complications.[147,166–168] In both ACAS and NASCET, women had a higher risk for surgical mortality, neurologic morbidity, recurrent stenosis, or gaining little to no benefit from surgery.[19,138]

There are insufficient data to determine the effects of ethnicity on outcomes.[39]

Anatomic considerations

Several factors that affect patient anatomy must be taken into account when considering the safety and technical challenges associated with CEA. Unfavorable factors include:

- High carotid bifurcation or arterial stenosis above the level of the second cervical vertebra
- Arterial stenosis below the clavicle (intrathoracic)
- Contralateral carotid occlusion
- Contralateral vocal cord paralysis
- Previous ipsilateral CEA
- Prior radical neck surgery or radiation
- Prior tracheostomy

A high carotid bifurcation or arterial stenosis above the level of the second vertebra may require high cervical exposure, which increases the risk for cranial nerve injury.[169,170] The risk for cranial nerve injury is also higher in patients with prior radical neck surgery or tracheostomy. In these cases, there usually is added difficulty in exposing the artery and increased risk for perioperative infection. Contralateral laryngeal nerve palsy is a relative contraindication for CEA because bilateral laryngeal nerve palsy can lead to significant compromise of the airway.[171] Prior radiation can make CEA technically challenging, but several series have shown that CEA can still be performed safely.[172] Although in this situation CAS may be a safer option, the rate of restenosis is high, ranging from 18% to 80% over 3 years.[173–175]

Technical considerations

There have been considerable variations in surgical technique with CEA over the past 50 years. Local anesthesia was initially recommended to permit observation of patients' level of consciousness during temporary carotid artery clamping. Several investigators also advocated local anesthesia because of the possibility of less perioperative adverse cardiac events.[39] However, there have been no significant data demonstrating an advantage of local anesthesia over general anesthesia.

Patients undergoing general anesthesia for CEA should undergo intraoperative monitoring of cerebral function to determine the need for shunting during arterial clamping.[176–178] Selective shunting of patients is preferable, owing to the potential complications associated with shunting such as mechanical injury to distal ICA, air embolism, or thromboembolism through the shunt, and obscuring the distal arterial anatomy during endarterectomy.[39] Intraoperative monitoring includes:

- Electroencephalography (EEG)
- Somatosensory evoked potential (SSEP)
- Transcranial Doppler US
- Computed topographic brain mapping, measurement of residual collateral perfusion pressure, or ICA back pressure

Shunting was generally indicated when EEG abnormalities associated with ischemia appeared.[179] In the authors' institution, shunts are used when a depression of at least 50% of EEG amplitude or SSEP P25 amplitude is observed. Shunts are used in all patients with contralateral carotid occlusion.

Patch closure of the arteriotomy may reduce the incidence of residual or recurrent stenosis. However, there is increased operative time and increased carotid clamp time. Multiple studies have failed to demonstrate a consistent difference in outcomes between patch closure and primary closure.[180–190] A Cochrane meta-analysis of the combined results of 10 trials showed that patch closure reduces the risk of perioperative arterial ooolusion and ipsilateral stroke. There was also reduction in the subsequent risk of restenosis, death, or stroke.[179] As such, most surgeons now advocate for patch closure. Several different patch materials have been described in the literature, including the use of bovine pericardium, vein, polyethylene terephthalate, and polytertrafluoroethyelene.[191–194] However, the outcomes have appeared to be similar independent of the patch material used.

The use of perioperative antiplatelet therapy such as aspirin or clopidogrel reduces the risk for adverse cardiac and neurologic events without a significant increase in risk for postoperative bleeding.[195,196] However, perioperative combination therapy consisting of aspirin and clopidogrel was associated with increased risk for postoperative bleeding or incisional hematoma.[197,198]

Perioperative management

Antiplatelet therapy with aspirin 81 to 325 mg daily is recommended before CEA, and should be continued indefinitely postoperatively.[71,199] In the Acetylsalicylic Acid and Carotid Endarterectomy (ACE) study, where 2849 patients were randomized to 4 different daily doses of aspirin, the risk of stroke, MI, and death within 30 days and 3 months after CEA was higher in patients taking higher doses of aspirin (650 or 1300 mg daily) compared with those taking lower doses (81 mg or 325 mg daily). The risk at 30 days was 7.0% vs 5.4%, (RR 1.31, 95% CI 0.98–1.75), and at 3 months 8.4% vs 6.2%, (RR 1.34, 95% CI 1.03–1.75).[199] Clopidogrel 75 mg daily or a combination of low-dose aspirin plus extended-release dipyridamole 25 to 200 mg twice daily are reasonable alternatives.[72,74,80]

The use of perioperative lipid-lowering drugs such as statins for prevention of ischemic events regardless of serum lipid levels after CEA is reasonable.[200] However, the optimum agents and doses for prevention of restenosis have not been established. A retrospective review of 1566 patients undergoing CEA at a single large academic center performed by 13 surgeons revealed that receiving statin medication at least 1 week before surgery (42% of total patients reviewed) was associated with lower rates of:

- Perioperative stroke (1.2% vs 4.5%; $P<.01$)
- TIA (1.5% vs 3.6%; $P<.01$)
- All causes of mortality (0.3% vs 2.1%; $P<.01$)
- Median (interquartile range) length of hospitalization (2 days [2–5 days] vs 3 days [2–7 days]; $P<.05$)

Antihypertensive medication is recommended before CEA and should be resumed postoperatively.[39]

Perioperative management pearls based on the authors' institutional experience are as follows:

- General anesthesia
- Continue EEG and SSEP monitoring
- Discuss with anesthesia the potential need for barbiturates in the reduction of cerebral metabolic demand
- Intravenous antibiotics: cefazolin or vancomycin
- Patient is kept normocapnic (35–45 mm Hg)
- Patient is kept normotensive with permissive hypertension to 20% above baseline during carotid clamping
- Strict control of blood pressure to avoid hypertension is initiated immediately after removal of carotid clamps
- Patient is kept nomothermic
- Goal hematocrit of at least 30%
- Shunt is used with any reduction in 50% in EEG amplitude or 50% in the P25 median nerve SSEP activity, or in cases of contralateral occlusion
- A single dose of intravenous heparin is given before cross-clamping, usually 5000 U. In

smaller patients or more heavy-set patients, an alternative dose of 85 U/kg can be used
- During dissection of the carotid bulb, arrhythmias may occur. Atropine or glycopyrrolate should be ready

Complications

Complications associated with CEA are listed here, and include neurologic and nonneurologic complications[201]:

- Cranial nerve palsy
- Infection
- Hemorrhage
- Stroke
- Venous thromboembolism
- Acute arterial occlusion
- Arterial restenosis
- MI
- Hemodynamic instability (hypertension or hypotension)
- Death

Risk factors associated with increased perioperative stroke and death include[201–203]:

- Symptomatic before CEA (OR 1.62, $P<.0001$)
- Hemispheric symptoms (OR 2.31, $P<.001$ vs retinal symptoms)
- Urgent operations (OR 4.9, $P<.001$)
- Reoperation (OR 1.95, $P<.018$)
- Contralateral carotid arterial occlusion (RR 2.2, CI 1.1–4.5)

A large, retrospective, cohort study reviewing CEAs performed at 6 different hospitals by 64 different surgeons in a 2-year period revealed a 30-day postoperative stroke or death rate of 2.28% in asymptomatic patients, 2.93% in patients with TIA, and 7.11% among patients presenting with stroke.[204] These results were similar to those of NASCET, which had a 30-day postoperative stroke or mortality rate of 6.7% among symptomatic patients.[19] The pooled analysis of NASCET, ECST, and VACS revealed a 30-day stroke and death rate after CEA of 7.1%.[150] The results for asymptomatic patients were also similar to those of prospective trials such as ACAS and ACST, which had 30-day stroke and mortality rates of 2.3% and 3.1%, respectively.[21,138] High-risk anatomic criteria, such as restenosis after CEA and contralateral carotid occlusion, further increase this risk, as seen in NASCET and ACAS.[138,201] The perioperative stroke and death rate have been reported to be as high as 19.9% in patients undergoing reoperative CEA and 14.3% among patients with contralateral carotid occlusion.[205]

However, more recent reports suggest a much lower risk than was previously reported. Case volume and surgical training are important factors in determining the clinical outcomes after a CEA. A population-based study in the state of Virginia investigating all CEAs performed from 1997 to 2001, with approximately 14,000 procedures, reported a cumulative stroke rate of 1.0% and mortality rate of 0.5%.[206] There was a progressive decline in these rates in each successive year. Similar results were found in Maryland from 1994 to 2003, which included 23,237 CEA procedures. The cumulative stroke rate was 0.73%; 2.12% in 1994, 1.47% in 1995, and 0.29% to 0.65% from 1996 to 2003.[207] The cumulative stroke rate in California from 1999 to 2003 was similar, at 0.54%. During this time 51,231 CEA procedures were performed.[207] Mortality rates in both states were relatively stable over the reported years.

Intracerebral hemorrhage can also occur as a result of hyperperfusion syndrome despite adequate control of blood pressure, which occurs in less than 1% of patients with a stable preoperative blood pressure and well-managed blood pressure perioperatively.[208–211]

Cranial nerve injury occurs in up to 7% of patients undergoing CEA; however, permanent injury remained in less than 1% of patients.[150,171,212] Cranial neuropathy typically appeared early in the postoperative period, with most patients showing complete resolution over time.[171] Only 3.7% had residual cranial nerve deficits. In decreasing order of frequency, cranial nerves or their branches involved are[171,201,213–215]:

1. Hypoglossal
2. Marginal mandibular
3. Recurrent laryngeal
4. Spinal accessory
5. Cervical sympathetic chain (Horner syndrome)

Cardiovascular events have been reported in up 20% of patients undergoing CEA, with hypotension occurring in 5%, hypertension in 20%, and perioperative MI in 1%.[39] Local anesthesia and cervical block may lessen cardiovascular instability in selected patient groups.[216] Myocardial ischemia, including nonfatal MI, is a major cause of morbidity in patients undergoing CEA because carotid bifurcation atherosclerosis is commonly associated with coronary atherosclerosis.[39] In NASCET and ECST, respectively, the incidence of MI was 0.3% and 0.2%.[19,147] The risk for cardiopulmonary complications is associated with[217–219]:

- Advanced age
- Active angina pectoris

- New York Heart Association (NYHA) functional class III or IV heart failure
- Left ventricular ejection fraction 30% or less
- MI within 30 days
- Urgent cardiac surgery 30 days prior
- Severe chronic lung disease
- Severe renal insufficiency

Wound infections occur in 1% or fewer patients.[220,221] Wound hematoma occurred in 5% or fewer patients and was associated with perioperative antiplatelet therapy,[222] duration of surgery, perioperative use of heparin and protamine, and other factors.[39]

Carotid Angioplasty and Stenting

CAS has shown varying outcome differences when compared with CEA, based on different patient factors. CAS seems to be a good alternative to CEA in certain patient groups, such as those with unfavorable surgical anatomy (noted previously). When performed with an embolic protection device (EPD), the risk associated with CAS may be lower than that of CEA in patients at increased risk for surgical complications.

Carotid angioplasty and stenting in asymptomatic patients

CAS has been reported to have superior outcomes when compared with CEA in patients at high surgical risk. In a selected group of asymptomatic patients with unfavorable surgical anatomy and significant comorbidities, it is reasonable to recommend CAS over CEA when intervention is indicated. Patients at high surgical risk were defined as having 1 or more of following criteria[223,224]:

- NYHA class III or IV heart failure
- Chronic obstructive pulmonary disease
- Greater than 50% contralateral carotid artery stenosis
- Prior CEA or CAS
- Prior coronary artery bypass graft surgery

The Stenting and Angioplasty with Protection in Patients at High Risk for Endarterectomy (SAPHIRE) trial randomized high-risk patients into CEA and CAS with EPD groups, with inclusion criteria of symptomatic stenosis greater than 50% or asymptomatic stenosis greater than 80%. The primary end point was defined as death, stroke, or MI within 30 days plus death from neurologic causes or ipsilateral stroke between 31 days and 1 year. The secondary end point was defined as the primary end point events plus death or ipsilateral stroke between 1 and 3 years. Technical success was achieved in 95.6% of patients who underwent CAS. However, the study incurred a selection bias by excluding patients from the CEA arm who were considered a priori to have exceedingly high risk for complication. The trial was stopped before completion after randomizing 334 patients, owing to a sharp decline in enrollment rate. Three-year follow-up data were available for only 85.6% of patients.[143,144] In asymptomatic patients, the occurrence of the primary end point was greater after CEA (21.5%) than after CAS (9.9%). The periprocedural death, MI, or stroke rate was also greater after CEA (10.2%) than after CAS (5.4%). The 3-year stroke rates were comparable between CEA and CAS, at 9.2% and 10.3%, respectively.

CAS does not appear to be superior to CEA in asymptomatic patients with conventional surgical risk for intervention. The Carotid Revascularization Endarterectomy versus Stenting Trial (CREST) was a multicenter, randomized trial comparing CAS with CEA in both symptomatic (carotid stenosis >50%) and asymptomatic (carotid stenosis >60%) patients.[141,225,226] Among 2502 patients followed for 2 years, the estimated 4-year rate of stroke, death, or MI was similar in both CAS and CEA (7.2% and 6.8%, respectively; stenting hazard ratio [HR] 1.11, 95% CI 0.81–1.51; $P = .51$). However, periprocedural stroke alone was more frequent after CAS (4.1% vs 2.3%; $P = .01$), whereas periprocedural MI alone was more frequent after CEA (2.3% vs 1.1%; $P = .03$). In the subgroup of asymptomatic patients, the 4-year stroke and death rates were higher after CAS (4.5% and 2.7%, respectively; HR 1.86, $P = .07$). In addition, CREST also showed that quality of life was significantly affected by major and minor stroke but not by MI, based on quality-of-life studies done at 1 year. The outcomes with CEA and CAS also appeared to be affected by age, with a crossover occurring at approximately 70 years. CEA showed greater efficacy at older ages and CAS at younger ages.[141] The comparative primary results did not vary by sex or symptom status. As seen in previous randomized trials, cranial nerve palsy was more common after CEA.

The Asymptomatic Carotid Surgery Trial 2 (ACST-2) is an ongoing, large, multicenter, randomized trial comparing CAS with CEA in asymptomatic patients with severe carotid stenosis. The trial aims to randomize 5000 patients. After randomizing 986 patients, interim safety results show that the combined CAS and CEA outcome is on a par with other recent trials; however, comparison results between CAS and CEA are not currently available.[227] CREST-2 is another study that will evaluate intensive medical management versus CEA or CAS in asymptomatic patients.

The study is designed as two independent, multi-center, randomized controlled trials evaluating medical management versus CEA in one and CAS in the other.[228]

Carotid angioplasty and stenting in symptomatic patients

In symptomatic patients, CEA has been reported to have superior outcomes over CAS in patients at both conventional and high surgical risk. In symptomatic patients at high surgical risk, SA-PHIRE showed that despite a similar occurrence of the primary end point at 1 year (CAS 16.8% vs CEA 16.5%), the secondary end point at 3 years was higher after CAS (32% vs 21.7%). Of note, a smaller proportion of symptomatic patients underwent 3-year follow-up in comparison with asymptomatic patients.[143,144]

Several studies have compared the outcomes of CEA and CAS in symptomatic patients with conventional surgical risk. One of the most comprehensive and better designed is CREST, a multicenter, randomized trial comparing CAS with CEA in both symptomatic (carotid stenosis >50%) and asymptomatic (carotid stenosis >60%) patients.[141,225,226] The 4-year stroke and death rate was higher after CAS in symptomatic patients (8.0% vs 6.4%, HR 1.37; $P = .14$). As mentioned earlier, although periprocedural MI was more frequent after CEA, the study showed that quality of life was significantly affected by major and minor stroke but not by MI.

Other studies comparing CAS with CEA in symptomatic patients with conventional surgical risk for intervention include the Carotid and Vertebral Artery Transluminal Angioplasty Study (CAVA-TAS), which was a multicenter randomized trial comparing CAS with CEA. A total of 504 patients were randomized, 90% of whom were symptomatic.[229–231] Of note, EPDs were not used and only 22% of CAS patients were stented. The combined stroke and death rate at 30 days was similar in both groups (10%). However, cranial neuropathy occurred more frequently in CEA patients (8.7% vs 0%; $P<.0001$). Major incisional hematoma after CEA occurred more frequently than access-site hematoma after CAS (6.7% vs 1.2%; $P<.0015$). The rate of ipsilateral stroke after 3 years of follow-up was similar in both groups (adjusted HR 1.04, 95% CI 0.63–1.70; $P = .9$). However, the 8-year incidence and HR for ipsilateral non-perioperative stroke was 11.3% versus 8.6% (HR 1.22, 95% CI 0.59–2.54). There was also a higher rate of restenosis associated with CAS, with an estimated 5-year incidence of 30.7% compared with 10.5% after CEA. The investigators found that several factors were associated with the higher incidence of restenosis, including longer segments of stenosis at baseline and performing a balloon angioplasty alone without stenting.[231,232]

The Endarterectomy Versus Angioplasty in Symptomatic Severe Carotid Stenosis (EVA-3S) trial randomized patients with a completed stroke or TIA within the past 120 days and an ipsilateral carotid stenosis greater than 60%.[233] Patients with disabling stroke were excluded from the trial (mRS >3). After randomizing 520 patients, the trial was stopped before completion for reasons of safety and futility. The 30-day incidence of stroke or death was 9.6% after CAS versus 3.9% after CEA, with an RR of 2.5 (95% CI 0.5–4.2). However, there were several factors in the EVA-3S trial that may have confounded its results, including inadequate training requirements for operators performing CAS and no uniform requirement for the use of EPDs.[234] In addition, 5 different carotid stent devices and 7 EPDs were used. Although experts have agreed that the EVA-3S trial results should not affect management guidelines, the trial has highlighted the importance of rigorous and standardized training criteria required for interventionists performing carotid stent placement.[234]

The Stent-Protected Angioplasty versus Carotid Endarterectomy (SPACE) study was a randomized, noninferiority trial comparing CAS with CEA in symptomatic patients with a stroke or TIA within the past 180 days and ipsilateral carotid stenosis greater than 70%.[142,235] Patients with severe disabling stroke (mRS >3) were excluded. The initial planned sample size of 1900 was not met; only 1214 patients were successfully randomized owing to the inability to further enroll patients. Surgeons were required to have at least 25 CEAs done with acceptable rates of mortality and morbidity in the past year; and CAS operators were required to have performed at least 25 successful angioplasties or stenting procedures, although not necessarily in the carotid artery. The rate of ipsilateral stroke and death were similar in both groups within 30 days (6.8% CAS vs 6.3% CEA) and also within 2 years (9.5% vs 8.8%, HR 1.10, 95%, CI 0.75–1.61). Recurrent stenosis of at least 70% was more frequent in CAS patients than in CEA patients (10.7% vs 4.6%; $P = .0009$).

The International Carotid Stenting Study (ICSS) is a multicenter randomized trial comparing the safety and efficacy of CAS and CEA in symptomatic patients with ipsilateral carotid stenosis of 50% and greater.[236] The clinical phase of the trial is complete. In ICSS, participating centers were classified into experienced or supervised. Experienced centers were defined as having at least 1 surgeon and 1 interventionist who have performed 50 CEA (minimum of 10 per year) or 50 CAS (at least 10 involving the carotid), respectively. Supervised centers were designated as experienced after randomization and treatment of 20 cases of CEA or CAS, if the results were acceptable to a proctor and credentialing committee. In total, 88% of patients were treated at an experienced center. Interim safety analysis reported that the risk for stroke and death by all causes was higher in the CAS group (stroke: 7.6% after CAS vs 4.1% after CEA, HR 1.92, 95% CI 1.27–2.89; death: 2.2% vs 0.8%, HR 2.76, 95% CI 1.16–6.56). In the MRI substudy, CAS was associated with more acute and persisting ischemic brain lesions.[237] Periprocedural hemodynamic instability, including bradycardia, asystole, or hypotension requiring treatment, were more likely to cause ischemic brain lesions in CAS patients than in CEA patients (RR 3.36; 95% CI 1.73–6.50).[238]

Anatomic considerations

Several anatomic factors are considered to be unfavorable for endovascular intervention, including[239]:

- Type II or III aortic arch
- Arch vessel origin stenosis greater than 50%
- Common and ICA tortuosity greater than 30°
- Significant plaque calcifications
- Long segment stenosis

These factors increase the technical difficulty of CAS, and also increase the risk for perioperative stroke; they are more prevalent in the elderly (>80 years of age), but may also be found in patients of all ages.

Prevention of cerebral embolism

The outcomes associated with the use of EPDs have not been studied in randomized trials. Several observational studies have suggested that EPDs, when used by experienced operators, lead to reduced rates of adverse events, including major and minor strokes.[240,241] An international survey involving 53 sites with a total of 11,392 CAS procedures performed by experienced operators reported a combined stroke and death rate of 2.8% when EPDs were used and 6.2% when they were not.[240] Several other studies have also shown an improvement in outcome with the use of EPDs.[143,144,242–244]

However, when used by operators who are not experienced with the device, EPDs have been associated with worse clinical outcome[229,233,235] and increased incidence of ischemic abnormalities seen on postprocedural brain imaging.[245] The AC-CULINK for Revascularization of Carotids in High-Risk Patients (ARCHeR) trial, a nonrandomized, multiphase trial that included experienced operators, did not show an improvement in outcome with the use of EPDs.

Periprocedural management

Dual-antiplatelet therapy consisting of aspirin 81 to 325 mg daily and clopidogrel 75 mg daily is recommended before CAS and for a minimum of 30 days after CAS, after which at least 1 antiplatelet agent should be continued long term. Ticlopidine 250 mg twice daily is an acceptable alternative for patients intolerant of clopidogrel. Adequate intraprocedural anticoagulation can be achieved with unfractionated heparin with a target activated clotting time of 250 to 300 seconds. Alternatively bivalirudin may be used, which has an added advantage over heparin in that there is no need to monitor activated clotting time.[246,247]

CAS is associated with hemodynamic instability, including hypotension and vasovagal responses. Several intraprocedural steps can be taken to minimize the associated risk[39]:

- Continuous electrocardiogram and blood pressure monitoring
- Adequate hydration and adjustment of antihypertensive medication immediately before CAS to avoid persistent intraprocedural hypotension
- Prophylactic administration of atropine 0.5 to 1 mg intravenously before angioplasty and stenting
- Temporary transvenous pacemaker for persistent bradycardia
- Phenylephrine 1 to 10 µg/kg/min or dopamine 5 to 15 µg/kg/min for persistent hypotension
- To minimize risk of intracerebral hemorrhage or hyperperfusion syndrome, the SBP should be maintained at below 180 mm Hg before and during the procedure. In the authors' experience, strict control of SBP lower than 140 mm Hg immediately after revascularization has consistently prevented hemorrhages.

Complications

Complications associated with CAS include:

- Cardiovascular: baroreflex responses, MI, arterial dissection, target vessel perforation, vasospasm, restenosis
- Neurologic: TIA, stroke, hemorrhage, seizure
- Device failure
- Access-site injury

Baroreflex responses such as hypotension, bradycardia, and vasovagal reactions occur in 5% to 10% of cases, but have been reported to be as high as 33%.[248–250] Most are transient and do not require additional treatment after the

Table 1
Summary of key randomized clinical trials

Trial, Year[Ref.]	Study Population, Degree of Stenosis	Intervention	Comparison	No. of Patients Treatment Group	No. of Patients Comparison Group	Event	Events (%) Treatment Group	Events (%) Control Group
NASCET, 1991[140]	S (70%–90% by angio)	CEA	Med	328	321	Ipsilateral stroke at 2 y	9.00	26.00
NASCET, 1998[8]	S (50%–69% by angio)	CEA	Med	320	428	Ipsilateral stroke at 5 y	15.70	22.20
ECST, 2003[151]	S (70%–99% by angio)	CEA	Med	429	850	Stroke or surgical death	6.80	NA
	S (50%–69% by angio)	CEA	Med	646	850	Stroke or surgical death	10.00	NA
ACAS, 1995[138]	AS (>60% by angio)	CEA	Med	825	834	Ipsilateral stroke, periprocedural stroke, or death	5.10	11.0
ACST, 2004[139]	AS (>60% by angio)	Immediate CEA	Delayed CEA	1560	1560	5-y stroke risk	3.8	11.0
SPACE, 2008[142]	S (≥70% by US)	CEA	CAS	589	607	All stroke at 2 y	10.10	10.90
						All periprocedural strokes or deaths and ipsilateral strokes up to 2 y	8.80	9.50
						Ipsilateral stroke between 31 d and 2 y	1.90	2.20
EVA-3S, 2008[145]	S (≥60%)	CEA	CAS	262	265	All stroke at 4 y	3.40	9.10
						Ipsilateral stroke at 4 y	1.50	1.50
						All periprocedural stroke, death, and nonprocedural ipsilateral stroke at 4 y	6.20	11.10
SAPHIRE, 2004 and 2008[143,144]	S (≥50% by US) + AS (≥80% by US)	CEA	CAS	167	167	All strokes at 1 y	7.90	6.20
						Ipsilateral stroke at 1 y	4.80	4.20
						All stroke, death, or MI within 30 d of procedure, ipsilateral stroke between 31 d and 1 y	20.10	12.20
						All strokes at 3 y	9.00	9.00
						Ipsilateral stroke at 3 y	5.40	6.60
						All stroke, death, or MI within 30 d of procedure, ipsilateral stroke between 31 and 1080 d	26.90	24.60

Trial	Subgroup			N		Outcome	CEA	CAS
ICSS, 2010[146]	S (≥50% by angio or 2 noninvasive imaging)	CEA	CAS	858	855	All strokes within 30 d of randomization	3.30	7.00
						All strokes within 120 d of randomization	4.10	7.70
CREST, 2010[141]	S (≥50% by angio, ≥70% by US)	CEA	CAS	653	688	All periprocedural strokes, MI, death, and postprocedural ipsilateral strokes up to 4 y	8.40	8.60
						All periprocedural strokes, death, and postprocedural ipsilateral strokes up to 4 y	6.40	8.00
						All periprocedural strokes and postprocedural ipsilateral strokes up to 4 y	6.40	7.60
	AS (≥60% by angio, ≥70% by US)	CEA	CAS	587	594	All periprocedural strokes, MI, death, and postprocedural ipsilateral strokes up to 4 y	4.90	5.60
						All periprocedural strokes, death, and postprocedural ipsilateral strokes up to 4 y	2.70	4.50
						All periprocedural strokes and postprocedural ipsilateral strokes up to 4 y	2.70	4.50
	S + AS	CEA	CAS	1240	1262	All strokes up to 4 y	7.90	10.20

Abbreviations: angio, catheter angiography; AS, asymptomatic; CAS, carotid angioplasty and stenting; CEA, carotid endarterectomy; d, days; Med, medical therapy; MI, myocardial infarction; NA, no data available; S, symptomatic; US, ultrasonography; y, years

procedure. With the introduction of appropriate preprocedural management, rates can be kept in the lower range.[249,251–256]

The risk for MI is approximately 1%, with rates as low as 0.9%, as reported in the CAPTURE registry of 3500 patients. However, this may be higher among high-risk patients, with up to 2.4% reported in the ARCHeR trial.[154,250,257–266]

In one study, the risk for arterial dissection or thrombosis was less than 1% and the risk for target vessel perforation was also less than 1%.[39] External carotid stenosis or occlusion occurred in 5% to 10% of cases, but were usually benign, with no further intervention required.[154,250,257–264,267] Transient vasospasm occurred in 10% to 15% of cases and was associated with vessel manipulation by guide wires, catheters, and capture devices. This occurrence is also more common among smokers and patients with hypertension.[268–271] Restenosis occurs in 3% to 5% of cases, and can be minimized by avoiding multiple or high-pressure balloon angioplasties, particularly in heavily calcified vessels.[174,272–289]

The CAPTURE registry reported an overall stroke rate of 4.9%, with disabling strokes occurring in 2% of patients.[267,290–298] The ARCHeR trial reported similar results, with an overall stroke rate of 5.5% and disabling strokes occurring in 1.5% of patients.[154,258–260,262,263,265,266] TIA occurs in up to 1% to 2% of patients undergoing CAS. Subclinical ischemic injury detected by MRI has also been reported.[146,299,300]

Intracranial hemorrhage associated with hyperperfusion, hypertension, and anticoagulation occurs in less than 1% of cases.[301–304] Seizures, which are predominantly associated with hyperperfusion, occur in less than 1% of cases.[305]

Device malfunction occurs in less than 1% of procedures and includes[268,269,306,307]:

- Stent malformation
- Stent migration
- Failure of deployment of device
- EPD failure (inability to deliver EPD to target zone, reduced steerability, and ischemia caused by EPD overloaded by embolic material)

EPDs can reduce the stroke risk associated with CAS, but the device itself is also associated with failures.[244,266,267,306,308–314] The use of appropriately sized EPDs is crucial, because undersized EPDs may allow passage of debris into distal circulation while oversized EPDs may cause endothelial injury or vasospasm.

Access-site injuries occur in up to 5% of cases and mostly consist of local pain and hematoma, which are largely self-limited and require no further intervention.[315–318] Other access-site injuries include:

- Groin infection (<1%)
- Pseudoaneurysm (1%–2%)
- Puncture-site bleeding or retroperitoneal hematoma requiring blood transfusion (2%–3%)

Contrast nephropathy is rare and has been reported in less than 1% of cases, largely because CAS is generally avoided in patients with severe renal dysfunction.[319]

EVALUATION FOR RECURRENCE AND RECURRENCE MANAGEMENT

Noninvasive imaging at the 1-month interval, followed by the 6-month interval, and then annually after revascularization, is recommended for both CAS and CEA patients. Regular imaging allows for adequate assessment of ipsilateral carotid patency and to exclude development of contralateral lesions. Once stability has been established, surveillance at longer intervals may be appropriate. Surveillance may not be indicated when the patient is no longer a candidate for intervention.

The mechanism responsible for arterial restenosis after CEA is related to the postoperative interval. Early stenosis within 2 years is largely attributed to intimal hyperplasia, whereas later restenosis is usually due to progression of the atherosclerotic disease. Very early stenosis, detected on the first postoperative duplex US, usually represents an unsatisfactory or incomplete CEA, which usually occurs in less than 1% of cases and can be minimized by using intraoperative duplex US or a completion angiography.[39]

The CAVATAS investigators reported that long-segment carotid stenosis (>0.65 times common carotid artery diameter) was associated with an increased risk for long-term restenosis. The risk for restenosis in long-segment carotid stenosis was significantly greater in CAS patients than in CEA patients.[231,232] In CAS patients, performing an angioplasty alone without stenting was also associated with increased rates of restenosis.[231,232]

The reported incidence of recurrent stenosis depends on the methods used for detection. When assessed by US, the rate of restenosis has been reported to be 5% to 10%. However, in more recent series where patch closures were used, the restenosis rate has consistently been less than 5%.[191,192,203,215,320–323] When duplex US was used, hemodynamically significant restenosis occurred in 5% to 7% of cases.[181,188,189,203,321,324–339]

Comparison data on restenosis after CAS and CEA should be interpreted with caution.[39] Most studies use US as the follow-up imaging modality, which introduces potential bias. Although stent placement has been shown to be associated with decreased rates of restenosis,[231,232] the role of stent-generated artifacts in US velocity measurements have yet to be resolved with angiographic comparison. In the authors' experience, this effect may be partially overcome by performing intraprocedural carotid US immediately after CAS, which allows for a direct comparison of carotid US results with postprocedural catheter angiography results for future reference. In the CAVATAS study, a carotid US at 1 year detected 70% to 99% stenosis in 4% of CEA patients and 14% of CAS patients (P<.001). Of note, only 22% of CAS patients had stent placement.[229–231] In the SAPHIRE trial, where all CAS patients had stent placement, carotid US at 1 year was available in 218 patients (96 CEA, 122 CAS), and the rate of restenosis greater than 70% was 4.2% in CEA patients and 0.8% in CAS patients (P = .17).[143,144] In the SPACE trial, carotid US at 1 year showed recurrent stenosis greater than 70% in 4.6% of CEA patients and 10.7% of CAS patients (P = .0009).[142,235]

In patients with recurrent symptomatic carotid stenosis, a repeat CEA or CAS can be considered, using the same criteria as recommended for initial revascularization (see earlier discussion). Repeat intervention is also recommended when duplex US and additional confirmatory imaging (MRA, CTA, or catheter angiography) shows rapidly progressive restenosis, indicating risk of complete occlusion.[39] A repeat CEA can be considered under the hands of an experienced surgeon. CAS is an alternative to repeat CEA in patients with recurrent stenosis after CEA, and may be appropriate in asymptomatic patients with restenosis greater than 80% or symptomatic restenosis greater than 50%. Repeat intervention can also be considered in patients with asymptomatic recurrent stenosis, using the same criteria for initial intervention, but should not be performed in patients with less than 70% stenosis.

SUMMARY

There are several imaging modalities available for the screening and diagnosis of carotid atherosclerotic disease, and treatment consists mainly of medical and interventional management.

Carotid US has a relatively low cost, minimal side effects and discomfort, and is widely available. It should be used as the initial screening tool for both symptomatic and asymptomatic patients with suspected carotid disease. Other more advanced noninvasive imaging, such as MRA and CTA, can be used when US yields equivocal results or is not available. MRA and CTA are helpful in determining the exact severity of stenosis and anatomic details in patients undergoing interventional management. Catheter angiography remains the gold standard for diagnosing carotid atherosclerotic disease and for grading the degree of stenosis. However, owing to its inherent cost and risk for complications such as ischemic strokes, it should be reserved for patients in whom noninvasive imaging is contraindicated, inconclusive, does not provide adequate delineation of the disease, or yields discordant results.

Medical therapy consists mainly of antithrombotic therapy and risk-factor modification. Dual-antiplatelet combination therapy has not been

Table 2 Factors influencing the decision of CEA versus CAS	
CEA	**CAS**
Anatomic factors	
• Normal location of carotid bifurcation • Independent of aortic arch • Independent of vessel tortuosity	• High (cervical) or low (intrathoracic) carotid bifurcation • Type I aortic arch • Reduced vessel tortuosity (<30°)
Plaque factors	
• Independent of aortic arch atherosclerosis • Independent of length of segment occlusion[a] • Independent of degree of calcification • Independent of stability of the plaque • Independent of presence of acute thrombus	• No arch atherosclerosis • Short segment stenosis • Lack of extensive circumferential calcification • Stable plaque • Absence of acute thrombus
Patient factors	
• Independent of age (up to 80 y old) • Male gender • Low cardiac risk • Independent of patient's renal function	• Younger patients • Independent of gender • Prior CEA • Prior neck surgery or tracheostomy • Prior neck radiation

[a] As long as distal segment can be surgically reached below the angle of the mandible.

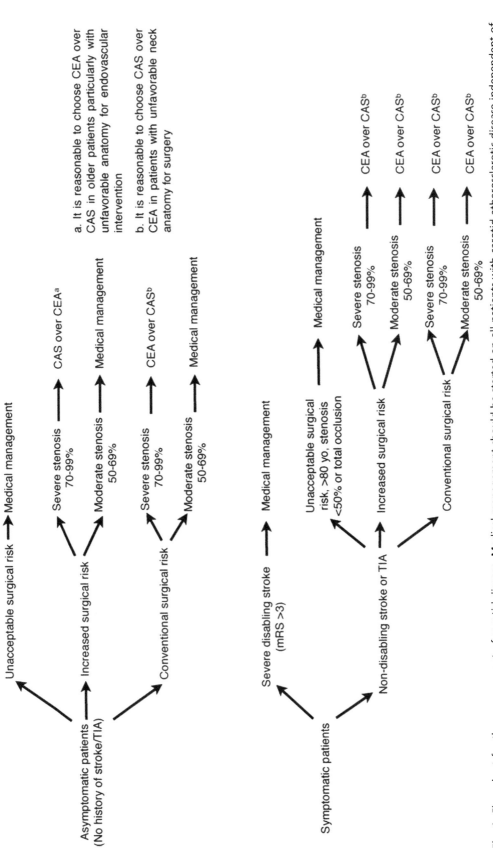

Fig. 1. Flow chart for the management of carotid disease. Medical management should be started on all patients with carotid atherosclerotic disease independent of intervention. Carotid endarterectomy (CEA) should be considered in all patients who require intervention. Carotid angioplasty and stenting (CAS) may be a better alternative to CEA in asymptomatic patients with severe stenosis and increased risk for surgery. mRS, modified Rankin Scale; TIA, transient ischemic attack; yo, years old.

shown to be superior to single agents. Anticoagulation with warfarin, along with its potential risk for increased hemorrhagic complications, also has not been shown to be superior to antiplatelet agents. Comprehensive risk-factor management should be used in these patients, including blood pressure control, cholesterol management, diabetes management, weight loss, cessation of smoking, and other lifestyle modifications.

Randomized trials such as NASCET, ECST, ACAS, ACST, SPACE, EVA-3S, SAPHIRE, and CREST (**Table 1**) have shown that revascularization decreases the long-term risk for adverse ischemic events in both asymptomatic patients with nonocclusive severe stenosis (>70%) and symptomatic patients without a devastating stroke (mRS >3), and with moderate to severe stenosis (>50%). However, patient comorbidities, overall life expectancy, and risk for periprocedural complications such as ischemic stroke, MI, and death must be taken into account (**Table 2**). The decision-making algorithm for medical treatment and types of revascularization is presented in **Fig. 1**.

REFERENCES

1. States U, Bureau TU, Participation P, et al. Prevalence of disabilities and associated health conditions among adults—United States, 1999. MMWR Morb Mortal Wkly Rep 2001;50(7):120–5. Available at: http://www.ncbi.nlm.nih.gov/pubmed/11300401.

2. Broderick J, Brott T, Kothari R, et al. The Greater Cincinnati/Northern Kentucky Stroke Study: preliminary first-ever and total incidence rates of stroke among blacks. Stroke 1998;29(2):415–21. Available at: http://www.ncbi.nlm.nih.gov/pubmed/9472883. Accessed July 15, 2014.

3. Wolf PA, Kannel WB, Sorlie P, et al. Asymptomatic carotid bruit and risk of stroke. The Framingham study. JAMA 1981;245(14):1442–5. Available at: http://www.ncbi.nlm.nih.gov/pubmed/7206146. Accessed July 23, 2014.

4. Chambless LE, Folsom AR, Clegg LX, et al. Carotid wall thickness is predictive of incident clinical stroke: the Atherosclerosis Risk in Communities (ARIC) study. Am J Epidemiol 2000;151(5): 478 87. Available at: http://www.ncbi.nlm.nih.gov/pubmed/10707916. Accessed July 23, 2014.

5. Heiss G, Sharrett AR, Barnes R, et al. Carotid atherosclerosis measured by B-mode ultrasound in populations: associations with cardiovascular risk factors in the ARIC study. Am J Epidemiol 1991; 134(3):250–6. Available at: http://www.ncbi.nlm.nih.gov/pubmed/1877584. Accessed July 23, 2014.

6. Rosamond W, Flegal K, Furie K, et al. Heart disease and stroke statistics—2008 update: a report from the American Heart Association Statistics Committee and Stroke Statistics Subcommittee. Circulation 2008;117(4):e25–146. http://dx.doi.org/10.1161/CIRCULATIONAHA.107.187998.

7. Muntner P, Garrett E, Klag MJ, et al. Trends in stroke prevalence between 1973 and 1991 in the US population 25 to 74 years of age. Stroke 2002;33(5):1209–13. Available at: http://www.ncbi.nlm.nih.gov/pubmed/11988592. Accessed July 9, 2014.

8. Barnett HJ, Taylor DW, Eliasziw M, et al. Benefit of carotid endarterectomy in patients with symptomatic moderate or severe stenosis. North American Symptomatic Carotid Endarterectomy Trial Collaborators. N Engl J Med 1998;339(20):1415–25. http://dx.doi.org/10.1056/NEJM199811123392002.

9. Taylor TN, Davis PH, Torner JC, et al. Lifetime cost of stroke in the United States. Stroke 1996;27(9): 1459–66. Available at: http://www.ncbi.nlm.nih.gov/pubmed/8784113. Accessed July 15, 2014.

10. Wolf PA, Clagett GP, Easton JD, et al. Preventing ischemic stroke in patients with prior stroke and transient ischemic attack: a statement for healthcare professionals from the Stroke Council of the American Heart Association. Stroke 1999;30(9): 1991–4. Available at: http://www.ncbi.nlm.nih.gov/pubmed/10471455. Accessed July 22, 2014.

11. Fine-Edelstein JS, Wolf PA, O'Leary DH, et al. Precursors of extracranial carotid atherosclerosis in the Framingham Study. Neurology 1994;44(6): 1046–50. Available at: http://www.ncbi.nlm.nih.gov/pubmed/8208307. Accessed July 22, 2014.

12. O'Leary DH, Polak JF, Kronmal RA, et al. Distribution and correlates of sonographically detected carotid artery disease in the Cardiovascular Health Study. The CHS Collaborative Research Group. Stroke 1992;23(12):1752–60. Available at: http://www.ncbi.nlm.nih.gov/pubmed/1448826. Accessed July 22, 2014.

13. White H, Boden-Albala B, Wang C, et al. Ischemic stroke subtype incidence among whites, blacks, and Hispanics: the Northern Manhattan Study. Circulation 2005;111(10):1327–31. http://dx.doi.org/10.1161/01.CIR.0000157736.19739.D0.

14. Petty GW, Brown RD, Whisnant JP, et al. Ischemic stroke subtypes: a population-based study of incidence and risk factors. Stroke 1999;30(12):2513–6. Available at: http://www.ncbi.nlm.nih.gov/pubmed/10582970. Accessed July 23, 2014.

15. Sacco RL, Kargman DE, Gu Q, et al. Race-ethnicity and determinants of intracranial atherosclerotic cerebral infarction. The Northern Manhattan Stroke Study. Stroke 1995;26(1):14–20. Available at: http://www.ncbi.nlm.nih.gov/pubmed/7839388. Accessed July 22, 2014.

16. Wityk RJ, Lehman D, Klag M, et al. Race and sex differences in the distribution of cerebral

atherosclerosis. Stroke 1996;27(11):1974–80. Available at: http://www.ncbi.nlm.nih.gov/pubmed/8898801. Accessed July 22, 2014.

17. Rincon F, Sacco RL, Kranwinkel G, et al. Incidence and risk factors of intracranial atherosclerotic stroke: the Northern Manhattan Stroke Study. Cerebrovasc Dis 2009;28(1):65–71. http://dx.doi.org/10.1159/000219299.

18. Gonzalez NR, Liebeskind DS, Dusick JR, et al. Intracranial arterial stenoses: current viewpoints, novel approaches, and surgical perspectives. Neurosurg Rev 2013;36(2):175–84. http://dx.doi.org/10.1007/s10143-012-0432-z [discussion: 184–5].

19. Clinical alert: benefit of carotid endarterectomy for patients with high-grade stenosis of the internal carotid artery. National Institute of Neurological Disorders and Stroke Stroke and Trauma Division. North American Symptomatic Carotid Endarterectomy Trial (NASCET) investigators. Stroke 1991; 22(6):816–7. Available at: http://www.ncbi.nlm.nih.gov/pubmed/2057984. Accessed July 22, 2014.

20. Young B, Moore WS, Robertson JT, et al. An analysis of perioperative surgical mortality and morbidity in the Asymptomatic Carotid Atherosclerosis Study. ACAS Investigators. Asymptomatic Carotid Atherosclerosis Study. Stroke 1996;27(12):2216–24. Available at: http://www.ncbi.nlm.nih.gov/pubmed/8969784. Accessed July 22, 2014.

21. Halliday AW, Thomas D, Mansfield A. The Asymptomatic Carotid Surgery Trial (ACST). Rationale and design. Steering Committee. Eur J Vasc Surg 1994; 8(6):703–10. Available at: http://www.ncbi.nlm.nih.gov/pubmed/7828747. Accessed July 22, 2014.

22. Fisher M, Paganini-Hill A, Martin A, et al. Carotid plaque pathology: thrombosis, ulceration, and stroke pathogenesis. Stroke 2005;36(2):253–7. http://dx.doi.org/10.1161/01.STR.0000152336.71224.21.

23. Lal BK, Hobson RW, Pappas PJ, et al. Pixel distribution analysis of B-mode ultrasound scan images predicts histologic features of atherosclerotic carotid plaques. J Vasc Surg 2002;35(6):1210–7. Available at: http://www.ncbi.nlm.nih.gov/pubmed/12042733. Accessed July 21, 2014.

24. Redgrave JN, Coutts SB, Schulz UG, et al. Systematic review of associations between the presence of acute ischemic lesions on diffusion-weighted imaging and clinical predictors of early stroke risk after transient ischemic attack. Stroke 2007;38(5):1482–8. http://dx.doi.org/10.1161/STROKEAHA.106.477380.

25. Takaya N, Yuan C, Chu B, et al. Association between carotid plaque characteristics and subsequent ischemic cerebrovascular events: a prospective assessment with MRI–initial results. Stroke 2006;37(3):818–23. http://dx.doi.org/10.1161/01.STR.0000204638.91099.91.

26. Spagnoli LG, Mauriello A, Sangiorgi G, et al. Extracranial thrombotically active carotid plaque as a risk factor for ischemic stroke. JAMA 2004; 292(15):1845–52. http://dx.doi.org/10.1001/jama.292.15.1845.

27. Redgrave JN, Lovett JK, Gallagher PJ, et al. Histological assessment of 526 symptomatic carotid plaques in relation to the nature and timing of ischemic symptoms: the Oxford plaque study. Circulation 2006;113(19):2320–8. http://dx.doi.org/10.1161/CIRCULATIONAHA.105.589044.

28. Rudd JH, Warburton EA, Fryer TD, et al. Imaging atherosclerotic plaque inflammation with [18F]-fluorodeoxyglucose positron emission tomography. Circulation 2002;105(23):2708–11. Available at: http://www.ncbi.nlm.nih.gov/pubmed/12057982. Accessed July 22, 2014.

29. Tawakol A, Migrino RQ, Bashian GG, et al. In vivo 18F-fluorodeoxyglucose positron emission tomography imaging provides a noninvasive measure of carotid plaque inflammation in patients. J Am Coll Cardiol 2006;48(9):1818–24. http://dx.doi.org/10.1016/j.jacc.2006.05.076.

30. Alvarez B, Ruiz C, Chacón P, et al. Serum values of metalloproteinase-2 and metalloproteinase-9 as related to unstable plaque and inflammatory cells in patients with greater than 70% carotid artery stenosis. J Vasc Surg 2004;40(3):469–75. http://dx.doi.org/10.1016/j.jvs.2004.06.023.

31. Arthurs ZM, Andersen C, Starnes BW, et al. A prospective evaluation of C-reactive protein in the progression of carotid artery stenosis. J Vasc Surg 2008;47(4):744–50. http://dx.doi.org/10.1016/j.jvs.2007.11.066 [discussion: 751].

32. Alvarez Garcia B, Ruiz C, Chacon P, et al. High sensitivity C-reactive protein in high-grade carotid stenosis: risk marker for unstable carotid plaque. J Vasc Surg 2003;38(5):1018–24. http://dx.doi.org/10.1016/S0741-5214(03)00709-2.

33. Howard G, Baker WH, Chambless LE, et al. An approach for the use of Doppler ultrasound as a screening tool for hemodynamically significant stenosis (despite heterogeneity of Doppler performance). A multicenter experience. Asymptomatic Carotid Atherosclerosis Study Investigators. Stroke 1996;27(11):1951–7. Available at: http://www.ncbi.nlm.nih.gov/pubmed/8898797. Accessed July 22, 2014.

34. Kuntz KM, Polak JF, Whittemore AD, et al. Duplex ultrasound criteria for the identification of carotid stenosis should be laboratory specific. Stroke 1997;28(3):597–602. Available at: http://www.ncbi.nlm.nih.gov/pubmed/9056618. Accessed July 22, 2014.

35. Alexandrov AV. Ultrasound and angiography in the selection of patients for carotid endarterectomy. Curr Cardiol Rep 2003;5(2):141–7. Available

at: http://www.ncbi.nlm.nih.gov/pubmed/125838 59. Accessed July 23, 2014.

36. Paciaroni M, Caso V, Cardaioli G, et al. Is ultrasound examination sufficient in the evaluation of patients with internal carotid artery severe stenosis or occlusion? Cerebrovasc Dis 2003;15(3):173–6. http://dx.doi.org/10.1159/000068832.

37. Filis KA, Arko FR, Johnson BL, et al. Duplex ultrasound criteria for defining the severity of carotid stenosis. Ann Vasc Surg 2002;16(4):413–21. http://dx.doi.org/10.1007/s10016-001-0175-8.

38. Mattos MA, Hodgson KJ, Faught WE, et al. Carotid endarterectomy without angiography: is color-flow duplex scanning sufficient? Surgery 1994;116(4): 776–82 [discussion: 782–3]. Available at: http://www.ncbi.nlm.nih.gov/pubmed/7940178. Accessed July 22, 2014.

39. Brott TG, Halperin JL, Abbara S, et al. 2011 ASA/ ACCF/AHA/AANN/AANS/ACR/ASNR/CNS/SAIP/ SCAI/SIR/SNIS/SVM/SVS guideline on the management of patients with extracranial carotid and vertebral artery disease. A report of the American College of Cardiology Foundation/American Heart Association Task Force on Practice Guidelines, and the American Stroke Association, American Association of Neuroscience Nurses, American Association of Neurological Surgeons, American College of Radiology, American Society of Neuroradiology, Congress of Neurological Surgeons, Society of Atherosclerosis Imaging and Prevention, Society for Cardiovascular Angiography and Interventions, Society of Interventional Radiology, Society of Neurointerventional Surgery, Society for Vascular Medicine, and Society for Vascular Surgery. Circulation 2011;124(4):e54–130. http://dx. doi.org/10.1161/CIR.0b013e31820d8c98.

40. Goldstein LB, Adams R, Alberts MJ, et al. Primary prevention of ischemic stroke: a guideline from the American Heart Association/American Stroke Association Stroke Council: cosponsored by the Atherosclerotic Peripheral Vascular Disease Interdisciplinary Working Group; Cardiovascular Nursing Council; Nutrition, Physical Activity, and Metabolism Council; and the Quality of Care and Outcomes Research Interdisciplinary Working Group. Circulation 2006;113(24):e873–923. http:// dx.doi.org/10.1161/01.STR.0000223048.70103.F1.

41. Whitty CJ, Sudlow CL, Warlow CP. Investigating individual subjects and screening populations for asymptomatic carotid stenosis can be harmful. J Neurol Neurosurg Psychiatry 1998;64(5): 619–23. Available at: http://www.pubmedcentral. nih.gov/articlerender.fcgi?artid=2170073&tool= pmcentrez&rendertype=abstract. Accessed July 22, 2014.

42. Grant EG, Benson CB, Moneta GL, et al. Carotid artery stenosis: gray-scale and Doppler US

diagnosis—Society of Radiologists in Ultrasound Consensus Conference. Radiology 2003;229(2): 340–6. http://dx.doi.org/10.1148/radiol.2292030516.

43. Blakeley DD, Oddone EZ, Hasselblad V, et al. Noninvasive carotid artery testing. A meta-analytic review. Ann Intern Med 1995;122(5):360–7. Available at: http://www.ncbi.nlm.nih.gov/pubmed/ 7847648. Accessed July 22, 2014.

44. AbuRahma AF, Robinson PA, Strickler DL, et al. Proposed new duplex classification for threshold stenoses used in various symptomatic and asymptomatic carotid endarterectomy trials. Ann Vasc Surg 1998;12(4):349–58. http://dx.doi.org/10. 1007/s100169900166.

45. Busuttil SJ, Franklin DP, Youkey JR, et al. Carotid duplex overestimation of stenosis due to severe contralateral disease. Am J Surg 1996;172(2): 144–7. http://dx.doi.org/10.1016/S0002-9610(96) 00137-7 [discussion: 147–8].

46. Comerota AJ, Salles-Cunha SX, Daoud Y, et al. Gender differences in blood velocities across carotid stenoses. J Vasc Surg 2004;40(5):939–44. http://dx.doi.org/10.1016/j.jvs.2004.08.030.

47. Chi YW, White CJ, Woods TC, et al. Ultrasound velocity criteria for carotid in-stent restenosis. Catheter Cardiovasc Interv 2007;69(3):349–54. http:// dx.doi.org/10.1002/ccd.21032.

48. Utter GH, Hollingworth W, Hallam DK, et al. Sixteen-slice CT angiography in patients with suspected blunt carotid and vertebral artery injuries. J Am Coll Surg 2006;203(6):838–48. http://dx.doi. org/10.1016/j.jamcollsurg.2006.08.003.

49. Jahromi AS, Cinà CS, Liu Y, et al. Sensitivity and specificity of color duplex ultrasound measurement in the estimation of internal carotid artery stenosis: a systematic review and meta-analysis. J Vasc Surg 2005;41(6):962–72. http://dx.doi.org/10. 1016/j.jvs.2005.02.044.

50. Nederkoorn PJ, van der Graaf Y, Hunink MG. Duplex ultrasound and magnetic resonance angiography compared with digital subtraction angiography in carotid artery stenosis: a systematic review. Stroke 2003;34(5):1324–32. http://dx.doi. org/10.1161/01.STR.0000068367.08991.A2.

51. DeMarco JK, Huston J, Bernstein MA. Evaluation of classic 2D time-of-flight MR angiography in the depiction of severe carotid stenosis. AJR Am J Roentgenol 2004;183(3):787–93. http://dx.doi.org/ 10.2214/ajr.183.3.1830787.

52. Belsky M, Gaitini D, Goldsher D, et al. Color-coded duplex ultrasound compared to CT angiography for detection and quantification of carotid artery stenosis. Eur J Ultrasound 2000;12(1):49–60. Available at: http://www.ncbi.nlm.nih.gov/pubmed/ 10996770. Accessed July 22, 2014.

53. Grønholdt ML. B-mode ultrasound and spiral CT for the assessment of carotid atherosclerosis.

Neuroimaging Clin N Am 2002;12(3):421–35. Available at: http://www.ncbi.nlm.nih.gov/pubmed/12486830. Accessed July 22, 2014.

54. Hollingworth W, Nathens AB, Kanne JP, et al. The diagnostic accuracy of computed tomography angiography for traumatic or atherosclerotic lesions of the carotid and vertebral arteries: a systematic review. Eur J Radiol 2003;48(1):88–102. Available at: http://www.ncbi.nlm.nih.gov/pubmed/14511863. Accessed July 22, 2014.

55. Koelemay MJ, Nederkoorn PJ, Reitsma JB, et al. Systematic review of computed tomographic angiography for assessment of carotid artery disease. Stroke 2004;35(10):2306–12. http://dx.doi.org/10.1161/01.STR.0000141426.63959.cc.

56. Enterline DS, Kapoor G. A practical approach to CT angiography of the neck and brain. Tech Vasc Interv Radiol 2006;9(4):192–204. http://dx.doi.org/10.1053/j.tvir.2007.03.003.

57. Clevert DA, Johnson T, Jung EM, et al. Color Doppler, power Doppler and B-flow ultrasound in the assessment of ICA stenosis: comparison with 64-MD-CT angiography. Eur Radiol 2007;17(8):2149–59. http://dx.doi.org/10.1007/s00330-006-0488-7.

58. Wutke R, Lang W, Fellner C, et al. High-resolution, contrast-enhanced magnetic resonance angiography with elliptical centric k-space ordering of supra-aortic arteries compared with selective X-ray angiography. Stroke 2002;33(6):1522–9. Available at: http://www.ncbi.nlm.nih.gov/pubmed/12052985. Accessed July 22, 2014.

59. Alvarez-Linera J, Benito-León J, Escribano J, et al. Prospective evaluation of carotid artery stenosis: elliptic centric contrast-enhanced MR angiography and spiral CT angiography compared with digital subtraction angiography. AJNR Am J Neuroradiol 2003;24(5):1012–9. Available at: http://www.ncbi.nlm.nih.gov/pubmed/12748115. Accessed July 22, 2014.

60. Remonda L, Senn P, Barth A, et al. Contrast-enhanced 3D MR angiography of the carotid artery: comparison with conventional digital subtraction angiography. AJNR Am J Neuroradiol 2002;23(2):213–9. Available at: http://www.ncbi.nlm.nih.gov/pubmed/11847044. Accessed July 22, 2014.

61. Cosottini M, Pingitore A, Puglioli M, et al. Contrast-enhanced three-dimensional magnetic resonance angiography of atherosclerotic internal carotid stenosis as the noninvasive imaging modality in revascularization decision making. Stroke 2003;34(3):660–4. http://dx.doi.org/10.1161/01.STR.0000057462.02141.6F.

62. Yucel EK, Anderson CM, Edelman RR, et al. AHA scientific statement. Magnetic resonance angiography: update on applications for extracranial arteries. Circulation 1999;100(22):2284–301.

Available at: http://www.ncbi.nlm.nih.gov/pubmed/10578005. Accessed July 22, 2014.

63. Josephson SA, Bryant SO, Mak HK, et al. Evaluation of carotid stenosis using CT angiography in the initial evaluation of stroke and TIA. Neurology 2004;63(3):457–60. Available at: http://www.ncbi.nlm.nih.gov/pubmed/15304575. Accessed July 22, 2014.

64. Glor FP, Ariff B, Crowe LA, et al. Carotid geometry reconstruction: a comparison between MRI and ultrasound. Med Phys 2003;30(12):3251–61. Available at: http://www.ncbi.nlm.nih.gov/pubmed/14713092. Accessed July 22, 2014.

65. Teng MM, Tsai F, Liou AJ, et al. Three-dimensional contrast-enhanced magnetic resonance angiography of carotid artery after stenting. J Neuroimaging 2004;14(4):336–41. http://dx.doi.org/10.1177/1051228404267620.

66. Chen CJ, Lee TH, Hsu HL, et al. Multi-slice CT angiography in diagnosing total versus near occlusions of the internal carotid artery: comparison with catheter angiography. Stroke 2004;35(1):83–5. http://dx.doi.org/10.1161/01.STR.0000106139.38566.B2.

67. Kaufmann TJ, Huston J, Mandrekar JN, et al. Complications of diagnostic cerebral angiography: evaluation of 19,826 consecutive patients. Radiology 2007;243(3):812–9. http://dx.doi.org/10.1148/radiol.2433060536.

68. Thiex R, Norbash AM, Frerichs KU. The safety of dedicated-team catheter-based diagnostic cerebral angiography in the era of advanced noninvasive imaging. AJNR Am J Neuroradiol 2010;31(2):230–4. http://dx.doi.org/10.3174/ajnr.A1803.

69. Antithrombotic Trialists' Collaboration. Collaborative meta-analysis of randomised trials of antiplatelet therapy for prevention of death, myocardial infarction, and stroke in high risk patients. BMJ 2002;324(7329):71–86. Available at: http://www.pubmedcentral.nih.gov/articlerender.fcgi?artid=64503&tool=pmcentrez&rendertype=abstract. Accessed July 14, 2014.

70. Adams RJ, Albers G, Alberts MJ, et al. Update to the AHA/ASA recommendations for the prevention of stroke in patients with stroke and transient ischemic attack. Stroke 2008;39(5):1647–52. http://dx.doi.org/10.1161/STROKEAHA.107.189063.

71. A randomized trial of aspirin and sulfinpyrazone in threatened stroke. The Canadian Cooperative Study Group. N Engl J Med 1978;299(2):53–9. http://dx.doi.org/10.1056/NEJM197807132990201.

72. CAPRIE Steering Committee. A randomised, blinded, trial of clopidogrel versus aspirin in patients at risk of ischaemic events (CAPRIE). CAPRIE Steering Committee. Lancet 1996;348(9038):1329–39. Available at: http://www.ncbi.nlm.nih.gov/pubmed/8918275. Accessed July 22, 2014.

73. Diener HC, Bogousslavsky J, Brass LM, et al. Aspirin and clopidogrel compared with clopidogrel

alone after recent ischaemic stroke or transient ischaemic attack in high-risk patients (MATCH): randomised, double-blind, placebo-controlled trial. Lancet 2004;364(9431):331–7. http://dx.doi.org/10.1016/S0140-6736(04)16721-4.

74. Bhatt DL, Fox KA, Hacke W, et al. Clopidogrel and aspirin versus aspirin alone for the prevention of atherothrombotic events. N Engl J Med 2006;354(16):1706–17. http://dx.doi.org/10.1056/NEJMoa060989.

75. Diener HC, Cunha L, Forbes C, et al. European Stroke Prevention Study. 2. Dipyridamole and acetylsalicylic acid in the secondary prevention of stroke. J Neurol Sci 1996;143(1–2):1–13. Available at: http://www.ncbi.nlm.nih.gov/pubmed/8981292. Accessed July 22, 2014.

76. Sacco RL, Diener HC, Yusuf S, et al. Aspirin and extended-release dipyridamole versus clopidogrel for recurrent stroke. N Engl J Med 2008;359(12):1238–51. http://dx.doi.org/10.1056/NEJMoa0805002.

77. Alberts MJ, Bergman DL, Molner E, et al. Antiplatelet effect of aspirin in patients with cerebrovascular disease. Stroke 2004;35(1):175–8. http://dx.doi.org/10.1161/01.STR.0000106763.46123.F6.

78. Chen LC, Ashcroft DM. Do selective COX-2 inhibitors increase the risk of cerebrovascular events? A meta-analysis of randomized controlled trials. J Clin Pharm Ther 2006;31(6):565–76. http://dx.doi.org/10.1111/j.1365-2710.2006.00774.x.

79. Côté R, Battista RN, Abrahamowicz M, et al. Lack of effect of aspirin in asymptomatic patients with carotid bruits and substantial carotid narrowing. The Asymptomatic Cervical Bruit Study Group. Ann Intern Med 1995;123(9):649–55. Available at: http://www.ncbi.nlm.nih.gov/pubmed/7574219. Accessed July 22, 2014.

80. Mohr JP, Thompson JL, Lazar RM, et al. A comparison of warfarin and aspirin for the prevention of recurrent ischemic stroke. N Engl J Med 2001;345(20):1444–51. http://dx.doi.org/10.1056/NEJMoa011258.

81. Adams HP, del Zoppo G, Alberts MJ, et al. Guidelines for the early management of adults with ischemic stroke: a guideline from the American Heart Association/American Stroke Association Stroke Council, Clinical Cardiology Council, Cardiovascular Radiology and Intervention Council, and the Atheros. Stroke 2007;38(5):1655–711. http://dx.doi.org/10.1161/STROKEAHA.107.181486.

82. Woessner R, Grauer M, Bianchi O, et al. Treatment with anticoagulants in cerebral events (TRACE). Thromb Haemost 2004;91(4):690–3. http://dx.doi.org/10.1267/THRO04040690.

83. Low molecular weight heparinoid, ORG 10172 (danaparoid), and outcome after acute ischemic stroke: a randomized controlled trial. The Publications Committee for the Trial of ORG 10172 in Acute Stroke Treatment (TOAST) Investigators. JAMA 1998;279(16):1265–72. Available at: http://www.ncbi.nlm.nih.gov/pubmed/9565006. Accessed July 22, 2014.

84. Risk factors for stroke and efficacy of antithrombotic therapy in atrial fibrillation. Analysis of pooled data from five randomized controlled trials. Arch Intern Med 1994;154(13):1449–57. Available at: http://www.ncbi.nlm.nih.gov/pubmed/8018000. Accessed July 20, 2014.

85. Lawes CM, Bennett DA, Feigin VL, et al. Blood pressure and stroke: an overview of published reviews. Stroke 2004;35(3):776–85. http://dx.doi.org/10.1161/01.STR.0000116869.64771.5A.

86. Neal B, MacMahon S, Chapman N. Effects of ACE inhibitors, calcium antagonists, and other blood-pressure-lowering drugs: results of prospectively designed overviews of randomised trials. Blood Pressure Lowering Treatment Trialists' Collaboration. Lancet 2000;356(9246):1955–64. Available at: http://www.ncbi.nlm.nih.gov/pubmed/11130523. Accessed July 22, 2014.

87. Rashid P, Leonardi-Bee J, Bath P. Blood pressure reduction and secondary prevention of stroke and other vascular events: a systematic review. Stroke 2003;34(11):2741–8. http://dx.doi.org/10.1161/01.STR.0000092488.40085.15.

88. MacMahon S, Rodgers A. Blood pressure, antihypertensive treatment and stroke risk. J Hypertens Suppl 1994;12(10):S5–14. Available at: http://www.ncbi.nlm.nih.gov/pubmed/7769492. Accessed July 22, 2014.

89. Sacco RL, Adams R, Albers G, et al. Guidelines for prevention of stroke in patients with ischemic stroke or transient ischemic attack: a statement for healthcare professionals from the American Heart Association/American Stroke Association Council on Stroke: co-sponsored by the Council on Cardiovascular Radiology and Intervention: the American Academy of Neurology affirms the value of this guideline. Stroke 2006;37(2):577–617. http://dx.doi.org/10.1161/01.STR.0000199147.30016.74.

90. PROGRESS Collaborative Group. Randomised trial of a perindopril-based blood-pressure-lowering regimen among 6,105 individuals with previous stroke or transient ischaemic attack. Lancet 2001;358(9287):1033–41. http://dx.doi.org/10.1016/S0140-6736(01)06178-5.

91. Yusuf S, Sleight P, Pogue J, et al. Effects of an angiotensin-converting-enzyme inhibitor, ramipril, on cardiovascular events in high-risk patients. The Heart Outcomes Prevention Evaluation Study Investigators. N Engl J Med 2000;342(3):145–53. http://dx.doi.org/10.1056/NEJM200001203420301.

92. Silvestrini M, Vernieri F, Pasqualetti P, et al. Impaired cerebral vasoreactivity and risk of stroke in patients with asymptomatic carotid artery stenosis. JAMA 2000;283(16):2122–7. Available at: http://www.ncbi.nlm.nih.gov/pubmed/10791504. Accessed July 22, 2014.

93. Amarenco P, Bogousslavsky J, Callahan A, et al. High-dose atorvastatin after stroke or transient ischemic attack. N Engl J Med 2006;355(6):549–59. http://dx.doi.org/10.1056/NEJMoa061894.

94. National Cholesterol Education Program (NCEP) Expert Panel on Detection, Evaluation, and Treatment of High Blood Cholesterol in Adults (Adult Treatment Panel III). Third report of the National Cholesterol Education Program (NCEP) Expert Panel on Detection, Evaluation, and Treatment of High Blood Cholesterol in Adults (Adult Treatment Panel III) final report. Circulation 2002; 106(25):3143–421. Available at: http://www.ncbi.nlm.nih.gov/pubmed/12485966. Accessed July 10, 2014.

95. Kris-Etherton PM, Harris WS, Appel LJ. Fish consumption, fish oil, omega-3 fatty acids, and cardiovascular disease. Circulation 2002;106(21): 2747–57. Available at: http://www.ncbi.nlm.nih.gov/pubmed/12438303. Accessed July 22, 2014.

96. Brown BG, Zhao XQ, Chait A, et al. Simvastatin and niacin, antioxidant vitamins, or the combination for the prevention of coronary disease. N Engl J Med 2001;345(22):1583–92. http://dx.doi.org/10.1056/NEJMoa011090.

97. Frick MH, Elo O, Haapa K, et al. Helsinki Heart Study: primary-prevention trial with gemfibrozil in middle-aged men with dyslipidemia. Safety of treatment, changes in risk factors, and incidence of coronary heart disease. N Engl J Med 1987; 317(20):1237–45. http://dx.doi.org/10.1056/NEJM198711123172001.

98. Rubins HB, Robins SJ, Collins D, et al. Gemfibrozil for the secondary prevention of coronary heart disease in men with low levels of high-density lipoprotein cholesterol. Veterans Affairs High-Density Lipoprotein Cholesterol Intervention Trial Study Group. N Engl J Med 1999;341(6):410–8. http://dx.doi.org/10.1056/NEJM199908053410604.

99. Sacco RL, Roberts JK, Boden-Albala B, et al. Race-ethnicity and determinants of carotid atherosclerosis in a multiethnic population. The Northern Manhattan Stroke Study. Stroke 1997;28(5): 929–35. Available at: http://www.ncbi.nlm.nih.gov/pubmed/9158627. Accessed July 22, 2014.

100. O'Leary DH, Polak JF, Kronmal RA, et al. Thickening of the carotid wall. A marker for atherosclerosis in the elderly? Cardiovascular Health Study Collaborative Research Group. Stroke 1996;27(2): 224–31. Available at: http://www.ncbi.nlm.nih.gov/pubmed/8571414. Accessed July 22, 2014.

101. Sharrett AR, Patsch W, Sorlie PD, et al. Associations of lipoprotein cholesterols, apolipoproteins A-I and B, and triglycerides with carotid atherosclerosis and coronary heart disease. The Atherosclerosis Risk in Communities (ARIC) Study. Arterioscler Thromb 1994;14(7):1098–104. Available at: http://www.ncbi.nlm.nih.gov/pubmed/8018665. Accessed July 22, 2014.

102. Briel M, Studer M, Glass TR, et al. Effects of statins on stroke prevention in patients with and without coronary heart disease: a meta-analysis of randomized controlled trials. Am J Med 2004;117(8): 596–606. http://dx.doi.org/10.1016/j.amjmed.2004.04.022.

103. Amarenco P, Labreuche J, Lavallée P, et al. Statins in stroke prevention and carotid atherosclerosis: systematic review and up-to-date meta-analysis. Stroke 2004;35(12):2902–9. http://dx.doi.org/10.1161/01.STR.0000147965.52712.fa.

104. Baigent C, Keech A, Kearney PM, et al. Efficacy and safety of cholesterol-lowering treatment: prospective meta-analysis of data from 90,056 participants in 14 randomised trials of statins. Lancet 2005;366(9493):1267–78. http://dx.doi.org/10.1016/S0140-6736(05)67394-1.

105. Smilde TJ, van Wissen S, Wollersheim H, et al. Effect of aggressive versus conventional lipid lowering on atherosclerosis progression in familial hypercholesterolaemia (ASAP): a prospective, randomised, double-blind trial. Lancet 2001; 357(9256):577–81. Available at: http://www.ncbi.nlm.nih.gov/pubmed/11558482. Accessed July 11, 2014.

106. Taylor AJ, Sullenberger LE, Lee HJ, et al. Arterial Biology for the Investigation of the Treatment Effects of Reducing Cholesterol (ARBITER) 2: a double-blind, placebo-controlled study of extended-release niacin on atherosclerosis progression in secondary prevention patients treated with statins. Circulation 2004;110(23): 3512–7. http://dx.doi.org/10.1161/01.CIR.0000148955.19792.8D.

107. Crouse JR, Raichlen JS, Riley WA, et al. Effect of rosuvastatin on progression of carotid intima-media thickness in low-risk individuals with subclinical atherosclerosis: the METEOR Trial. JAMA 2007; 297(12):1344–53. http://dx.doi.org/10.1001/jama.297.12.1344.

108. Canner PL, Berge KG, Wenger NK, et al. Fifteen year mortality in Coronary Drug Project patients: long-term benefit with niacin. J Am Coll Cardiol 1986;8(6):1245–55. Available at: http://www.ncbi.nlm.nih.gov/pubmed/3782631. Accessed July 22, 2014.

109. Keech A, Simes RJ, Barter P, et al. Effects of long-term fenofibrate therapy on cardiovascular events in 9795 people with type 2 diabetes mellitus

(the FIELD study): randomised controlled trial. Lancet 2005;366(9500):1849–61. http://dx.doi.org/10.1016/S0140-6736(05)67667-2.

110. Bloomfield Rubins H, Davenport J, Babikian V, et al. Reduction in stroke with gemfibrozil in men with coronary heart disease and low HDL cholesterol: the Veterans Affairs HDL Intervention Trial (VA-HIT). Circulation 2001;103(23):2828–33. Available at: http://www.ncbi.nlm.nih.gov/pubmed/11401940. Accessed July 22, 2014.

111. Kastelein JJP, Akdim F, Stroes ES, et al. Simvastatin with or without ezetimibe in familial hypercholesterolemia. N Engl J Med 2008;358(14):1431–43. http://dx.doi.org/10.1056/NEJMoa0800742.

112. Blankenhorn DH, Selzer RH, Crawford DW, et al. Beneficial effects of colestipol-niacin therapy on the common carotid artery. Two- and four-year reduction of intima-media thickness measured by ultrasound. Circulation 1993;88(1):20–8. Available at: http://www.ncbi.nlm.nih.gov/pubmed/8319334. Accessed July 22, 2014.

113. Smith NL, Barzilay JI, Shaffer D, et al. Fasting and 2-hour postchallenge serum glucose measures and risk of incident cardiovascular events in the elderly: the Cardiovascular Health Study. Arch Intern Med 2002;162(2):209–16. Available at: http://www.ncbi.nlm.nih.gov/pubmed/11802755. Accessed July 22, 2014.

114. Manson JE, Colditz GA, Stampfer MJ, et al. A prospective study of maturity-onset diabetes mellitus and risk of coronary heart disease and stroke in women. Arch Intern Med 1991;151(6):1141–7. Available at: http://www.ncbi.nlm.nih.gov/pubmed/2043016. Accessed July 22, 2014.

115. Karapanayiotides T, Piechowski-Jozwiak B, van Melle G, et al. Stroke patterns, etiology, and prognosis in patients with diabetes mellitus. Neurology 2004;62(9):1558–62. Available at: http://www.ncbi.nlm.nih.gov/pubmed/15136681. Accessed July 22, 2014.

116. Folsom AR, Rasmussen ML, Chambless LE, et al. Prospective associations of fasting insulin, body fat distribution, and diabetes with risk of ischemic stroke. The Atherosclerosis Risk in Communities (ARIC) Study Investigators. Diabetes Care 1999;22(7):1077–83. Available at: http://www.ncbi.nlm.nih.gov/pubmed/10388971. Accessed July 22, 2014.

117. Dobs AS, Nieto FJ, Szklo M, et al. Risk factors for popliteal and carotid wall thicknesses in the Atherosclerosis Risk in Communities (ARIC) Study. Am J Epidemiol 1999;150(10):1055–67. Available at: http://www.ncbi.nlm.nih.gov/pubmed/10568620. Accessed July 24, 2014.

118. Wagenknecht LE, D'Agostino R, Savage PJ, et al. Duration of diabetes and carotid wall thickness. The Insulin Resistance Atherosclerosis Study (IRAS). Stroke 1997;28(5):999–1005. Available at: http://www.ncbi.nlm.nih.gov/pubmed/9158641. Accessed July 22, 2014.

119. Haffner SM, Agostino RD, Saad MF, et al. Carotid artery atherosclerosis in type-2 diabetic and nondiabetic subjects with and without symptomatic coronary artery disease (The Insulin Resistance Atherosclerosis Study). Am J Cardiol 2000;85(12):1395–400. Available at: http://www.ncbi.nlm.nih.gov/pubmed/10856382. Accessed July 22, 2014.

120. Wagenknecht LE, Zaccaro D, Espeland MA, et al. Diabetes and progression of carotid atherosclerosis: the insulin resistance atherosclerosis study. Arterioscler Thromb Vasc Biol 2003;23(6):1035–41. http://dx.doi.org/10.1161/01.ATV.0000072273.67342.6D.

121. Chambless LE, Folsom AR, Davis V, et al. Risk factors for progression of common carotid atherosclerosis: the Atherosclerosis Risk in Communities Study, 1987-1998. Am J Epidemiol 2002;155(1):38–47. Available at: http://www.ncbi.nlm.nih.gov/pubmed/11772783. Accessed July 22, 2014.

122. Nathan DM, Lachin J, Cleary P, et al. Intensive diabetes therapy and carotid intima-media thickness in type 1 diabetes mellitus. N Engl J Med 2003;348(23):2294–303. http://dx.doi.org/10.1056/NEJMoa022314.

123. Langenfeld MR, Forst T, Hohberg C, et al. Pioglitazone decreases carotid intima-media thickness independently of glycemic control in patients with type 2 diabetes mellitus: results from a controlled randomized study. Circulation 2005;111(19):2525–31. http://dx.doi.org/10.1161/01.CIR.0000165072.01672.21.

124. Mazzone T, Meyer PM, Feinstein SB, et al. Effect of pioglitazone compared with glimepiride on carotid intima-media thickness in type 2 diabetes: a randomized trial. JAMA 2006;296(21):2572–81. http://dx.doi.org/10.1001/jama.296.21.joc60158.

125. Shinton R, Beevers G. Meta-analysis of relation between cigarette smoking and stroke. BMJ 1989;298(6676):789–94. Available at: http://www.pubmedcentral.nih.gov/articlerender.fcgi?artid=1836102&tool=pmcentrez&rendertype=abstract. Accessed July 24, 2014.

126. Kawachi I, Colditz GA, Stampfer MJ, et al. Smoking cessation and decreased risk of stroke in women. JAMA 1993;269(2):232–6. Available at: http://www.ncbi.nlm.nih.gov/pubmed/8417241. Accessed July 22, 2014.

127. Robbins AS, Manson JE, Lee IM, et al. Cigarette smoking and stroke in a cohort of U.S. male physicians. Ann Intern Med 1994;120(6):458–62. Available at: http://www.ncbi.nlm.nih.gov/pubmed/8311368. Accessed July 13, 2014.

128. Wannamethee SG, Shaper AG, Whincup PH, et al. Smoking cessation and the risk of stroke in

middle-aged men. JAMA 1995;274(2):155–60. Available at: http://www.ncbi.nlm.nih.gov/pubmed/7596004. Accessed July 22, 2014.

129. Rohr J, Kittner S, Feeser B, et al. Traditional risk factors and ischemic stroke in young adults: the Baltimore-Washington Cooperative Young Stroke Study. Arch Neurol 1996;53(7):603–7. Available at: http://www.ncbi.nlm.nih.gov/pubmed/8929167. Accessed July 22, 2014.

130. Howard G, Wagenknecht LE, Cai J, et al. Cigarette smoking and other risk factors for silent cerebral infarction in the general population. Stroke 1998; 29(5):913–7. Available at: http://www.ncbi.nlm.nih.gov/pubmed/9596234. Accessed July 22, 2014.

131. Lu M, Ye W, Adami HO, et al. Stroke incidence in women under 60 years of age related to alcohol intake and smoking habit. Cerebrovasc Dis 2008; 25(6):517–25. http://dx.doi.org/10.1159/000131669.

132. Wilson PW, Hoeg JM, D'Agostino RB, et al. Cumulative effects of high cholesterol levels, high blood pressure, and cigarette smoking on carotid stenosis. N Engl J Med 1997;337(8):516–22. http://dx.doi.org/10.1056/NEJM199708213370802.

133. Tell GS, Rutan GH, Kronmal RA, et al. Correlates of blood pressure in community-dwelling older adults. The Cardiovascular Health Study. Cardiovascular Health Study (CHS) Collaborative Research Group. Hypertension 1994;23(1):59–67. Available at: http://www.ncbi.nlm.nih.gov/pubmed/8282331. Accessed July 22, 2014.

134. Wolf PA, D'Agostino RB, Kannel WB, et al. Cigarette smoking as a risk factor for stroke. The Framingham Study. JAMA 1988;259(7):1025–9. Available at: http://www.ncbi.nlm.nih.gov/pubmed/3339799. Accessed July 22, 2014.

135. Winter Y, Rohrmann S, Linseisen J, et al. Contribution of obesity and abdominal fat mass to risk of stroke and transient ischemic attacks. Stroke 2008;39(12):3145–51. http://dx.doi.org/10.1161/STROKEAHA.108.523001.

136. Sacco RL, Gan R, Boden-Albala B, et al. Leisure-time physical activity and ischemic stroke risk: the Northern Manhattan Stroke Study. Stroke 1998; 29(2):380–7. Available at: http://www.ncbi.nlm.nih.gov/pubmed/9472878. Accessed July 22, 2014.

137. Hankey GJ. Potential new risk factors for ischemic stroke: what is their potential? Stroke 2006;37(8): 2181–8. http://dx.doi.org/10.1161/01.STR.0000229883.72010.e4.

138. Endarterectomy for asymptomatic carotid artery stenosis. Executive Committee for the Asymptomatic Carotid Atherosclerosis Study. JAMA 1995;273(18): 1421–8. Available at: http://www.ncbi.nlm.nih.gov/pubmed/7723155. Accessed July 22, 2014.

139. Halliday A, Mansfield A, Marro J, et al. Prevention of disabling and fatal strokes by successful carotid endarterectomy in patients without recent neurological symptoms: randomised controlled trial. Lancet 2004;363(9420):1491–502. http://dx.doi.org/10.1016/S0140-6736(04)16146-1.

140. North American Symptomatic Carotid Endarterectomy Trial Collaborators. Beneficial effect of carotid endarterectomy in symptomatic patients with high-grade carotid stenosis. N Engl J Med 1991;325(7):445–53. http://dx.doi.org/10.1056/NEJM199108153250701.

141. Brott TG, Hobson RW, Howard G, et al. Stenting versus endarterectomy for treatment of carotid-artery stenosis. N Engl J Med 2010;363(1):11–23. http://dx.doi.org/10.1056/NEJMoa0912321.

142. Eckstein HH, Ringleb P, Allenberg JR, et al. Results of the Stent-Protected Angioplasty versus Carotid Endarterectomy (SPACE) study to treat symptomatic stenoses at 2 years: a multinational, prospective, randomised trial. Lancet Neurol 2008;7(10):893–902. http://dx.doi.org/10.1016/S1474-4422(08)70196-0.

143. Gurm HS, Yadav JS, Fayad P, et al. Long-term results of carotid stenting versus endarterectomy in high-risk patients. N Engl J Med 2008;358(15):1572–9. http://dx.doi.org/10.1056/NEJMoa0708028.

144. Yadav JS, Wholey MH, Kuntz RE, et al. Protected carotid-artery stenting versus endarterectomy in high-risk patients. N Engl J Med 2004;351(15): 1493–501. http://dx.doi.org/10.1056/NEJMoa040127.

145. Mas JL, Trinquart L, Leys D, et al. Endarterectomy versus angioplasty in patients with symptomatic severe carotid stenosis (EVA-3S) trial: results up to 4 years from a randomised, multicentre trial. Lancet Neurol 2008;7(10):885–92. http://dx.doi.org/10.1016/S1474-4422(08)70195-9.

146. Bonati LH, Jongen LM, Haller S, et al. New ischaemic brain lesions on MRI after stenting or endarterectomy for symptomatic carotid stenosis: a substudy of the International Carotid Stenting Study (ICSS). Lancet Neurol 2010;9(4):353–62. http://dx.doi.org/10.1016/S1474-4422(10)70057-0.

147. Randomised trial of endarterectomy for recently symptomatic carotid stenosis: final results of the MRC European Carotid Surgery Trial (ECST). Lancet 1998;351(9113):1379–87. Available at: http://www.ncbi.nlm.nih.gov/pubmed/9593407. Accessed July 22, 2014.

148. Rothwell PM, Slattery J, Warlow CP. A systematic review of the risks of stroke and death due to endarterectomy for symptomatic carotid stenosis. Stroke 1996;27(2):260–5. Available at: http://www.ncbi.nlm.nih.gov/pubmed/8571420. Accessed July 22, 2014.

149. Rothwell PM, Eliasziw M, Gutnikov SA, et al. Endarterectomy for symptomatic carotid stenosis in relation to clinical subgroups and timing of surgery. Lancet 2004;363(9413):915–24. http://dx.doi.org/10.1016/S0140-6736(04)15785-1.

150. Rothwell PM, Eliasziw M, Gutnikov SA, et al. Analysis of pooled data from the randomised controlled trials of endarterectomy for symptomatic carotid stenosis. Lancet 2003;361(9352):107–16. Available at: http://www.ncbi.nlm.nih.gov/pubmed/12531577. Accessed July 22, 2014.

151. Rothwell PM, Gutnikov SA, Warlow CP. Reanalysis of the final results of the European Carotid Surgery Trial. Stroke 2003;34(2):514–23. http://dx.doi.org/10.1161/01.STR.0000054671.71777.C7.

152. Mayberg MR, Wilson SE, Yatsu F, et al. Carotid endarterectomy and prevention of cerebral ischemia in symptomatic carotid stenosis. Veterans Affairs Cooperative Studies Program 309 Trialist Group. JAMA 1991;266(23):3289–94. Available at: http://www.ncbi.nlm.nih.gov/pubmed/1960828. Accessed July 22, 2014.

153. Hobson RW, Weiss DG, Fields WS, et al. Efficacy of carotid endarterectomy for asymptomatic carotid stenosis. The Veterans Affairs Cooperative Study Group. N Engl J Med 1993;328(4):221–7. http://dx.doi.org/10.1056/NEJM199301283280401.

154. Gray WA, Hopkins LN, Yadav S, et al. Protected carotid stenting in high-surgical-risk patients: the ARCHeR results. J Vasc Surg 2006;44(2):258–68. http://dx.doi.org/10.1016/j.jvs.2006.03.044.

155. Katzen BT, Criado FJ, Ramee SR, et al. Carotid artery stenting with emboli protection surveillance study: thirty-day results of the CASES-PMS study. Catheter Cardiovasc Interv 2007;70(2):316–23. http://dx.doi.org/10.1002/ccd.21222.

156. Rothwell PM, Goldstein LB. Carotid endarterectomy for asymptomatic carotid stenosis: Asymptomatic Carotid Surgery Trial. Stroke 2004; 35(10):2425–7. http://dx.doi.org/10.1161/01.STR.0000141706.50170.a7.

157. Role of carotid endarterectomy in asymptomatic carotid stenosis. A Veterans Administration Cooperative Study. Stroke 1986;17(3):534–9. Available at: http://www.ncbi.nlm.nih.gov/pubmed/2872740. Accessed July 22, 2014.

158. Towne JB, Weiss DG, Hobson RW. First phase report of cooperative Veterans Administration asymptomatic carotid stenosis study—operative morbidity and mortality. J Vasc Surg 1990;11(2):252–8 [discussion: 258–9]. Available at: http://www.ncbi.nlm.nih.gov/pubmed/2405197. Accessed July 22, 2014.

159. Cowan JA, Dimick JB, Thompson BG, et al. Surgeon volume as an indicator of outcomes after carotid endarterectomy: an effect independent of specialty practice and hospital volume. J Am Coll Surg 2002;195(6):814–21. Available at: http://www.ncbi.nlm.nih.gov/pubmed/12495314. Accessed July 23, 2014.

160. Killeen SD, Andrews EJ, Redmond HP, et al. Provider volume and outcomes for abdominal aortic aneurysm repair, carotid endarterectomy, and lower extremity revascularization procedures. J Vasc Surg 2007;45(3):615–26. http://dx.doi.org/10.1016/j.jvs.2006.11.019.

161. Holt PJ, Poloniecki JD, Loftus IM, et al. Meta-analysis and systematic review of the relationship between hospital volume and outcome following carotid endarterectomy. Eur J Vasc Endovasc Surg 2007;33(6):645–51. http://dx.doi.org/10.1016/j.ejvs.2007.01.014.

162. Kennedy J, Quan H, Buchan AM, et al. Statins are associated with better outcomes after carotid endarterectomy in symptomatic patients. Stroke 2005; 36(10):2072–6. http://dx.doi.org/10.1161/01.STR.0000183623.28144.32.

163. Kazmers A, Perkins AJ, Huber TS, et al. Carotid surgery in octogenarians in Veterans Affairs medical centers. J Surg Res 1999;81(1):87–90. http://dx.doi.org/10.1006/jsre.1998.5459.

164. Wennberg DE, Lucas FL, Birkmeyer JD, et al. Variation in carotid endarterectomy mortality in the Medicare population: trial hospitals, volume, and patient characteristics. JAMA 1998;279(16): 1278–81. Available at: http://www.ncbi.nlm.nih.gov/pubmed/9565008. Accessed July 22, 2014.

165. Debing E, Van den Brande P. Carotid endarterectomy in the elderly: are the patient characteristics, the early outcome, and the predictors the same as those in younger patients? Surg Neurol 2007; 67(5):467–71. http://dx.doi.org/10.1016/j.surneu.2006.08.084 [discussion: 471].

166. Hellings WE, Pasterkamp G, Verhoeven BA, et al. Gender associated differences in plaque phenotype of patients undergoing carotid endarterectomy. J Vasc Surg 2007;45(2):289–96. http://dx.doi.org/10.1016/j.jvs.2006.09.051 [discussion: 296–7].

167. Debing E, Von Kemp K, Van den Brande P. Gender differences in cardiovascular risk factors in a carotid endarterectomy population. Int Angiol 2006; 25(1):18–25. Available at: http://www.ncbi.nlm.nih.gov/pubmed/16520720. Accessed July 22, 2014.

168. Alamowitch S, Eliasziw M, Barnett HJ. The risk and benefit of endarterectomy in women with symptomatic internal carotid artery disease. Stroke 2005; 36(1):27–31. http://dx.doi.org/10.1161/01.STR.0000149622.12636.1f.

169. Bryant MF. Anatomic considerations in carotid endarterectomy. Surg Clin North Am 1974;54(6): 1291–6. Available at: http://www.ncbi.nlm.nih.gov/pubmed/4432208. Accessed July 22, 2014.

170. Hans SS, Shah S, Hans B. Carotid endarterectomy for high plaques. Am J Surg 1989;157(4):431–4 [discussion: 434–5]. Available at: http://www.ncbi.nlm.nih.gov/pubmed/2929868. Accessed July 22, 2014.

171. Bond R, Warlow CP, Naylor AR, et al. Variation in surgical and anaesthetic technique and associations with operative risk in the European Carotid

Surgery Trial: implications for trials of ancillary techniques. Eur J Vasc Endovasc Surg 2002;23(2): 117–26. http://dx.doi.org/10.1053/ejvs.2001.1566.

172. Kashyap VS, Moore WS, Quinones-Baldrich WJ. Carotid artery repair for radiation-associated atherosclerosis is a safe and durable procedure. J Vasc Surg 1999;29(1):90–6 [discussion: 97–9]. Available at: http://www.ncbi.nlm.nih.gov/pubmed/9882793. Accessed July 22, 2014.

173. Harrod-Kim P, Kadkhodayan Y, Derdeyn CP, et al. Outcomes of carotid angioplasty and stenting for radiation-associated stenosis. AJNR Am J Neuroradiol 2005;26(7):1781–8. Available at: http://www.ncbi.nlm.nih.gov/pubmed/16091530. Accessed July 22, 2014.

174. Protack CD, Bakken AM, Saad WE, et al. Radiation arteritis: a contraindication to carotid stenting? J Vasc Surg 2007;45(1):110–7. http://dx.doi.org/10.1016/j.jvs.2006.08.083.

175. Favre JP, Nourissat A, Duprey A, et al. Endovascular treatment for carotid artery stenosis after neck irradiation. J Vasc Surg 2008;48(4):852–8. http://dx.doi.org/10.1016/j.jvs.2008.05.069.

176. Baker JD, Gluecklich B, Watson CW, et al. An evaluation of electroencephalographic monitoring for carotid study. Surgery 1975;78(6):787–94. Available at: http://www.ncbi.nlm.nih.gov/pubmed/1188621. Accessed July 23, 2014.

177. Elmore JR, Eldrup-Jorgensen J, Leschey WH, et al. Computerized topographic brain mapping during carotid endarterectomy. Arch Surg 1990;125(6): 734–7 [discussion: 738]. Available at: http://www.ncbi.nlm.nih.gov/pubmed/2088317. Accessed July 23, 2014.

178. Moore WS, Yee JM, Hall AD. Collateral cerebral blood pressure. An index of tolerance to temporary carotid occlusion. Arch Surg 1973;106(4):521–3. Available at: http://www.ncbi.nlm.nih.gov/pubmed/4696724. Accessed July 23, 2014.

179. Rerkasem K, Rothwell PM. Patch angioplasty versus primary closure for carotid endarterectomy. Cochrane Database Syst Rev 2009;(4):CD000160. http://dx.doi.org/10.1002/14651858.CD000160.pub3.

180. Golledge J, Cuming R, Davies AH, et al. Outcome of selective patching following carotid endarterectomy. Eur J Vasc Endovasc Surg 1996;11(4): 458–63. Available at: http://www.ncbi.nlm.nih.gov/pubmed/8846183. Accessed July 23, 2014.

181. Gelabert HA, el-Massry S, Moore WS. Carotid endarterectomy with primary closure does not adversely affect the rate of recurrent stenosis. Arch Surg 1994;129(6):648–54. Available at: http://www.ncbi.nlm.nih.gov/pubmed/8204041. Accessed July 23, 2014.

182. Myers SI, Valentine RJ, Chervu A, et al. Saphenous vein patch versus primary closure for carotid endarterectomy: long-term assessment of a randomized prospective study. J Vasc Surg 1994; 19(1):15–22. Available at: http://www.ncbi.nlm.nih.gov/pubmed/8301727. Accessed July 23, 2014.

183. De Letter JA, Moll FL, Welten RJ, et al. Benefits of carotid patching: a prospective randomized study with long-term follow-up. Ann Vasc Surg 1994; 8(1):54–8. http://dx.doi.org/10.1007/BF02133406.

184. Fietsam R, Ranval T, Cohn S, et al. Hemodynamic effects of primary closure versus patch angioplasty of the carotid artery. Ann Vasc Surg 1992;6(5): 443–9. http://dx.doi.org/10.1007/BF02007000.

185. Rosenthal D, Archie JP, Garcia-Rinaldi R, et al. Carotid patch angioplasty: immediate and long-term results. J Vasc Surg 1990;12(3):326–33. Available at: http://www.ncbi.nlm.nih.gov/pubmed/2144599. Accessed July 23, 2014.

186. Vanmaele R, Van Schil P, De Maeseneer M. Closure of the internal carotid artery after endarterectomy: the advantages of patch angioplasty without its disadvantages. Ann Vasc Surg 1990;4(1):81–4. http://dx.doi.org/10.1007/BF02042696.

187. Clagett GP, Patterson CB, Fisher DF, et al. Vein patch versus primary closure for carotid endarterectomy. A randomized prospective study in a selected group of patients. J Vasc Surg 1989; 9(2):213–23. Available at: http://www.ncbi.nlm.nih.gov/pubmed/2645441. Accessed July 23, 2014.

188. Eikelboom BC, Ackerstaff RG, Hoeneveld H, et al. Benefits of carotid patching: a randomized study. J Vasc Surg 1988;7(2):240–7. Available at: http://www.ncbi.nlm.nih.gov/pubmed/3276933. Accessed July 23, 2014.

189. Hertzer NR, Beven EG, O'Hara PJ, et al. A prospective study of vein patch angioplasty during carotid endarterectomy. Three-year results for 801 patients and 917 operations. Ann Surg 1987; 206(5):628–35. Available at: http://www.pubmedcentral.nih.gov/articlerender.fcgi?artid=1493295&tool=pmcentrez&rendertype=abstract. Accessed July 23, 2014.

190. Katz MM, Jones GT, Degenhardt J, et al. The use of patch angioplasty to alter the incidence of carotid restenosis following thromboendarterectomy. J Cardiovasc Surg (Torino) 1987;28(1):2–8. Available at: http://www.ncbi.nlm.nih.gov/pubmed/3805106. Accessed July 23, 2014.

191. Bond R, Rerkasem K, Naylor R, et al. Patches of different types for carotid patch angioplasty. Cochrane Database Syst Rev 2004;(2): CD000071. http://dx.doi.org/10.1002/14651858.CD000071.pub2.

192. Matsagas MI, Bali C, Arnaoutoglou E, et al. Carotid endarterectomy with bovine pericardium patch angioplasty: mid-term results. Ann Vasc Surg 2006; 20(5):614–9. http://dx.doi.org/10.1007/s10016-006-9102-3.

193. Mannheim D, Weller B, Vahadim E, et al. Carotid endarterectomy with a polyurethane patch versus primary closure: a prospective randomized study. J Vasc Surg 2005;41(3):403–7. http://dx.doi.org/10.1016/j.jvs.2004.11.036 [discussion: 407–8].

194. Krishnan S, Clowes AW. Dacron patch infection after carotid endarterectomy: case report and review of the literature. Ann Vasc Surg 2006; 20(5):672–7. http://dx.doi.org/10.1007/s10016-006-9064-5.

195. Schoenefeld E, Donas K, Radicke A, et al. Perioperative use of aspirin for patients undergoing carotid endarterectomy. Vasa 2012;41(4):282–7. http://dx.doi.org/10.1024/0301-1526/a000204.

196. Stone DH, Goodney PP, Schanzer A, et al. Clopidogrel is not associated with major bleeding complications during peripheral arterial surgery. J Vasc Surg 2011;54(3):779–84. http://dx.doi.org/10.1016/j.jvs.2011.03.003.

197. Rosenbaum A, Rizvi AZ, Alden PB, et al. Outcomes related to antiplatelet or anticoagulation use in patients undergoing carotid endarterectomy. Ann Vasc Surg 2011;25(1):25–31. http://dx.doi.org/10.1016/j.avsg.2010.06.007.

198. Oldag A, Schreiber S, Schreiber S, et al. Risk of wound hematoma at carotid endarterectomy under dual antiplatelet therapy. Langenbecks Arch Surg 2012;397(8):1275–82. http://dx.doi.org/10.1007/s00423-012-0967-z.

199. Taylor DW, Barnett HJ, Haynes RB, et al. Low-dose and high-dose acetylsalicylic acid for patients undergoing carotid endarterectomy: a randomised controlled trial. ASA and Carotid Endarterectomy (ACE) Trial Collaborators. Lancet 1999;353(9171):2179–84. Available at: http://www.ncbi.nlm.nih.gov/pubmed/10392981. Accessed July 23, 2014.

200. LaMuraglia GM, Stoner MC, Brewster DC, et al. Determinants of carotid endarterectomy anatomic durability: effects of serum lipids and lipid-lowering drugs. J Vasc Surg 2005;41(5):762–8. http://dx.doi.org/10.1016/j.jvs.2005.01.035.

201. Ferguson GG, Eliasziw M, Barr HW, et al. The North American Symptomatic Carotid Endarterectomy Trial: surgical results in 1415 patients. Stroke 1999;30(9):1751–8. Available at: http://www.ncbi.nlm.nih.gov/pubmed/10471419. Accessed July 23, 2014.

202. Bond R, Rerkasem K, Cuffe R, et al. A systematic review of the associations between age and sex and the operative risks of carotid endarterectomy. Cerebrovasc Dis 2005;20(2):69–77. http://dx.doi.org/10.1159/000086509.

203. Bond R, Rerkasem K, Naylor AR, et al. Systematic review of randomized controlled trials of patch angioplasty versus primary closure and different types of patch materials during carotid endarterectomy. J Vasc Surg 2004;40(6):1126–35. http://dx.doi.org/10.1016/j.jvs.2004.08.048.

204. Halm EA, Hannan EL, Rojas M, et al. Clinical and operative predictors of outcomes of carotid endarterectomy. J Vasc Surg 2005;42(3):420–8. http://dx.doi.org/10.1016/j.jvs.2005.05.029.

205. Mericle RA, Kim SH, Lanzino G, et al. Carotid artery angioplasty and use of stents in high-risk patients with contralateral occlusions. J Neurosurg 1999; 90(6):1031–6. http://dx.doi.org/10.3171/jns.1999.90.6.1031.

206. Harthun NL, Baglioni AJ, Kongable GL, et al. Carotid endarterectomy: update on the gold standard treatment for carotid stenosis. Am Surg 2005;71(8): 647–51 [discussion: 651–2]. Available at: http://www.ncbi.nlm.nih.gov/pubmed/16217946. Accessed July 23, 2014.

207. Matsen SL, Chang DC, Perler BA, et al. Trends in the in-hospital stroke rate following carotid endarterectomy in California and Maryland. J Vasc Surg 2006;44(3):488–95. http://dx.doi.org/10.1016/j.jvs.2006.05.017.

208. Gupta AK, Purkayastha S, Unnikrishnan M, et al. Hyperperfusion syndrome after supraaortic vessel interventions and bypass surgery. J Neuroradiol 2005;32(5):352–8. Available at: http://www.ncbi.nlm.nih.gov/pubmed/16424839. Accessed July 23, 2014.

209. Van Mook WN, Rennenberg RJ, Schurink GW, et al. Cerebral hyperperfusion syndrome. Lancet Neurol 2005;4(12):877–88. http://dx.doi.org/10.1016/S1474-4422(05)70251-9.

210. Nouraei SA, Al-Rawi PG, Sigaudo-Roussel D, et al. Carotid endarterectomy impairs blood pressure homeostasis by reducing the physiologic baroreflex reserve. J Vasc Surg 2005;41(4):631–7. http://dx.doi.org/10.1016/j.jvs.2005.01.009.

211. Posner SR, Boxer L, Proctor M, et al. Uncomplicated carotid endarterectomy: factors contributing to blood pressure instability precluding safe early discharge. Vascular 2004;12(5):278–84. Available at: http://www.ncbi.nlm.nih.gov/pubmed/15765908. Accessed July 23, 2014.

212. Maroulis J, Karkanevatos A, Papakostas K, et al. Cranial nerve dysfunction following carotid endarterectomy. Int Angiol 2000;19(3):237–41. Available at: http://www.ncbi.nlm.nih.gov/pubmed/11201592. Accessed July 23, 2014.

213. Stoner MC, Cambria RP, Brewster DC, et al. Safety and efficacy of reoperative carotid endarterectomy: a 14-year experience. J Vasc Surg 2005;41(6):942–9. http://dx.doi.org/10.1016/j.jvs.2005.02.047.

214. Sajid MS, Vijaynagar B, Singh P, et al. Literature review of cranial nerve injuries during carotid endarterectomy. Acta Chir Belg 2007;107(1):25–8. Available at: http://www.ncbi.nlm.nih.gov/pubmed/17405594. Accessed July 23, 2014.

215. Cunningham EJ, Bond R, Mayberg MR, et al. Risk of persistent cranial nerve injury after carotid endarterectomy. J Neurosurg 2004;101(3):445–8. http://dx.doi.org/10.3171/jns.2004.101.3.0445.

216. Sternbach Y, Illig KA, Zhang R, et al. Hemodynamic benefits of regional anesthesia for carotid endarterectomy. J Vasc Surg 2002;35(2):333–9. Available at: http://www.ncbi.nlm.nih.gov/pubmed/11854732. Accessed July 23, 2014.

217. Cywinski JB, Koch CG, Krajewski LP, et al. Increased risk associated with combined carotid endarterectomy and coronary artery bypass graft surgery: a propensity-matched comparison with isolated coronary artery bypass graft surgery. J Cardiothorac Vasc Anesth 2006;20(6):796–802. http://dx.doi.org/10.1053/j.jvca.2006.01.022.

218. Stoner MC, Abbott WM, Wong DR, et al. Defining the high-risk patient for carotid endarterectomy: an analysis of the prospective National Surgical Quality Improvement Program database. J Vasc Surg 2006;43(2):285–95. http://dx.doi.org/10.1016/j.jvs.2005.10.069 [discussion: 295–6].

219. Debing E, Van den Brande P. Does the type, number or combinations of traditional cardiovascular risk factors affect early outcome after carotid endarterectomy? Eur J Vasc Endovasc Surg 2006;31(6):622–6. http://dx.doi.org/10.1016/j.ejvs.2005.12.013.

220. Asciutto G, Geier B, Marpe B, et al. Dacron patch infection after carotid angioplasty. A report of 6 cases. Eur J Vasc Endovasc Surg 2007;33(1):55–7. http://dx.doi.org/10.1016/j.ejvs.2006.07.017.

221. Borazjani BH, Wilson SE, Fujitani RM, et al. Postoperative complications of carotid patching: pseudoaneurysm and infection. Ann Vasc Surg 2003;17(2):156–61. http://dx.doi.org/10.1007/s10016-001-0400-5.

222. Moore M, Power M. Perioperative hemorrhage and combined clopidogrel and aspirin therapy. Anesthesiology 2004;101(3):792–4. Available at: http://www.ncbi.nlm.nih.gov/pubmed/15329606. Accessed July 23, 2014.

223. CARESS Steering Committee. Carotid Revascularization using Endarterectomy or Stenting Systems (CARESS): phase I clinical trial. J Endovasc Ther 2003;10(6):1021–30. http://dx.doi.org/10.1583/1545-1550(2003)010<1021:CRUEOS>2.0.CO;2.

224. CARESS Steering Committee. Carotid Revascularization Using Endarterectomy or Stenting Systems (CARESS) phase I clinical trial: 1-year results. J Vasc Surg 2005;42(2):213–9. http://dx.doi.org/10.1016/j.jvs.2005.04.023.

225. Hobson RW. CREST (Carotid Revascularization Endarterectomy versus Stent Trial): background, design, and current status. Semin Vasc Surg 2000;13(2):139–43. Available at: http://www.ncbi.nlm.nih.gov/pubmed/10879554. Accessed July 23, 2014.

226. Hobson RW, Howard VJ, Roubin GS, et al. Carotid artery stenting is associated with increased complications in octogenarians: 30-day stroke and death rates in the CREST lead-in phase. J Vasc Surg 2004;40(6):1106–11. http://dx.doi.org/10.1016/j.jvs.2004.10.022.

227. Halliday A, Bulbulia R, Gray W, et al. Status update and interim results from the asymptomatic carotid surgery trial-2 (ACST-2). Eur J Vasc Endovasc Surg 2013;46(5):510–8. http://dx.doi.org/10.1016/j.ejvs.2013.07.020.

228. Carotid revascularization for primary prevention of stroke - Full text view - ClinicalTrials.gov. Available at: http://clinicaltrials.gov/ct2/show/study/NCT02089217?term=CREST+2&rank=1. Accessed August 13, 2014.

229. Endovascular versus surgical treatment in patients with carotid stenosis in the Carotid and Vertebral Artery Transluminal Angioplasty Study (CAVATAS): a randomised trial. Lancet 2001;357(9270):1729–37. Available at: http://www.ncbi.nlm.nih.gov/pubmed/11403808. Accessed July 23, 2014.

230. Ederle J, Bonati LH, Dobson J, et al. Endovascular treatment with angioplasty or stenting versus endarterectomy in patients with carotid artery stenosis in the Carotid and Vertebral Artery Transluminal Angioplasty Study (CAVATAS): long-term follow-up of a randomised trial. Lancet Neurol 2009;8(10):898–907. http://dx.doi.org/10.1016/S1474-4422(09)70228-5.

231. Bonati LH, Ederle J, McCabe DJ, et al. Long-term risk of carotid restenosis in patients randomly assigned to endovascular treatment or endarterectomy in the Carotid and Vertebral Artery Transluminal Angioplasty Study (CAVATAS): long-term follow-up of a randomised trial. Lancet Neurol 2009;8(10):908–17. http://dx.doi.org/10.1016/S1474-4422(09)70227-3.

232. Bonati LH, Ederle J, Dobson J, et al. Length of carotid stenosis predicts peri-procedural stroke or death and restenosis in patients randomized to endovascular treatment or endarterectomy. Int J Stroke 2014;9(3):297–305. http://dx.doi.org/10.1111/ijs.12084.

233. Mas JL, Chatellier G, Beyssen B, et al. Endarterectomy versus stenting in patients with symptomatic severe carotid stenosis. N Engl J Med 2006;355(16):1660–71. http://dx.doi.org/10.1056/NEJMoa061752.

234. Qureshi AI. Carotid angioplasty and stent placement after EVA-3S trial. Stroke 2007;38(6):1993–6. http://dx.doi.org/10.1161/STROKEAHA.107.484352.

235. Ringleb PA, Allenberg J, Brückmann H, et al. 30 day results from the SPACE trial of stent-protected angioplasty versus carotid endarterectomy in symptomatic patients: a randomised non-inferiority trial.

Lancet 2006;368(9543):1239–47. http://dx.doi.org/10.1016/S0140-6736(06)69122-8.

236. Ederle J, Dobson J, Featherstone RL, et al. Carotid artery stenting compared with endarterectomy in patients with symptomatic carotid stenosis (International Carotid Stenting Study): an interim analysis of a randomised controlled trial. Lancet 2010; 375(9719):985–97. http://dx.doi.org/10.1016/S0140-6736(10)60239-5.

237. Rostamzadeh A, Zumbrunn T, Jongen LM, et al. Predictors of acute and persisting ischemic brain lesions in patients randomized to carotid stenting or endarterectomy. Stroke 2014;45(2):591–4. http://dx.doi.org/10.1161/STROKEAHA.113.003605.

238. Altinbas A, Algra A, Bonati LH, et al. Periprocedural hemodynamic depression is associated with a higher number of new ischemic brain lesions after stenting in the International Carotid Stenting Study-MRI Substudy. Stroke 2014;45(1):146–51. http://dx.doi.org/10.1161/STROKEAHA.113.003397.

239. Lam RC, Lin SC, DeRubertis B, et al. The impact of increasing age on anatomic factors affecting carotid angioplasty and stenting. J Vasc Surg 2007; 45(5):875–80. http://dx.doi.org/10.1016/j.jvs.2006.12.059.

240. Wholey MH, Al-Mubarek N, Wholey MH. Updated review of the global carotid artery stent registry. Catheter Cardiovasc Interv 2003;60(2):259–66. http://dx.doi.org/10.1002/ccd.10645.

241. Kastrup A, Gröschel K, Krapf H, et al. Early outcome of carotid angioplasty and stenting with and without cerebral protection devices: a systematic review of the literature. Stroke 2003;34(3):813–9. http://dx.doi.org/10.1161/01.STR.0000058160.53040.5F.

242. Roubin GS, New G, Iyer SS, et al. Immediate and late clinical outcomes of carotid artery stenting in patients with symptomatic and asymptomatic carotid artery stenosis: a 5-year prospective analysis. Circulation 2001;103(4):532–7. Available at: http://www.ncbi.nlm.nih.gov/pubmed/11157718. Accessed July 23, 2014.

243. White CJ, Iyer SS, Hopkins LN, et al. Carotid stenting with distal protection in high surgical risk patients: the BEACH trial 30 day results. Catheter Cardiovasc Interv 2006;67(4):503–12. http://dx.doi.org/10.1002/ccd.20689.

244. Safian RD, Bresnahan JF, Jaff MR, et al. Protected carotid stenting in high-risk patients with severe carotid artery stenosis. J Am Coll Cardiol 2006; 47(12):2384–9. http://dx.doi.org/10.1016/j.jacc.2005.12.076.

245. Barbato JE, Dillavou E, Horowitz MB, et al. A randomized trial of carotid artery stenting with and without cerebral protection. J Vasc Surg 2008;47(4):760–5. http://dx.doi.org/10.1016/j.jvs.2007.11.058.

246. Katzen BT, Ardid MI, MacLean AA, et al. Bivalirudin as an anticoagulation agent: safety and efficacy in peripheral interventions. J Vasc Interv Radiol 2005; 16(9):1183–7. http://dx.doi.org/10.1097/01.RVI.0000171694.01237.26 [quiz: 1187].

247. Schneider LM, Polena S, Roubin G, et al. Carotid stenting and bivalirudin with and without vascular closure: 3-year analysis of procedural outcomes. Catheter Cardiovasc Interv 2010;75(3):420–6. http://dx.doi.org/10.1002/ccd.22322.

248. Cayne NS, Faries PL, Trocciola SM, et al. Carotid angioplasty and stent-induced bradycardia and hypotension: impact of prophylactic atropine administration and prior carotid endarterectomy. J Vasc Surg 2005;41(6):956–61. http://dx.doi.org/10.1016/j.jvs.2005.02.038.

249. Leisch F, Kerschner K, Hofmann R, et al. Carotid sinus reactions during carotid artery stenting: predictors, incidence, and influence on clinical outcome. Catheter Cardiovasc Interv 2003;58(4):516–23. http://dx.doi.org/10.1002/ccd.10483.

250. Coward LJ, Featherstone RL, Brown MM. Percutaneous transluminal angioplasty and stenting for carotid artery stenosis. Cochrane Database Syst Rev 2004;(2):CD000515. http://dx.doi.org/10.1002/14651858.CD000515.pub2.

251. Bak S, Andersen M, Tsiropoulos I, et al. Risk of stroke associated with nonsteroidal anti-inflammatory drugs: a nested case-control study. Stroke 2003;34(2):379–86. Available at: http://www.ncbi.nlm.nih.gov/pubmed/12574540. Accessed July 23, 2014.

252. Criado E, Doblas M, Fontcuberta J, et al. Carotid angioplasty with internal carotid artery flow reversal is well tolerated in the awake patient. J Vasc Surg 2004;40(1):92–7. http://dx.doi.org/10.1016/j.jvs.2004.03.034.

253. Sganzerla P, Bocciarelli M, Savasta C, et al. The treatment of carotid artery bifurcation stenoses with systematic stenting: experience of first 100 consecutive cardiological procedures. J Invasive Cardiol 2004;16(10):592–5. Available at: http://www.ncbi.nlm.nih.gov/pubmed/15505359. Accessed July 23, 2014.

254. Tan KT, Cleveland TJ, Berczi V, et al. Timing and frequency of complications after carotid artery stenting: what is the optimal period of observation? J Vasc Surg 2003;38(2):236–43. Available at: http://www.ncbi.nlm.nih.gov/pubmed/12891103. Accessed July 23, 2014.

255. Srimahachota S, Singhatanadgige S, Boonyaratavej S, et al. Bilateral carotid stenting prior to coronary artery bypass graft: a case report. J Med Assoc Thai 2002;85(11):1232–5. Available at: http://www.ncbi.nlm.nih.gov/pubmed/12546322. Accessed July 23, 2014.

256. Leisch F, Kerschner K, Hofman R, et al. Carotid stenting: acute results and complications. Z Kardiol 1999;88(9):661–8 [in German]. Available at: http://www.ncbi.nlm.nih.gov/pubmed/10525928. Accessed July 23, 2014.

257. Illig KA, Zhang R, Tanski W, et al. Is the rationale for carotid angioplasty and stenting in patients excluded from NASCET/ACAS or eligible for ARCHeR justified? J Vasc Surg 2003;37(3):575–81. http://dx.doi.org/10.1067/mva.2003.79.

258. Coward LJ, Featherstone RL, Brown MM. Safety and efficacy of endovascular treatment of carotid artery stenosis compared with carotid endarterectomy: a Cochrane systematic review of the randomized evidence. Stroke 2005;36(4):905–11. http://dx.doi.org/10.1161/01.STR.0000158921.51037.64.

259. Back MR. Commentary. Protected carotid stenting in high-surgical-risk patients: the ARCHeR results. Perspect Vasc Surg Endovasc Ther 2006;18(4):349–51. Available at: http://www.ncbi.nlm.nih.gov/pubmed/17396364. Accessed July 23, 2014.

260. Coward LJ, Featherstone RL, Brown MM. Percutaneous transluminal angioplasty and stenting for vertebral artery stenosis. Cochrane Database Syst Rev 2005;(2):CD000516. http://dx.doi.org/10.1002/14651858.CD000516.pub2.

261. Crawley F, Brown MM. Percutaneous transluminal angioplasty and stenting for carotid artery stenosis. Cochrane Database Syst Rev 2000;(2):CD000515. http://dx.doi.org/10.1002/14651858.CD000515.

262. Gray WA. Endovascular treatment of extra-cranial carotid artery bifurcation disease. Minerva Cardioangiol 2005;53(1):69–77. Available at: http://www.ncbi.nlm.nih.gov/pubmed/15788981. Accessed July 23, 2014.

263. Gray WA. A cardiologist in the carotids. J Am Coll Cardiol 2004;43(9):1602–5. http://dx.doi.org/10.1016/j.jacc.2003.11.051.

264. Kasirajan K. What is the latest in inventory for carotid stenting and cerebral protection? Perspect Vasc Surg Endovasc Ther 2005;17(2):135–41. Available at: http://www.ncbi.nlm.nih.gov/pubmed/16110380. Accessed July 23, 2014.

265. Naylor AR. Regarding "Protected carotid stenting in high-surgical-risk patients: the ARCHeR results". J Vasc Surg 2007;45(1):222–3. http://dx.doi.org/10.1016/j.jvs.2006.08.089 [author reply: 223–4].

266. Schonholz CJ, Uflacker R, Parodi JC, et al. Is there evidence that cerebral protection is beneficial? Clinical data. J Cardiovasc Surg (Torino) 2006;47(2):137–41. Available at: http://www.ncbi.nlm.nih.gov/pubmed/16572087. Accessed July 23, 2014.

267. Gray WA, Yadav JS, Verta P, et al. The CAPTURE registry: results of carotid stenting with embolic protection in the post approval setting. Catheter Cardiovasc Interv 2007;69(3):341–8. http://dx.doi.org/10.1002/ccd.21050.

268. Kwon BJ, Han MH, Kang HS, et al. Protection filter-related events in extracranial carotid artery stenting: a single-center experience. J Endovasc Ther 2006;13(6):711–22. http://dx.doi.org/10.1583/06-1900.1.

269. Cardaioli P, Giordan M, Panfili M, et al. Complication with an embolic protection device during carotid angioplasty. Catheter Cardiovasc Interv 2004;62(2):234–6. http://dx.doi.org/10.1002/ccd.20061.

270. Van den Berg JC. The nature and management of complications in carotid artery stenting. Acta Chir Belg 2004;104(1):60–4. Available at: http://www.ncbi.nlm.nih.gov/pubmed/15053467. Accessed July 23, 2014.

271. Griewing B, Brassel F, von Smekal U, et al. Carotid artery stenting in patients at surgical high risk: clinical and ultrasound findings. Cerebrovasc Dis 2000;10(1):44–8.

272. Kadkhodayan Y, Moran CJ, Derdeyn CP, et al. Carotid angioplasty and stent placement for restenosis after endarterectomy. Neuroradiology 2007;49(4):357–64. http://dx.doi.org/10.1007/s00234-006-0206-9.

273. Kitta Y, Obata J, Takano H, et al. Echolucent carotid plaques predict in-stent restenosis after bare metal stenting in native coronary arteries. Atherosclerosis 2008;197(1):177–82. http://dx.doi.org/10.1016/j.atherosclerosis.2007.03.021.

274. Geary GG. The vascular therapist. Heart Lung Circ 2007;16(3):193–9. http://dx.doi.org/10.1016/j.hlc.2007.02.103.

275. Teng Z, Ji G, Chu H, et al. Does PGA external stenting reduce compliance mismatch in venous grafts? Biomed Eng Online 2007;6:12. http://dx.doi.org/10.1186/1475-925X-6-12.

276. Bosiers M, De Donato G, Deloose K, et al. Are there predictive risk factors for complications after carotid artery stenting? J Cardiovasc Surg (Torino) 2007;48(2):125–30. Available at: http://www.ncbi.nlm.nih.gov/pubmed/17410060. Accessed July 23, 2014.

277. Parodi JC, Schönholz C, Parodi FE, et al. Initial 200 cases of carotid artery stenting using a reversal-of-flow cerebral protection device. J Cardiovasc Surg (Torino) 2007;48(2):117–24. Available at: http://www.ncbi.nlm.nih.gov/pubmed/17410059. Accessed July 23, 2014.

278. Peynircioglu B, Geyik S, Yavuz K, et al. Exclusion of atherosclerotic plaque from the circulation using stent-grafts: alternative to carotid stenting with a protection device? Cardiovasc Intervent Radiol 2007;30(5):854–60. http://dx.doi.org/10.1007/s00270-007-9010-0.

279. Younis GA, Gupta K, Mortazavi A, et al. Predictors of carotid stent restenosis. Catheter Cardiovasc Interv 2007;69(5):673–82. http://dx.doi.org/10.1002/ccd.20809.

280. De Souza JM, Espinosa G, Santos Machado M, et al. Bilateral occlusion associated to steal phenomenon of internal carotid and left subclavian arteries: treatment by angioplasty and stenting. Surg Neurol 2007;67(3):298–302. http://dx.doi.org/10.1016/j.surneu.2006.04.013 [discussion: 302].

281. Chahwan S, Miller MT, Pigott JP, et al. Carotid artery velocity characteristics after carotid artery angioplasty and stenting. J Vasc Surg 2007;45(3):523–6. http://dx.doi.org/10.1016/j.jvs.2006.11.044.

282. de Borst GJ, Ackerstaff RG, de Vries JP, et al. Carotid angioplasty and stenting for postendarterectomy stenosis: long-term follow-up. J Vasc Surg 2007;45(1):118–23. http://dx.doi.org/10.1016/j.jvs.2006.09.013.

283. Ali ZA, Alp NJ, Lupton H, et al. Increased in-stent stenosis in ApoE knockout mice: insights from a novel mouse model of balloon angioplasty and stenting. Arterioscler Thromb Vasc Biol 2007;27(4):833–40. http://dx.doi.org/10.1161/01.ATV.0000257135.39571.5b.

284. Park B, Aiello F, Dahn M, et al. Follow-up results of carotid angioplasty with stenting as assessed by duplex ultrasound surveillance. Am J Surg 2006;192(5):583–8. http://dx.doi.org/10.1016/j.amjsurg.2006.08.025.

285. Gupta R, Al-Ali F, Thomas AJ, et al. Safety, feasibility, and short-term follow-up of drug-eluting stent placement in the intracranial and extracranial circulation. Stroke 2006;37(10):2562–6. http://dx.doi.org/10.1161/01.STR.0000242481.38262.7b.

286. Hauth EA, Drescher R, Jansen C, et al. Complications and follow-up after unprotected carotid artery stenting. Cardiovasc Intervent Radiol 2006;29(4):511–8. http://dx.doi.org/10.1007/s00270-005-0050-z.

287. Cao P, De Rango P, Vorzini F, et al. Outcome of carotid stenting versus endarterectomy: a case-control study. Stroke 2006;37(5):1221–6. http://dx.doi.org/10.1161/01.STR.0000217435.21051.60.

288. Lal BK, Hobson RW. Management of carotid restenosis. J Cardiovasc Surg (Torino) 2006;47(2):153–60. Available at: http://www.ncbi.nlm.nih.gov/pubmed/16572089. Accessed July 23, 2014.

289. Halabi M, Gruberg L, Pitchersky S, et al. Carotid artery stenting in surgical high-risk patients. Catheter Cardiovasc Interv 2006;67(4):513–8. http://dx.doi.org/10.1002/ccd.20640.

290. Maleux G, Demaerel P, Verbeken E, et al. Cerebral ischemia after filter-protected carotid artery stenting is common and cannot be predicted by the presence of substantial amount of debris captured by the filter device. AJNR Am J Neuroradiol 2006;

27(9):1830–3. Available at: http://www.ncbi.nlm.nih.gov/pubmed/17032852. Accessed July 23, 2014.

291. Reimers B, Tübler T, de Donato G, et al. Endovascular treatment of in-stent restenosis after carotid artery stenting: immediate and midterm results. J Endovasc Ther 2006;13(4):429–35. http://dx.doi.org/10.1583/06-1811.1.

292. Imai K, Mori T, Izumoto H, et al. Successful stenting seven days after atherothrombotic occlusion of the intracranial internal carotid artery. J Endovasc Ther 2006;13(2):254–9. http://dx.doi.org/10.1583/05-1742R.1.

293. Macdonald S. Is there any evidence that cerebral protection is beneficial? Experimental data. J Cardiovasc Surg (Torino) 2006;47(2):127–36. Available at: http://www.ncbi.nlm.nih.gov/pubmed/16572086. Accessed July 23, 2014.

294. Quan VH, Huynh R, Seifert PA, et al. Morphometric analysis of particulate debris extracted by four different embolic protection devices from coronary arteries, aortocoronary saphenous vein conduits, and carotid arteries. Am J Cardiol 2005;95(12):1415–9. http://dx.doi.org/10.1016/j.amjcard.2005.02.006.

295. Sprouse LR, Peeters P, Bosiers M. The capture of visible debris by distal cerebral protection filters during carotid artery stenting: is it predictable? J Vasc Surg 2005;41(6):950–5. http://dx.doi.org/10.1016/j.jvs.2005.02.048.

296. Ohki T, Veith FJ. Critical analysis of distal protection devices. Semin Vasc Surg 2003;16(4):317–25. Available at: http://www.ncbi.nlm.nih.gov/pubmed/14691774. Accessed July 23, 2014.

297. Grube E, Colombo A, Hauptmann E, et al. Initial multicenter experience with a novel distal protection filter during carotid artery stent implantation. Catheter Cardiovasc Interv 2003;58(2):139–46. http://dx.doi.org/10.1002/ccd.10348.

298. Sievert H, Rabe K. Role of distal protection during carotid stenting. J Interv Cardiol 2002;15(6):499–504. Available at: http://www.ncbi.nlm.nih.gov/pubmed/12476654. Accessed July 23, 2014.

299. Capoccia L, Speziale F, Gazzetti M, et al. Comparative study on carotid revascularization (endarterectomy vs stenting) using markers of cellular brain injury, neuropsychometric tests, and diffusion-weighted magnetic resonance imaging. J Vasc Surg 2010;51(3):584–91. http://dx.doi.org/10.1016/j.jvs.2009.10.079, 591.e1–3. [discussion: 592].

300. Tedesco MM, Lee JT, Dalman RL, et al. Postprocedural microembolic events following carotid surgery and carotid angioplasty and stenting. J Vasc Surg 2007;46(2):244–50. http://dx.doi.org/10.1016/j.jvs.2007.04.049.

301. Morrish W, Grahovac S, Douen A, et al. Intracranial hemorrhage after stenting and angioplasty of

extracranial carotid stenosis. AJNR Am J Neurora-diol 2000;21(10):1911–6. Available at: http://www.ncbi.nlm.nih.gov/pubmed/11110546. Accessed July 23, 2014.

302. Buhk JH, Cepek L, Knauth M. Hyperacute intracerebral hemorrhage complicating carotid stenting should be distinguished from hyperperfusion syndrome. AJNR Am J Neuroradiol 2006;27(7):1508–13. Available at: http://www.ncbi.nlm.nih.gov/pubmed/16908570. Accessed July 23, 2014.

303. Hartmann M, Weber R, Zoubaa S, et al. Fatal subarachnoid hemorrhage after carotid stenting. J Neuroradiol 2004;31(1):63–6. Available at: http://www.ncbi.nlm.nih.gov/pubmed/15026733. Accessed July 24, 2014.

304. Chuang YM, Wu HM. Early recognition of cerebral hyperperfusion syndrome after carotid stenting—a case report. Kaohsiung J Med Sci 2001;17(9):489–94. Available at: http://www.ncbi.nlm.nih.gov/pubmed/11842653. Accessed July 23, 2014.

305. Ho DS, Wang Y, Chui M, et al. Epileptic seizures attributed to cerebral hyperperfusion after percutaneous transluminal angioplasty and stenting of the internal carotid artery. Cerebrovasc Dis 2000;10(5):374–9. http://dx.doi.org/10.1159/000016093.

306. Eskandari MK, Najjar SF, Matsumura JS, et al. Technical limitations of carotid filter embolic protection devices. Ann Vasc Surg 2007;21(4):403–7. http://dx.doi.org/10.1016/j.avsg.2006.07.005.

307. Schillinger M, Exner M, Sabeti S, et al. Excessive carotid in-stent neointimal formation predicts late cardiovascular events. J Endovasc Ther 2004;11(3):229–39. http://dx.doi.org/10.1583/04-1214.1.

308. DeRubertis BG, Chaer RA, Gordon R, et al. Determining the quantity and character of carotid artery embolic debris by electron microscopy and energy dispersive spectroscopy. J Vasc Surg 2007;45(4):716–24. http://dx.doi.org/10.1016/j.jvs.2006.12.015 [discussion: 724–5].

309. Rapp JH, Wakil L, Sawhney R, et al. Subclinical embolization after carotid artery stenting: new lesions on diffusion-weighted magnetic resonance imaging occur postprocedure. J Vasc Surg 2007;45(5):867–72. http://dx.doi.org/10.1016/j.jvs.2006.12.058 [discussion: 872–4].

310. Hart JP, Peeters P, Verbist J, et al. Do device characteristics impact outcome in carotid artery stenting? J Vasc Surg 2006;44(4):725–30. http://dx.doi.org/10.1016/j.jvs.2006.06.029 [discussion: 730–1].

311. Powell RJ, Alessi C, Nolan B, et al. Comparison of embolization protection device-specific technical difficulties during carotid artery stenting. J Vasc Surg 2006;44(1):56–61. http://dx.doi.org/10.1016/j.jvs.2006.03.035.

312. Hamood H, Makhoul N, Hassan A, et al. Embolic protection: limitations of current technology and novel concepts. Int J Cardiovasc Intervent 2005;

7(4):176–82. http://dx.doi.org/10.1080/14628840500285038.

313. Gruberg L, Beyar R. Cerebral embolic protection devices and percutaneous carotid artery stenting. Int J Cardiovasc Intervent 2005;7(3):117–21. http://dx.doi.org/10.1080/14628840500280542.

314. Yadav JS. Embolic protection devices: methods, techniques, and data. Tech Vasc Interv Radiol 2004;7(4):190–3. http://dx.doi.org/10.1053/j.tvir.2005.03.008.

315. Cil BE, Türkbey B, Canyiğit M, et al. An unusual complication of carotid stenting: spontaneous rectus sheath hematoma and its endovascular management. Diagn Interv Radiol 2007;13(1):46–8. Available at: http://www.ncbi.nlm.nih.gov/pubmed/17354196. Accessed July 23, 2014.

316. Pipinos II, Johanning JM, Pham CN, et al. Transcervical approach with protective flow reversal for carotid angioplasty and stenting. J Endovasc Ther 2005;12(4):446–53. http://dx.doi.org/10.1583/05-1561.1.

317. Zorger N, Finkenzeller T, Lenhart M, et al. Safety and efficacy of the Perclose suture-mediated closure device following carotid artery stenting under clopidogrel platelet blockade. Eur Radiol 2004;14(4):719–22. http://dx.doi.org/10.1007/s00330-003-2143-x.

318. Gupta A, Bhatia A, Ahuja A, et al. Carotid stenting in patients older than 65 years with inoperable carotid artery disease: a single-center experience. Catheter Cardiovasc Interv 2000;50(1):1–8 [discussion: 9]. Available at: http://www.ncbi.nlm.nih.gov/pubmed/10816271. Accessed July 23, 2014.

319. Schneider LM, Roubin GS. Minimal contrast use in carotid stenting: avoiding contrast pitfalls. J Invasive Cardiol 2007;19(1):37–8. Available at: http://www.ncbi.nlm.nih.gov/pubmed/17297184. Accessed July 23, 2014.

320. Bond R, Rerkasem K, AbuRahma AF, et al. Patch angioplasty versus primary closure for carotid endarterectomy. Cochrane Database Syst Rev 2004;(2):CD000160. http://dx.doi.org/10.1002/14651858.CD000160.pub2.

321. Moore WS, Kempczinski RF, Nelson JJ, et al. Recurrent carotid stenosis: results of the asymptomatic carotid atherosclerosis study. Stroke 1998;29(10):2018–25. Available at: http://www.ncbi.nlm.nih.gov/pubmed/9756575. Accessed July 23, 2014.

322. Cunningham EJ, Bond R, Mehta Z, et al. Long-term durability of carotid endarterectomy for symptomatic stenosis and risk factors for late postoperative stroke. Stroke 2002;33(11):2658–63. Available at: http://www.ncbi.nlm.nih.gov/pubmed/12411657. Accessed July 23, 2014.

323. Cikrit DF, Larson DM, Sawchuk AP, et al. Discretionary carotid patch angioplasty leads to good

results. Am J Surg 2006;192(5):e46–50. http://dx.doi.org/10.1016/j.amjsurg.2006.08.027.

324. AbuRahma AF, Robinson PA, Saiedy S, et al. Prospective randomized trial of bilateral carotid endarterectomies: primary closure versus patching. Stroke 1999;30(6):1185–9. Available at: http://www.ncbi.nlm.nih.gov/pubmed/10356097. Accessed July 23, 2014.

325. Rockman CB, Halm EA, Wang JJ, et al. Primary closure of the carotid artery is associated with poorer outcomes during carotid endarterectomy. J Vasc Surg 2005;42(5):870–7. http://dx.doi.org/10.1016/j.jvs.2005.07.043.

326. Hansen F, Lindblad B, Persson NH, et al. Can recurrent stenosis after carotid endarterectomy be prevented by low-dose acetylsalicylic acid? A double-blind, randomised and placebo-controlled study. Eur J Vasc Surg 1993;7(4):380–5. Available at: http://www.ncbi.nlm.nih.gov/pubmed/8359292. Accessed July 23, 2014.

327. Petrik PV, Gelabert HA, Moore WS, et al. Cigarette smoking accelerates carotid artery intimal hyperplasia in a dose-dependent manner. Stroke 1995;26(8):1409–14. Available at: http://www.ncbi.nlm.nih.gov/pubmed/7631346. Accessed July 23, 2014.

328. Salvian A, Baker JD, Machleder HI, et al. Cause and noninvasive detection of restenosis after carotid endarterectomy. Am J Surg 1983;146(1):29–34. Available at: http://www.ncbi.nlm.nih.gov/pubmed/6869676. Accessed July 23, 2014.

329. AbuRahma AF, Robinson PA, Saiedy S, et al. Prospective randomized trial of carotid endarterectomy with primary closure and patch angioplasty with saphenous vein, jugular vein, and polytetrafluoroethylene: long-term follow-up. J Vasc Surg 1998;27(2):222–32 [discussion: 233–4]. Available at: http://www.ncbi.nlm.nih.gov/pubmed/9510277. Accessed July 23, 2014.

330. Lord RS, Raj TB, Stary DL, et al. Comparison of saphenous vein patch, polytetrafluoroethylene patch, and direct arteriotomy closure after carotid endarterectomy. Part I. Perioperative results. J Vasc Surg 1989;9(4):521–9. Available at: http://www.ncbi.nlm.nih.gov/pubmed/2709521. Accessed July 23, 2014.

331. Curley S, Edwards WS, Jacob TP. Recurrent carotid stenosis after autologous tissue patching. J Vasc Surg 1987;6(4):350–4. Available at: http://www.ncbi.nlm.nih.gov/pubmed/3309379. Accessed July 23, 2014.

332. Awad IA, Little JR. Patch angioplasty in carotid endarterectomy. Advantages, concerns, and controversies. Stroke 1989;20(3):417–22. Available at: http://www.ncbi.nlm.nih.gov/pubmed/2604762. Accessed July 23, 2014.

333. Bernstein EF, Torem S, Dilley RB. Does carotid restenosis predict an increased risk of late symptoms, stroke, or death? Ann Surg 1990;212(5):629–36. Available at: http://www.pubmedcentral.nih.gov/articlerender.fcgi?artid=1358192&tool=pmcentrez&rendertype=abstract. Accessed July 23, 2014.

334. Nicholls SC, Phillips DJ, Bergelin RO, et al. Carotid endarterectomy. Relationship of outcome to early restenosis. J Vasc Surg 1985;2(3):375–81. Available at: http://www.ncbi.nlm.nih.gov/pubmed/3889378. Accessed July 24, 2014.

335. O'Donnell TF, Callow AD, Scott G, et al. Ultrasound characteristics of recurrent carotid disease: hypothesis explaining the low incidence of symptomatic recurrence. J Vasc Surg 1985;2(1):26–41. Available at: http://www.ncbi.nlm.nih.gov/pubmed/3880832. Accessed July 23, 2014.

336. Zierler RE, Bandyk DF, Thiele BL, et al. Carotid artery stenosis following endarterectomy. Arch Surg 1982;117(11):1408–15. Available at: http://www.ncbi.nlm.nih.gov/pubmed/7138302. Accessed July 23, 2014.

337. Stoney RJ, String ST. Recurrent carotid stenosis. Surgery 1976;80(6):705–10. Available at: http://www.ncbi.nlm.nih.gov/pubmed/1006517. Accessed July 23, 2014.

338. Hertzer NR, Martinez BD, Benjamin SP, et al. Recurrent stenosis after carotid endarterectomy. Surg Gynecol Obstet 1979;149(3):360–4. Available at: http://www.ncbi.nlm.nih.gov/pubmed/472995. Accessed July 23, 2014.

339. DeGroote RD, Lynch TG, Jamil Z, et al. Carotid restenosis: long-term noninvasive follow-up after carotid endarterectomy. Stroke 1987;18(6):1031–6. Available at: http://www.ncbi.nlm.nih.gov/pubmed/3318001. Accessed July 23, 2014.

Critical Limb Ischemia

Sarah Elsayed, MD[a], Leonardo C. Clavijo, MD, PhD[b],*

KEYWORDS

• Critical limb ischemia • Diagnosis • Management • Endovascular • Guidelines • Review

KEY POINTS

- Certain patient populations should be screened for peripheral artery disease.
- Critical limb ischemia is becoming increasingly prevalent. A high index of suspicion is warranted and early referral is recommended.
- Meticulous history and physical examination are necessary.
- Arterial profile is performed for patients suspected with peripheral artery disease or critical limb ischemia.
- Once critical limb ischemia is confirmed, lesion location and severity should be promptly diagnosed.
- In addition to guideline-directed medical therapy, different revascularization options are weighed.
- Coronary artery disease is the major cause of death in the critical limb ischemia population.

DEFINITION AND PREVALENCE OF CRITICAL LIMB ISCHEMIA

Critical limb ischemia (CLI), the most advanced form of peripheral artery disease (PAD), carries grave implications with regard to morbidity and mortality. This article is a comprehensive review of CLI, including different treatment options and current review of the literature. PAD has been estimated to reduce quality of life in about 2 million symptomatic Americans, and millions more Americans without claudication are likely to suffer PAD-associated impairment.

This impairment leads to significant morbidity and health care expenditures. Perhaps, more importantly, PAD is a powerful independent predictor of coronary artery disease (CAD) and cerebrovascular disease events and mortality (**Fig. 1**).[1]

The incidence of CLI in the United States is estimated at 1% of the population aged ≥50 years and at approximately double that rate in those older than 70 years. Within 1 year of CLI diagnosis, 40% to 50% of diabetics will experience an amputation, and 20% to 25% will die. The estimated

cost for treating CLI in the United States alone is $10 to $20 billion per year, but just a 25% reduction in amputations could save $2.9 to $3.0 billion annually.[2]

CLI is defined as limb pain that occurs at rest or impending limb loss that is caused by severe compromise of blood flow to the affected extremity. The term *CLI* should be used for patients with chronic ischemic rest pain, ulcers, or gangrene attributable to objectively proven arterial occlusive disease. The term *CLI* implies chronicity and is to be distinguished from acute limb ischemia. CLI is defined by most vascular clinicians as those patients in whom the untreated natural history would lead to major limb amputation within 6 months.[3]

CAUSES OF CRITICAL LIMB ISCHEMIA

CLI is usually caused by atherosclerosis; however, it can also be caused by atheroembolic or thromboembolic disease, vasculitis, in situ thrombosis related to hypercoagulable states, thromboangiitis obliterans, cystic adventitial disease, or trauma.

[a] Vascular Medicine Graduated Fellow, Division of Cardiovascular Medicine, University of Southern California, 1510 San Pablo Street, Suite 322, Los Angeles, CA 90033, USA; [b] Interventional Cardiology Fellowship Program, Vascular Medicine and Peripheral Interventions, Division of Cardiovascular Medicine, University of Southern California, 1510 San Pablo Street, Suite 322, Los Angeles, CA 90033, USA
* Corresponding author.
E-mail address: lclavijo@usc.edu

Cardiol Clin 33 (2015) 37–47
http://dx.doi.org/10.1016/j.ccl.2014.09.008
0733-8651/15/$ – see front matter © 2015 Elsevier Inc. All rights reserved.

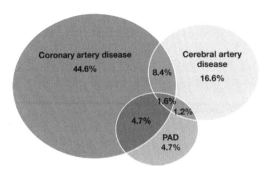

Fig. 1. Prevalence overlap of different vascular territories in peripheral arterial disease (PAD). (*From* Norgren L, Hiatt WR, Dormandy JA, et al. Inter-Society Consensus for the Management of Peripheral Arterial Disease (TASC II). J Vasc Surg 2007;45(Suppl S):S12A; with permission.)

Factors that increase the risk of limb loss in patients with CLI include:

- Factors that reduce blood supply
  - ○ Diabetes mellitus
  - ○ Severe renal failure
  - ○ Severe heart failure, shock
  - ○ Vasospastic diseases
  - ○ Smoking
- Factors that increase demand for blood flow to the microvascular bed
  - ○ Infection (cellulitis, osteomyelitis)
  - ○ Skin breakdown
  - ○ Trauma

CLASSIFICATION OF PERIPHERAL ARTERY DISEASE AND CRITICAL LIMB ISCHEMIA

Fontaine's Stages and Rutherford's Categories are used to classify the degree of ischemia and salvageability of the limb (**Table 1**). CLI is a component of the more advanced stages. Given the 3- to 5-fold increase in cardiovascular (CV)

mortality in patients with CLI compared to those without, this should prompt clinicians to recognize the ideal care strategies to optimize risk factors and be aware of the possibility of CAD, cerebrovascular disease, and aortic aneurysmal disease.

NEW CLASSIFICATION OF CRITICAL LIMB ISCHEMIA

CLI was first defined in 1982. The purpose of these 2 prior classification systems was to classify risk of amputation and benefit of revascularization. Over the last 40 years, diabetes has become increasingly prevalent, and there has been significant advent of revascularization strategies, especially endovascular therapy. The Society of Vascular Surgery Lower Extremity Guidelines Committee created a comprehensive new classification termed the *Society of Vascular Surgery (SVS) Lower Extremity Threatened Limb Classification System* (**Table 2**). This classification system includes 3 factors: wound, ischemia, and foot infection (SVS WIfI).[4]

The SVS grade from each table is then categorized into 5 clinical stages in ascending order: very low, low, moderate, high, and unsalvageable foot. These categories provide risk stratification of amputation risk at 1 year and estimated likelihood of benefit of revascularization (assuming infection can be controlled first).

EVALUATION OF CRITICAL LIMB ISCHEMIA PATIENTS
History

- Patients with CLI present with ischemic rest pain with or without skin changes, which is worse when supine and tends to lessen when the extremity is in the dependent position.

Table 1
Classification of peripheral arterial disease and critical limb ischemia

	Fontaine		Rutherford		
Stage	Clinical	Grade	Category		Clinical
I	Asymptomatic	0	0		Asymptomatic
IIa	Mild claudication	I	1		Mild claudication
IIb	Moderate-severe claudication	I	2		Moderate claudication
		I	3		Severe claudication
III	Rest pain	II	4		Rest pain
IV	Ulcers or gangrene	III	5		Minor tissue loss
		IV	6		Ulcers or gangrene

From Norgren L, Hiatt WR, Dormandy JA, et al. Inter-Society Consensus for the Management of Peripheral Arterial Disease (TASC II). J Vasc Surg 2007;45(Suppl S):S29A; with permission.

Table 2
Society of Vascular Surgery lower extremity threatened limb classification system

	Wound (W)	
Grade	Ulcer	Gangrene
0	No ulcer	No gangrene
1	Small shallow ulcer	No gangrene
2	Deeper ulcer with exposed bone, tendon	Gangrene limited to digits
3	Extensive deep ulcer full thickness	Extensive gangrene forefoot/midfoot

	Ischemia (I)		
Grade	ABI	Ankle Systolic Pressure	TP, TcPO2
0	$\geq$0.80	>100 mm Hg	$\geq$60 mm Hg
1	0.6–0.79	70–100 mm Hg	40–59 mm Hg
2	0.4–0.59	50–70 mm Hg	30–39 mm Hg
3	$\leq$0.39	<50 mm Hg	<30 mm Hg

Foot Infection (fI)		
Clinical Manifestation of Infection	SVS	Infection Severity
No symptoms or signs of infection	0	Uninfected
Infection present (at least 2 signs: local swelling, erythema, tenderness, warmth, purulent discharge) *Local skin and subcutaneous tissue* (no deep tissue involvement, no systemic signs)	1	Mild
Local Infection involving deeper tissues (no systemic signs)	2	Moderate
Local infection with systemic signs	3	Severe

Abbreviations: TcPO2, transcutaneous oximetry; TP, toe pressure.
Adapted from Mills J, Conte M, Armstrong D, et al. The Society for Vascular Surgery Lower Extremity Threatened Limb Classification System: risk stratification based on wound, ischemia, and foot infection (WIfI). J Vasc Surg 2014;59:220–34.

- Rest pain may be so severe that it has been described as worse than terminal cancer. This leads to severe decline in functional status.
- Individuals with diabetes may have concomitant neuropathy and may present with painless CLI and tissue loss, which is challenging to diagnose early.
- CLI may develop as progression of PAD or it may be the initial presentation, which may raise the suspicion for thromboembolic disease.

History is essential with regard to time course of CLI. Acute versus chronic presentation must be differentiated given different treatment and management approaches. Although patients with CLI (chronic) do not require immediate intervention, they will definitely need a thorough evaluation and likely early revascularization. A meticulous vascular history is warranted, which includes symptom assessment of coronary and cerebral circulations, and global atherosclerosis risk assessment that encompasses smoking, diabetes, hypertension, hypercholesterolemia, and elevated levels of C-reactive protein. Moreover, in individuals with elevated C-reactive protein, levels of soluble intercellular adhesion molecule-1, a leukocyte adhesion molecule that is upregulated by inflammatory cytokines, were independently associated with the future development of lower-extremity PAD. Precipitating factors such as trauma, removal of toenail, or infection should also be identified.

Physical Examination

- Physical examination should be thorough and aimed at palpating pulses at different levels to anticipate the level of obstruction.
- Physical examination should have a systematic approach and signs of chronic ischemia should be evaluated:
  - Rubor of the dependent extremity (**Fig. 2**)
  - Early pallor upon elevation of the extremity
  - Reduced capillary refill
  - Loss of hair and brittle nails of the extremity
  - Manifestations of atheroembolic disease as livedo reticularis

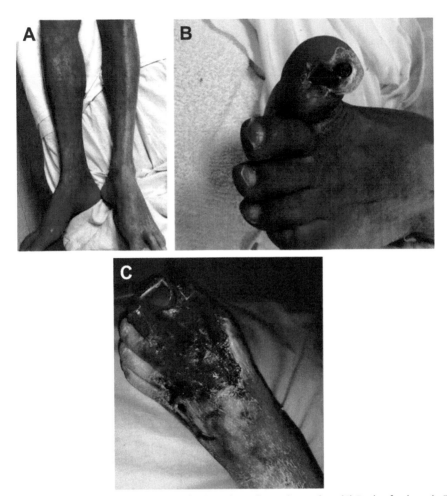

Fig. 2. Physical examination findings. (*A*) Rutherford grade 4, dependent rubor. (*B*) Rutherford grade 5. (*C*) Rutherford class 6.

- Motor and sensory assessment is always necessary.
- Source of infection should be detected.
- Distinction should be made between ulcers ischemic in origin (toes, foot) versus venous (often malleolar) versus neuropathic (foot, sole).
- Patients with a history of critical limb ischemia should be assessed at least biannually for recurrence by thorough physical examination and inspection of the feet.

DIAGNOSIS

Baseline investigations should be done, including hematologic and biochemical tests, such as complete blood count, fasting blood glucose level, hemoglobin A1c level, serum creatinine level, fasting lipid profile, and urinalysis (for glycosuria and proteinuria). Resting electrocardiogram is important for perioperative evaluation. Also, transthoracic echocardiography and nuclear stress test are often done to provide risk stratification before high-risk peripheral vascular surgery.

A single academic center performed a retrospective review of CLI patients undergoing bypass surgery using a contemporary preoperative evaluation. There was a low incidence of perioperative mortality and morbidity.[5]

Objectives for diagnostic evaluation of patients with CLI should be directed at:

- Confirmation of the diagnosis.
- Localization of the responsible lesion(s) with range of severity (usually multilevel disease).
- Assessment of the hemodynamic requirements for successful revascularization.
- Assessment of individual patient's endovascular or operative risk.

Arterial profile provides useful information, such as baseline ankle-brachial index (ABI), ankle or toe pressure measurement, toe-brachial index, waveform analysis, and localization of lesion (**Fig. 3**).

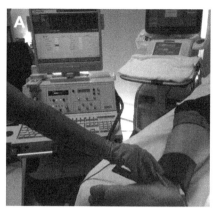
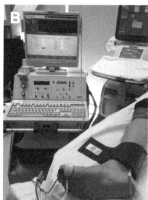

Fig. 3. Ankle-brachial index (*A*) and toe-brachial index (*B*), both with normal triphasic waveforms.

- ABI less than 1.0 is abnormal and greater than 1.4 is considered noncompressible (**Table 3**).[3]
- Generally, measurement of an absolute systolic blood pressure ≤50 mm Hg at the ankle and ≤30 mm Hg at the toe will often imply that spontaneous healing will not occur in the absence of successful revascularization. If there is major tissue loss, a toe pressure of 30 to 40 mm Hg may still not be sufficient to promote healing.
- ABI less than 0.90 is up to 95% sensitive and specific for detecting angiographic arterial disease, which was identified by the Trans Atlantic Inter-Society Consensus (TASC) working group in 2000.

The predictors of nonhealing were found to be insulin-dependent diabetes mellitus, end-stage renal disease dependent on hemodialysis, and major tissue loss after endovascular therapy.[6] Similar factors were found relevant after bypass surgery.[7] Some believe that angiosome-directed endovascular revascularization is more beneficial to promote wound healing.[8]

The next step is localization of the lesion(s) and identification of severity, which can be done invasively or noninvasively before endovascular or surgical intervention. Imaging of the lower limb arteries can be done using duplex ultrasound scan, digital subtraction angiography (DSA), magnetic resonance angiography, or computed tomographic angiography (**Table 4**).[9] DSA provides diagnostic and interventional opportunities and is the commonly performed method to identify lower extremity arterial anatomy.

On the other hand, individuals who present with clinical features to suggest atheroembolization, such as onset of signs and symptoms of CLI after recent catheter manipulation with associated systemic fatigue or muscle discomfort, symmetric bilateral limb symptoms, or increasing creatinine level, should be evaluated for more proximal aneurysmal disease such as aortoiliac, common femoral, or popliteal aneurysms.

MANAGEMENT

Management is optimally directed at:

- Increasing blood flow to the affected extremity to relieve rest pain.
- Healing ischemic ulcerations and wound care.
- Avoiding limb loss.

This management is achieved by guideline-directed medical therapy and risk factor modification. The mainstay of therapy remains to be revascularization by endovascular or surgical means for potential candidates.

Medical Therapy

Medical therapy strategies include the use of antiplatelet agents, anticoagulant medications, intravenous prostanoids, rheologic agents, and optimization of risk factors for all CLI patients,

Table 3	
Ankle-brachial index interpretation	
Ankle-Brachial Index	**Interpretation**
1.0–1.4	Normal
0.90–0.99	Borderline
0.7–.089	Mild
0.40–0.69	Moderate
≤0.40	Severe

From Rooke T, Hirsch A, Misra S, et al. 2011 ACCF/AHA focused update of the guideline for the management of patients with peripheral artery disease (updating the 2005 guideline). Circulation 2011;124:2025; with permission.

Table 4
Characteristics of imaging methods used to diagnose peripheral arterial disease

Characteristic	Duplex Ultrasound	Digital-Subtraction Angiography	Magnetic Resonance Angiography (MRA)	Computed Tomographic Angiography (CTA)
Advantages	• Noninvasive • Can visualize & quantitate severity.	• Gold Standard • High resolution • Can guide intervention	• Noninvasive • No radiation • No contrast • 3 D	• Noninvasive • Higher resolution than MRA • 3 D
Disadvantages	• Operator dependent • Limited by dense calcification	• Invasive • Radiation • Contrast • 2 dimensional	• Lower resolution than CTA • Claustrophobia • Image artifact if stent present	• Radiation (25% of dose with DSA) • Contrast • Limited by calcification

Adapted from White C. Intermittent claudication. N Engl J Med 2007;356:1246.

especially for those who are poor revascularization candidates because of multiple comorbidities.

However, few of these clinical interventions have been evaluated adequately or have been proven to offer predictable improvements in limb outcomes in prospective clinical trials. The 2011[10] and 2013[11] American College of Cardiology Foundation/American Heart Association (AHA) Guidelines for the Management of PAD address all therapies and emphasize the importance of screening for PAD. Currently, asymptomatic patients ≥65 years old should receive a resting ABI, as should patients ≥50 years old with a history of smoking or diabetes mellitus. This new recommendation stems from the German Epidemiologic Trial on ABI study group that included 6880 patients ≥65 years of age. In total, 21% of this cohort had asymptomatic or symptomatic PAD.

- Antiplatelet therapy with aspirin is currently recommended for symptomatic PAD patients (class 1).
- The Critical Limb Ischemia Prevention Study (CLIPS) showed direct evidence, for the first time, that PAD patients treated with low-dose aspirin had a decrease in major vascular events ($P = .022$) and CLI ($P = .014$).[10]
- The combination of aspirin and clopidogrel may be considered to reduce CV events in patients with symptomatic lower extremity PAD, low risk of bleeding events, and high CV risk (class IIb).
- In the Clopidogrel for High Atherothrombotic Risk and Ischemic Stabilization, Management, and Avoidance (CHARSIMA) trial, stable, high-CV-risk patients were randomly assigned to receive aspirin plus clopidogrel versus aspirin only and were followed up for

a mean of 2.3 years. The authors concluded that dual antiplatelet therapy did not confer a difference in primary outcome of CV death, myocardial infarction, or stroke compared with aspirin monotherapy. Interestingly, the symptomatic PAD cohort showed a benefit with clopidogrel (6.9% vs 7.9%; relative risk, 0.88; $P = .046$).
- β-blockers are recommended to treat hypertension in patients with PAD (class I).
- Angiotensin-converting enzyme inhibitors are recommended in patients with PAD to reduced adverse CV events (class IIa).
- Goal low-density lipoprotein is less than 100 mg/dL with use of statin (class I).
- Smoking cessation is also recommended (class I).
- Warfarin in addition to antiplatelet therapy is contraindicated in the absence of any other proven indication for warfarin in patients with PAD (class III).

The Project or Ex-Vivo Vein Graft Engineering via Transfection (PREVENT) III trial, a prospective, randomized controlled trial using molecular therapy to prevent vein graft failure in CLI patients undergoing infrainguinal bypass surgery, did a post-hoc analysis showing mortality benefit with statin in the CLI population.[12] Treatment of infection may decrease the metabolic demands that impede wound healing. Investigation of angiogenic therapies, via administration of gene or protein, to enhance collateral blood flow, has offered promise as a potential strategy to treat CLI, but further investigations are needed to prove their significant utility and cost effectiveness.

Parenteral administration of pentoxifylline is not useful in the treatment of CLI. Parenteral administration of prostaglandin E-1or iloprost for 7 to

28 days may be considered to reduce ischemic pain and facilitate ulcer healing in patients with CLI, but its efficacy is likely to be limited to a small percentage of patients as specifically mentioned in the 2006 American College of Cardiology (ACC)/AHA management of PAD guidelines. Oral iloprost is not an effective therapy to reduce the risk of amputation or death in patients with CLI. Cilostazol remains first-line medical treatment when applicable for patients with claudication to increase walking distance.

Mohler and Giri[13] reviewed the significant differences between the ACC/AHA management of PAD guidelines and the TASC II guidelines for treatment and diagnosis of PAD, which are mentioned briefly. In addition to slightly different evidence grading systems, HbA1c is recommended to be less than 7% by both guidelines but closer to 6% per TASC II. The TASC II guidelines recommend that the initial strategy for reducing lipid levels should focus on the use of dietary modifications, whereas the ACC/AHA guidelines recommend the use of statins as first-line therapy for lipid level reduction (**Table 5**).

The most recent 2013 ACC/AHA guidelines on the treatment of blood cholesterol to reduce atherosclerotic CV risk in adults advocate the use of high-intensity statin therapy in patients with PAD who are less than 75 years of age (class I recommendation). No specific low-density lipoprotein goal was recommended in this particular document.[14]

It is worth emphasizing that primary care physicians should refer patients with CLI in a timely fashion to vascular specialists to expedite treatment, prevent further deterioration, and reverse the ischemic process if feasible. In the PAD Awareness, Risk, and Treatment: New Resources for Survival (PARTNERS) Study, 6979 patients were enrolled in a multicenter cross-sectional study.

- The study investigators found that 83% of patients were aware of their PAD diagnosis but only 49% of physicians were aware.
- Hypertension and hyperlipidemia were treated less often in the PAD cohort (88% and 56%, respectively, $P<.001$) compared with the CAD group (95% and 73%, respectively, $P<.001$).
- Antiplatelet agents were prescribed in 54% of PAD patients compared with 71% of patients with CAD ($P<.001$). The authors concluded that PAD is underdiagnosed and subsequently undertreated in the primary care setting.[15]

Currently, the concept of aspirin plus clopidogrel high on treatment platelet reactivity "resistance" is evolving. This has been studied in the CAD population but was only recently shown in a CLI subgroup. Clopidogrel resistance was found in 75% of CLI patients and aspirin resistance in 28.5% in a small cohort of CLI patients.[16] In the Platelet Responsiveness to Clopidogrel Treatment after Peripheral Endovascular Procedures (PRECLOP) study, 100 patients were enrolled into a prospective study, and all received clopidogrel daily, before and after infrainguinal angioplasty or stenting. VerifyNow P2Y12 was used. Cox multivariate regression analysis identified high platelet reactivity (platelet reactivity units $\geq$234) as the only independent predictor of an increased number of adverse events (hazard ratio, 16.9; 95% confidence interval [CI], 5–55; $P<.0001$).[17] This may be the direction of tailoring treatment in CLI but it is not currently guideline driven.

The use of pneumatic compression devices is now emerging especially in patients with CLI and nonreconstructible anatomy. In a study of 171 patients, this device was found to be cost effective and clinically effective. The toe pressure increased

Table 5
Comparison between ACC/AHA and TASC II guidelines for management of peripheral arterial disease patients

	ACC/AHA	TASC II
Evidence grading system	ABC and Roman numeral classifications	ABC system
HbA1C Goal	<7%	Closer to 6%
Second-Line med to cilostazol in claudication	Pentoxifylline	Naftidrofuryl
Initial med for HTN	Not specified	Thiazide or ACEi
Initial strategy for hyperlipidemia	Statins	Dietary modification

Abbreviation: ACEi, angiotensin-converting enzyme inhibitor; HTN, hypertension.
Data from Mohler E, Giri J. Management of peripheral arterial disease patients: comparing the ACC/AHA and TASC-II guidelines. Curr Med Res Opin 2008;24:2511–13.

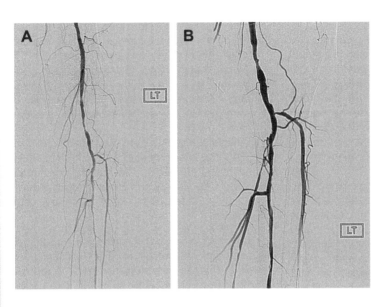

Fig. 4. Angiograms of patient with critical limb ischemia before (A) and after (B) revascularization.

from 39.9 to 54.2 mm Hg (P = .0001). Median amputation-free survival (AFS) was 18 months and limb salvage at 3.5 years was 94%.[18]

Endovascular and Surgical Treatment

The goal of revascularization in patients with CLI is to establish inline flow to the foot. Examples are shown in **Figs. 4** and **5**. If it is unclear whether hemodynamically significant inflow disease exists, intra-arterial pressure measurements across suprainguinal lesions should be measured with or without the administration of a vasodilator (given possible false low trans-stenotic pressure gradient in the setting of severe outflow disease). Catheter-based thrombolysis is generally reserved for patients with acute limb ischemia.

The Bypass versus Angioplasty in Severe Ischemia of the Leg (BASIL) trial evaluated patients with severe lower limb ischemia caused by infrainguinal disease who had a life expectancy of 2 years after an intervention and were randomly assigned

to receive bypass surgery first versus balloon angioplasty (PTA) first as revascularization strategies.[19] Of note, this trial was performed in the pre–drug-eluting stent (DES) era.

- Bradbury and colleagues[19] determined that the primary endpoint of AFS, as well as the secondary endpoint of overall survival (OS), was not different between the 2 strategies at 1 and 3 years.
- Considering the follow-up period as a whole, AFS and OS did not differ between treatments; however, for patients surviving beyond 2 years from randomization, bypass was associated with reduced hazard ratio (HR) for OS (HR, 0.61; 95% CI 0.50–0.75; P = .009) but not for AFS (HR, 0.85; 95% CI, 0.50–1.07; P = .108) during the subsequent follow-up period.
- Vein bypasses and angioplasties performed better than prosthetic bypasses.

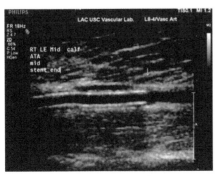
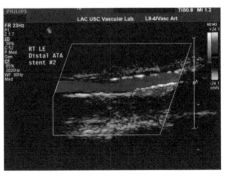

Fig. 5. Critical limb ischemia patient with patent stent in the anterior tibial artery on gray-scale duplex ultrasound scan (*left*) and with color Doppler (*right*). (Not the same patient shown in **Fig. 4**.)

Table 6
Comparison of outcomes between major trials

	TASC II[24]	PaRADISE[25]	BASIL[26]
Major amputation	30% at 1 y	6% at 3 y	11% at 1 y 18% at 3 y
Symptom relief FAILURE	20%	1%	—
Patient population	Benchmark	• All CLI • Older • Renal failure	• <25% CLI • Younger • Low risk

- These findings suggest that in patients with SLI caused by infrainguinal disease, the decision whether to perform bypass surgery or balloon angioplasty first appears to depend on anticipated life expectancy.
- Patients expected to live less than 2 years should usually be offered balloon angioplasty first, as it is associated with less morbidity and lower costs.
- Patients with longer expected longevity should be offered bypass surgery initially, but this depends on the individual comorbidities, since it is worth noting that the patients in the BASIL trial did not have significant comorbidities.

Thus, multiple survival prediction models were proposed to aid in clinical decision making according to multiple factors, including below-knee Bollinger angiogram score, body mass index, age, diabetes, serum creatinine level, and smoking status in the COX model. The Weibull model includes the same parameters in addition to presence of tissue loss, number of ankle pressure measurements detectable, maximum ankle pressure measured, a history of myocardial infarction or angina, and history of stroke or transient ischemic attack (but not diabetes). Furthermore, the Weibull model can be used to help predict outcomes for individuals and subsequent optimal decision making for choice of procedure.[20]

The Preventing Leg Amputations in Critical Limb Ischemia with Below-the-Knee Drug Eluting Stents (PARADISE) trial was a prospective, nonrandomized trial that investigated the efficacy and safety of DES in below-the-knee CLI.[21] CLI patients treated with DES had a 3-year limb salvage rate of 94%, which exceeded historic controls of balloon angioplasty and bypass surgery (**Table 6**). The randomized, controlled trials for DES in CLI are summarized in **Table 7**.

Egorova and colleagues[22] analyzed data from inpatient hospitalizations and outpatient surgeries discharge databases from 1998 to 2007 and found

Table 7
Summary of prospective randomized controlled trials in CLI: balloon expandable DES versus PTA versus bare metal stents (BMS) and the PREVENT III trial (surgical bypass)

Trial	Intervention	n	Death (%)	Patency (%)	TLR (%)	Amputation (%)
Achilles DES[a]	Cypher	200	10	77.6	10	13.8
Achilles PTA[a]	Balloon	—	12	58.1	16.5	20
Destiny DES[b]	Xcience	140	16	85	9	2.4
Destiny BMS[b]	Vision	—	16	54	34	2.4
Yukon DES[c]	Sirolimus	161	17.1	80.6	9.7	3.4
Yukon BMS[c]	BMS	—	14	55.6	17.5	4.3
Prevent III[d]	Bypass	1400	16	61	22.9	12

Abbreviation: TLR, target lesion revascularization.

[a] Scheinert D, Katsanos K, Zeller T, et al. A prospective randomized multicenter comparison of balloon angioplasty and infrapopliteal stenting with the sirolimus-eluting stent in patients with ischemic peripheral arterial disease: 1-year results from the achilles trial. J Am Coll Cardiol 2012;60(22):2290–5.

[b] Bosiers M, Scheinert D, Peeters P, et al. Randomized comparison of everolimus-eluting versus bare-metal stents in patients with critical limb ischemia and infrapopliteal arterial occlusive disease. J Vasc Surg 2012;55(2):390–8.

[c] Rastan A, Tepe G, Krankenberg H, et al. Sirolimus-eluting stents versus bare-metal stents for treatment of focal lesions in infrapopliteal arteries: a double-blind, multi-centre, randomized clinical trial. Eur Heart J 2011;32(18):2274–81.

[d] Conte MS, Bandyk DF, Clowes AW, et al. Results of PREVENT III: a multicenter, randomized trial of edifoligide for the prevention of vein graft failure in lower extremity bypass surgery. J Vasc Surg 2006;43(4):742–51.

that the volume of major amputations decreased by 38% as a result of endovascular lower extremity revascularization (LER) techniques, as its use doubled during this time. The volume of open LER decreased by 67% from 1998 to 2007. It is worth noting that interventions declined by 20% for CLI but increased by nearly 50% for claudication. Although patients today have more comorbidities, regardless of whether treated for claudication or CLI, the rates of amputation, the procedural morbidity and mortality, and the length of hospital stay have all significantly decreased. Infrainguinal surgical bypass with at least 3 mm vein conduit at 1 year has a primary, assisted primary, and secondary patency of 68.4%, 93.3%, and 95.2%, respectively.[23]

Primary Amputation

Patients who have significant necrosis of the weight-bearing portions of the foot (in ambulatory patients), an uncorrectable flexion contracture, paresis of the extremity, refractory ischemic rest pain, sepsis, or a limited life expectancy because of comorbid conditions should be evaluated for primary amputation of the leg. Surgical or endovascular intervention is not indicated in patients with severe decrements in limb perfusion (ie, ABI <0.4) in the absence of clinical symptoms of CLI. It is worth noting that active progressive infection may lead to wet gangrene and guillotine amputation.

SUMMARY

The long-term prognosis of patients with PAD is worse than in patients with CAD. Vascular patients receive fewer medications than do CAD patients. Cardiovascular and cerebrovascular complications are the major causes of death. We need to close the survival gap in PAD patients, which can be facilitated by a multidisciplinary team including vascular medicine, vascular surgery, interventional cardiology, and primary care.

REFERENCES

1. Golomb B, Dang T, Criqui M. Contemporary reviews in cardiovascular medicine, peripheral arterial disease, morbidity and mortality implications. Circulation 2006;114:688–99.
2. Allie DE, Hebert CJ, Ingraldi A, et al. 24-carat gold, 14-carat gold, or platinum standards in the treatment of critical limb ischemia: bypass surgery or endovascular intervention? J Endovasc Ther 2009; 16(Suppl 1):I134–46.
3. Hirsch A, Haskal Z, Hertzer N, et al. ACC/AHA 2005 practice guidelines for the management of patients with peripheral arterial disease (Lower Extremity, Renal, Mesenteric, and Abdominal Aortic): A Collaborative Report from the American Association for Vascular Surgery/Society for Vascular Surgery, Society for Cardiovascular Angiography and Interventions, Society for Vascular Medicine and Biology, Society of Interventional Radiology, and the ACC/AHA Task Force on Practice Guidelines (Writing Committee to Develop Guidelines for the Management of Patients With Peripheral Arterial Disease): Endorsed by the American Association of Cardiovascular and Pulmonary Rehabilitation; National Heart, Lung, and Blood Institute; Society for Vascular Nursing; TransAtlantic Inter-Society Consensus; and Vascular Disease Foundation. Circulation 2006;113:e463–654.
4. Mills J, Conte M, Armstrong D, et al. The Society for Vascular Surgery Lower Extremity Threatened Limb Classification System: risk stratification based on wound, ischemia, and foot infection (WIfI). J Vasc Surg 2014;59:220–34.
5. Elsayed S, Theophanous C, Upadhyay R, et al. Contemporary preoperative evaluation of patients with critical limb ischemia undergoing vascular surgery. Catheter Cardiovasc Interv 2014;83(S1):S76.
6. Kobayashi N, Hirano K, Nakano M, et al. Predictors of non-healing in patients with critical limb ischemia and tissue loss following successful endovascular therapy. Catheter Cardiovasc Interv 2014. [Epub ahead of print].
7. McPhee J, Barshes N, Ho K, et al. Predictors factors of 30-day unplanned readmission after lower extremity bypass. J Vasc Surg 2013;57:955–62.
8. Iida O, Soga Y, Hirano K, et al. Long-term results of direct and indirect endovascular revascularization based on the angiosome concept in patients with critical limb ischemia presenting with isolated below-the-knee lesions. J Vasc Surg 2012;55: 363–70.
9. White C. Intermittent claudication. N Engl J Med 2007;356:1241–50.
10. Rooke T, Hirsch A, Misra S, et al. 2011 ACCF/AHA focused update of the guideline for the management of patients with peripheral artery disease (updating the 2005 guideline). Circulation 2011;124:2020–45.
11. Anderson J, Halperin J, Albert N, et al. Management of patients with peripheral artery disease (compilation of 2005 and 2011 ACCF/AHA guideline recommendations): a report of the American College of Cardiology Foundation/American Heart Association Task Force on Practice Guidelines. Circulation 2013;127:1425–43.
12. Conte M, Bandyk D, Clowes A, et al. Results of PREVENT III: a multicenter, randomized trial of edifoligide for the prevention of vein graft failure in lower extremity bypass surgery. J Vasc Surg 2006;43:742–51.

13. Mohler E, Giri J. Management of peripheral arterial disease patients: comparing the ACC/AHA and TASC-II guidelines. Curr Med Res Opin 2008;24: 2509–22.

14. Stone N, Robinson J, Lichtenstein A, et al. 2013 ACC/AHA guideline on the treatment of blood cholesterol to reduce atherosclerotic cardiovascular risk in adults. Circulation 2014;129(25 Suppl 2):S1–45.

15. Hirsch A, Criqui M, Treat-Jacobson D, et al. Peripheral arterial disease detection, awareness, and treatment in primary care. JAMA 2001;286:1317–24.

16. Elsayed S, Shavelle D, Matthews R, et al. Aspirin and clopidogrel high on treatment platelet reactivity "resistance" in critical limb ischemia. J Am Coll Cardiol 2012;59(13s1):E2114.

17. Spiliopoulos S, Pastromas G, Katsanos K, et al. Platelet responsiveness to clopidogrel treatment after peripheral endovascular procedures: the PRECLOP study: clinical impact and optimal cutoff value of on-treatment high platelet reactivity. J Am Coll Cardiol 2013;61:2428–34.

18. Sultan S, Hamada N, Soylu E, et al. Sequential compression biomechanical device in patients with critical limb ischemia and nonreconstructible peripheral vascular disease. J Vasc Surg 2011;54:440–6.

19. Bradbury A, Adam D, Bell J, et al. Bypass versus angioplasty in severe ischaemia of the leg (BASIL) trial: an intention-to-treat analysis of amputation-free and overall survival in patients randomized to a bypass surgery-first or a balloon angioplasty-first revascularization strategy. J Vasc Surg 2010;51:5S–17S.

20. Bradbury A, Adam D, Bell J, et al. Bypass versus angioplasty in severe ischaemia of the leg (BASIL) trial: a survival prediction model to facilitate clinical decision making. J Vasc Surg 2010;51(5 Suppl): 52S–68S.

21. Feiring A, Krahn M, Nelson L, et al. Preventing leg amputations in critical limb ischemia with below-the-knee drug-eluting stents. The PaRADISE (PReventing Amputations using Drug eluting StEnts) Trial. J Am Coll Cardiol 2010;55:1580–9.

22. Egorova N, Guillerme S, Gelijns A, et al. An analysis of the outcomes of a decade of experience with lower extremity revascularization including limb salvage, lengths of stay, and safety. J Vasc Surg 2010;51:878–85, 885.e1.

23. Slim H, Tiwari A, Ritter J, et al. Outcome of infra-inguinal bypass grafts using vein conduit with less than 3 millimeters diameter in critical leg ischemia. J Vasc Surg 2011;53:421–5.

24. Norgren L, Hiatt WR, Dormandy JA, et al. Inter-Society Consensus for the Management of Peripheral Arterial Disease (TASC II). J Vasc Surg 2007; 45(Suppl S):S5–67.

25. Feiring A, Krahn M, Nelson L, et al. Preventing leg amputations in critical limb ischemia with below the-knee drug-eluting stents. The PaRADISE (PReventing Amputations using Drug eluting StEnts) Trial. J Am Coll Cardiol 2010;55:1580–9.

26. Bradbury A, Adam D, Bell J, et al. Bypass versus Angioplasty in Severe Ischaemia of the Leg (BASIL) trial: An intention-to-treat analysis of amputation-free and overall survival in patients randomized to a bypass surgery-first or a balloon angioplasty-first revascularization strategy. J Vasc Surg 2010;51: 5S–17S.

Contemporary Treatment of Venous Thromboembolic Disease

Taki Galanis, MD*, Geno J. Merli, MD

KEYWORDS

- Venous thromboembolism • Deep vein thrombosis • Pulmonary embolism • Anticoagulation
- Thrombolysis • Inferior vena cava filter

KEY POINTS

- The routine use of thrombolysis for lower-extremity deep vein thrombosis (DVT) is not recommended.
- Catheter-directed thrombolysis is suggested in patients with impending venous gangrene whose symptom duration is less than 14 days and who have a low risk of bleeding.
- Systemic thrombolysis, administered through a peripheral intravenous line, is recommended in patients with hemodynamic collapse (ie, persistent hypotension).
- The new target-specific oral anticoagulants have been shown to be as safe and effective as standard anticoagulation for the treatment of acute venous thromboembolism (VTE).
- Indefinite anticoagulation is suggested in patients with an unprovoked or recurrent VTE and in patients with an active malignancy.

INTRODUCTION

Venous thromboembolism (VTE) encompasses deep vein thrombosis (DVT) and pulmonary embolism (PE). The incidence of VTE is approximately 1 per 1000 person-years.[1,2] The case-fatality rate in patients presenting with an acute DVT and PE during the first 3 months of anticoagulation is 9.0% and 30.1%, respectively.[3] In addition to mortality, the cumulative incidence of chronic thromboembolic pulmonary hypertension is approximately 4% at 2 years following a diagnosis of PE.[4] Furthermore, postthrombotic syndrome (PTS) occurs in 20% to 50% of patients diagnosed with a symptomatic DVT.[5] The treatment of VTE is divided into 3 phases (**Fig. 1**).[6] Several target-specific oral anticoagulants (TSOACs) have been studied for the treatment of VTE during these phases of therapy (**Tables 1** and **2**) and have been shown to be as noninferior in safety and efficacy as conventional therapy. This article reviews the contemporary treatment of VTE.

RISK STRATIFICATION (INPATIENT VS OUTPATIENT TREATMENT)

A *Cochrane Review* of randomized controlled trials (RCTs) demonstrated the efficacy and safety of the outpatient treatment of DVT with low-molecular-weight heparin (LMWH) compared with inpatient anticoagulation.[7] Several clinical prediction rules have been established to stratify PE-related mortality risk,[8–10] of which the Pulmonary Embolism Severity Index seems to be the best validated

The authors have nothing to disclose.

Department of Surgery, Jefferson Vascular Center, Thomas Jefferson University Hospitals, 111 South 11th Street, Philadelphia, PA 19107, USA

* Corresponding author. Department of Surgery, Jefferson Vascular Center, Thomas Jefferson University Hospitals, 111 South 11th Street, Suite 6270, Gibbon Building, Philadelphia, PA 19107.

E-mail address: taki.galanis@jefferson.edu

0733-8651/15/$ – see front matter © 2015 Elsevier Inc. All rights reserved.

cardiology.theclinics.com

(Table 3).[6] The use of LMWH as outpatient treatment of patients with low-risk PE has been shown to be safe and effective in several RCTs and a systematic review.[11–13]

THROMBOLYSIS FOR LOWER EXTREMITY DEEP VEIN THROMBOSIS

There are no RCTs comparing catheter-directed thrombolysis (CDT) with systemic thrombolysis for lower-extremity DVT. Lower-quality evidence suggests that CDT is more effective in establishing vein patency and is associated with a lower risk of bleeding compared with systemic thrombolysis.[6] A meta-analysis of thrombolysis (either systemic or catheter-directed) for lower-extremity DVT demonstrated a significant difference in clot lysis, vein patency, and reduction of PTS in patients treated with lytic therapy compared with standard anticoagulation at the expense of more bleeding complications.[14] There are insufficient data to recommend one thrombolytic agent over others. CDT is suggested in patients with an ileofemoral DVT with the following criteria: impending venous gangrene, symptom duration less than 14 days, good functional capacity, life expectancy greater than 1 year, and low risk of bleeding. In the absence of impending limb gangrene, standard anticoagulation is an acceptable, initial form of treatment.[6] The use of venous stents following balloon angioplasty in patients with residual occlusion after CDT has not been studied in prospective, randomized trials.

THROMBOLYSIS FOR PULMONARY EMBOLISM

Features of right ventricular dysfunction as determined by echocardiography, CT scanning, or an elevation of cardiac biomarkers (ie, troponins, brain natriuretic peptide) are associated with worse outcomes in patients with an acute PE.[15] However, systemic thrombolysis was not associated with a reduction in mortality in patients with a submassive PE (abnormal right ventricular dysfunction without arterial hypotension) in 2 randomized, double-blind studies.[16,17] In the most recent RCT using thrombolysis in patients with a submassive PE, major bleeding and hemorrhagic stroke occurred in approximately 12% and 2%, respectively, in patients treated with thrombolysis (statistically significant).[17] Systemic thrombolysis is recommended in patients who experience hemodynamic compromise.[6] There is insufficient evidence to recommend the administration of

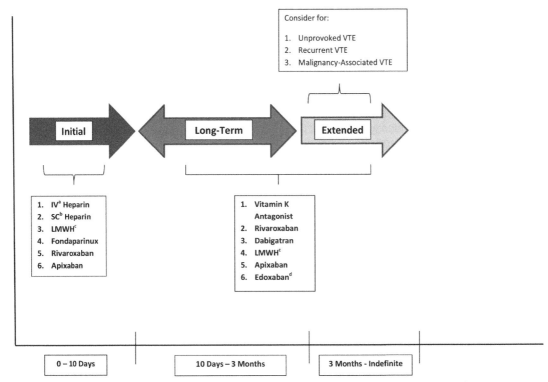

Fig. 1. Phases of anticoagulant treatment. (a) Intravenous; (b) subcutaneous; (c) LMWH, preferred in patients with a malignancy; (d) edoxaban has not yet been approved for VTE treatment.

Table 1
Clinical trials comparing the new oral anticoagulants to standard therapy in acute venous thromboembolism[a]

	Einstein-DVT	Einstein-PE	Amplify	Re-Cover	Re-Cover II	Hokusai-VTE
Trial design	Open-label, randomized	Open-label, randomized	Double-blind, randomized	Double-blind, randomized	Double-blind, randomized	Double-blind, randomized
Regimen	Rivaroxaban 15 mg BID × 3 wk, then 20 mg daily	Rivaroxaban 15 mg BID × 3 wk, then 20 mg daily	Apixaban 10 mg BID × 7 d, then 5 mg BID	Standard therapy for median 9 d, then Dabigatran 150 mg BID	Standard therapy for median 9 d, then Dabigatran 150 mg BID	Standard therapy for median 7 d, then edoxaban 60 mg daily (30 mg daily if CrCl 30–50 mL/min or weight ≤60 kg)
Average age	55–58 y old	58 y old	57 y old	54–55 y old	55 y old	56 y old
PE only	—	All patients	25%	21%	23%	30%
DVT + PE	All patients (no PE)	25%	8%–9%	10%	8%–9%	10%
Unprovoked VTE	61%–63%	64%–65%	90%	Undefined	Undefined	65%–66%
Prior VTE	19%	19%–20%	15%–17%	25%–26%	16%–19%	18%–19%
Malignancy	5%–7%	5%	3%	5%	4%	9%
Thrombophilia	6%–7%	5%–6%	2%–3%	Undefined	Undefined	Undefined
% TTR for INR[b]	57.7%	62.7%	61%	60%	57%	63.5%
Efficacy outcome[c]	Rivaroxaban: 2.1% Standard Tx: 3.0%	Rivaroxaban: 2.1% Standard Tx: 1.8%	Apixaban: 2.3% Standard Tx: 2.7%	Dabigatran: 2.4% Standard Tx: 2.1%	Dabigatran: 2.3% Standard Tx: 2.2%	Edoxaban: 3.2% Standard Tx: 3.5%
Major bleeding[d]	Rivaroxaban: 0.8% Standard Tx: 1.2%	Rivaroxaban: 1.1% Standard Tx: 2.2%	Apixaban: 0.6% Standard Tx: 1.8%	Dabigatran: 1.6% Standard Tx: 1.9%	Dabigatran: 1.2% Standard Tx: 1.7%	Edoxaban: 1.4% Standard Tx: 1.6%
Clinically relevant bleeding[e]	Rivaroxaban: 8.1% Standard Tx: 8.1%	Rivaroxaban: 10.3% Standard Tx: 11.4%	Apixaban: 4.3% Standard Tx: 9.7%	Dabigatran: 5.6% Standard Tx: 8.8%	Dabigatran: 5.0% Standard Tx: 7.9%	Edoxaban: 8.5% Standard Tx: 10.3%

Abbreviation: Amplify, Apixaban for the Initial Management of Pulmonary Embolism and Deep-Vein Thrombosis as First-Line Therapy.
[a] Standard therapy is defined as the use of a short-acting anticoagulant (ie, intravenous heparin, low-molecular-weight heparin) followed by a vitamin K antagonist.
[b] TTR is defined as time in therapeutic range for vitamin K antagonism.
[c] Efficacy outcome = symptomatic VTE.
[d] Major bleeding is defined as per the International Society of Thrombosis and Haemostasis guidelines.
[e] Clinically relevant bleeding is defined as the composite of major and clinically relevant nonmajor bleeding as per the International Society of Thrombosis and Haemostasis guidelines.

Table 2
Clinical trials investigating the new oral anticoagulants for the extended treatment of venous thromboembolism[a]

	Einstein-Ext	Amplify-Ext	Re-Medy	Re-Sonate
Trial design	Double-blind, randomized	Double-blind, randomized	Double-blind, randomized	Double-blind, randomized
Regimen	Rivaroxaban 20 mg daily vs Placebo	Apixaban 2.5 mg or 5 mg BID vs Placebo	Dabigatran 150 mg BID vs warfarin	Dabigatran 150 mg BID vs placebo
Average age	58 y old	56–57 y old	54–55 y old	56 y old
Index event[b]	DVT: 60%–64% PE: 36%–40%	DVT: 65%–67% PE: 34%–35%	DVT: 65%–66% PE: 34%–35%	DVT: 63%–67% PE: 32%
Unprovoked VTE	73%–74%	91%–93%	Undefined	Undefined
Prior VTE	14%–18%	12%–15%	52%–55%	2 patients
Malignancy	4%–5%	Excluded (1%–2%)	4%	Excluded
Thrombophilia	8%	Excluded (3%–4%)	18%	10%–13%
% TTR for INR[c]	—	—	65.3%	—
Efficacy outcome[d]	Rivaroxaban: 1.3%, Placebo: 7.1%	Apixaban 2.5 mg: 3.8%, Apixaban 5 mg: 4.2%, Placebo: 11.6%	Dabigatran: 1.8%, warfarin: 1.3%	Dabigatran: 0.4%, placebo: 5.6%
Major bleeding[e]	Rivaroxaban: 0.7%, Placebo: 0%	Apixaban 2.5 mg: 0.2%, Apixaban 5 mg: 0.1%, Placebo: 0.5%	Dabigatran: 0.9%, warfarin: 1.8%	Dabigatran: 0.3%, placebo: 0%
Clinically relevant bleeding[f]	Rivaroxaban: 6.0%, Placebo: 1.2%	Apixaban 2.5 mg: 3.2%, Apixaban 5 mg: 4.3%, Placebo: 2.7%	Dabigatran: 5.6%, warfarin: 10.2%	Dabigatran: 5.3%, placebo: 1.8%

[a] Patients were treated with either a standard anticoagulant or study drug for at least 3 months before being randomized in the extended treatment trials.
[b] PE = PE ± DVT, DVT = DVT only.
[c] TTR is defined as time in therapeutic range for vitamin K antagonism.
[d] Efficacy outcome = symptomatic VTE.
[e] Major bleeding is defined as per the International Society of Thrombosis and Haemostasis guidelines.
[f] Clinically relevant bleeding is defined as the composite of major and clinically relevant nonmajor bleeding as per the International Society of Thrombosis and Haemostasis guidelines.

Table 3
Simplified Pulmonary Embolism Severity Index

Variable	Points
Age >80 y	1
History of cancer	1
Chronic cardiopulmonary disease	1
Pulse ≥110 beats per minute	1
Systolic blood pressure <100 mm Hg	1
Pulse oximetry <90%	1
PE Risk	**Score**
Low risk	0
High risk	≥1

Adapted from Jimenez D, Aujesky D, Moores L, et al. Simplification of the pulmonary embolism severity index for prognostication in patients with acute symptomatic pulmonary embolism. Arch Intern Med 2010;170(15):1383–9.

thrombolysis through a pulmonary artery catheter rather than through a peripheral vein.

INITIAL PHASE OF TREATMENT (FIRST 5–10 DAYS)

A meta-analysis comparing LMWH versus adjusted-dose unfractionated heparin (UFH; intravenous or subcutaneous) for the initial treatment of VTE showed a statistically significant advantage of LMWH in preventing recurrent VTE, major bleeding, or death compared with UFH.[18] Furthermore, a meta-analysis comparing once-daily versus twice-daily LMWH revealed that the once-daily regimen was associated with less recurrent VTE and major hemorrhage. However, the difference for both endpoints did not reach statistical significance.[19] UFH is the drug of choice in patients with renal insufficiency given the renal excretion of LMWH, fondaparinux, and the TSOACs.

As shown in **Table 1**, several of the TSOACs have been studied for the treatment of an acute DVT and/or PE. In all of these trials, the new anticoagulants were shown to be at least as safe and effective as conventional therapy.[6] A recent, pooled analysis confirmed the noninferiority of rivaroxaban for the treatment of VTE compared with vitamin K antagonism. Rivaroxaban was associated with a statistically significant reduction in major bleeding compared with conventional therapy, and its efficacy as well as safety profile did not vary according to thrombus burden, patient frailty, or the presence of a malignancy.[20] Dabigatran was shown to be as effective and safe as warfarin for the treatment of VTE in a recent pooled analysis as well. Although the rate of clinically significant bleeding was significantly less in patients treated with dabigatran, there were numerically more acute coronary syndromes in patients treated with this new anticoagulant (which did not reach statistical significance).[21,22] A meta-analysis of noninferiority trials comparing dabigatran to various therapies, including placebo, in different populations showed a higher risk of acute coronary syndrome in patients exposed to the direct-thrombin inhibitor.[23]

Apixaban, edoxaban, and rivaroxaban were shown to be as safe and effective in patients with renal impairment (creatinine clearance <50 mL/min) for the treatment of VTE compared with vitamin K antagonism in a recent metaregression and meta-analysis. Data were not available for dabigatran in the VTE population. As shown in **Table 1**, the trial designs of the acute-phase studies differed. Although apixaban and rivaroxaban were started at the time of randomization, dabigatran and edoxaban were initiated after patients received lead-in therapy with a conventional anticoagulant for at least 5 days (ie, with LMWH). Of all the TSOACs studied for VTE, a subgroup analysis for drug efficacy in patients with a submassive PE was only provided for edoxaban. In this specific population, edoxaban was more effective than standard therapy in reducing the risk of symptomatic, recurrent VTE. At the time of this writing, apixaban, rivaroxaban, and dabigatran have been approved for the treatment of VTE during the initial phase of therapy. Based on the aforementioned differences in the trial designs, dabigatran should not be started for an acute VTE until the patient has been treated with a conventional anticoagulant for at least 5 days. On the other hand, apixaban and rivaroxaban can be immediately given at the time of diagnosis.

Although, historically, compression stockings were recommended in patients with symptomatic DVT to prevent PTS, a recent randomized, double-blind study of compression stockings did not reduce the risk of PTS.[24] Despite these results, compression therapy is generally recommended in patients with a symptomatic DVT to improve symptoms. In a systematic review, early ambulation led to a more rapid resolution of limb pain in patients with a DVT and potentially reduced the risk of PTS.[25] Thus, patients should be encouraged to ambulate during this phase of treatment.

LONG-TERM PHASE OF TREATMENT (DAY 10 TO 3 MONTHS)

In addition to the newly approved anticoagulants, warfarin remains a viable option for treatment during this phase of therapy, particularly in patients with renal insufficiency. Although there is evidence that a 10-mg loading dose of warfarin achieves a therapeutic level faster, there are insufficient data to recommend one specific nomogram for warfarin dosing. Pharmacogenetic testing to guide warfarin dosing is not recommended given the results of trials and high cost.[26] LMWH is recommended over vitamin K antagonism in patients with a malignancy for at least the first 3 months of therapy. The TSOACs have not been well-studied in patients with cancer and should likely not be used in this patient population until further evidence supports their use for this indication. A 3-month duration of anticoagulation is suggested in patients with a provoked VTE.[6]

EXTENDED TREATMENT PHASE (3 MONTHS TO INDEFINITELY)

Extended treatment is suggested in patients with unprovoked VTE, recurrent VTE, or malignancy.[6] Results demonstrating an increased risk of VTE recurrence in patients with thrombophilia are inconsistent.[6,27–29] Several meta-analyses and systematic reviews have confirmed the correlation of a positive d-dimer assay after stopping anticoagulation and a higher risk of VTE recurrence in patients with an unprovoked thrombotic event.[30–32] However, the presence of residual vein obstruction (RVO) has not been consistently shown to predict recurrence of VTE after withdrawal of anticoagulation, particularly in patients with unprovoked VTE.[33–35] These factors (hereditary and acquired thrombophilia, abnormal d-dimer testing, and RVO) do not appear individually to be strong enough risk factors to determine the duration of anticoagulation, whereas the combination of these factors may be more predictive.[6] Low-dose aspirin

(100 mg daily) has been studied for secondary prevention of VTE in patients with an unprovoked thrombotic event after completing at least 3 months of treatment.[36,37] The efficacy of aspirin for this indication has not been consistently demonstrated in pooled analyses.[38] Most recently, apixaban 2.5 mg twice daily has been approved for treatment during this phase of therapy based on the results of the Amplify-Extend trial. In this trial, apixaban was found to be more effective than and just as safe as placebo in preventing recurrent VTE in patients who completed the long-term phase of treatment (ie, at least 3 months of therapy).

INFERIOR VENA CAVA FILTERS

There are no randomized studies comparing the use of inferior vena cava (IVC) filters to anticoagulation. IVC filters are associated with a reduction in PE at the expense of an increased risk of a recurrent DVT over a period of 8 years.[39] Lower-quality evidence suggests a mortality benefit with IVC filters in patients with a massive PE (ie, with

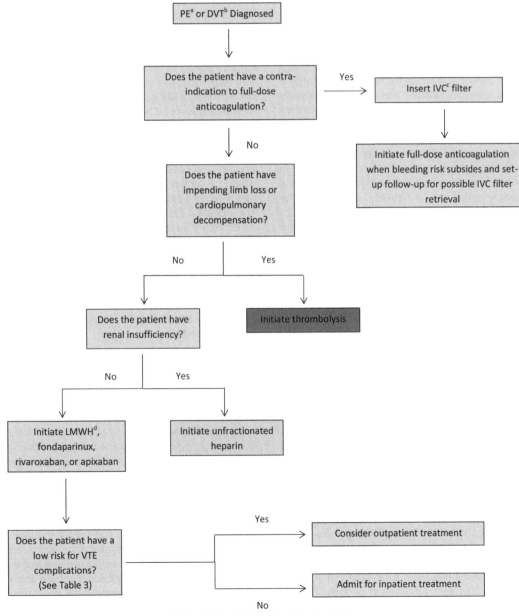

Fig. 2. Algorithm for treatment of VTE. (a) PE; (b) DVT; (c) IVC; (d) LMWH.

persistent hypotension) or in those patients with a PE who are receiving thrombolysis therapy.[40,41] In patients with a DVT or PE who have a contraindication to anticoagulation therapy, an IVC filter is indicated. Initiation of a conventional course of anticoagulation is suggested once the contraindication resolves.[6] The reported rates of filter complications vary widely. Of 921 complications listed in a 2010 report issued by the US Food and Drug Administration, the following complications were noted: 35.6% device migration, 15.8% filter embolization, 7.6% perforation of the IVC, and 6% filter fractures.[42] IVC filter thrombosis is also not an uncommon complication.[39] The risks and benefits of retrieving IVC filters should be reviewed. Institutional programs may increase the probability of successful filter retrieval.[43]

SUMMARY

The treatment armament for VTE has increased dramatically during recent years owing to the results of several phase III clinical trials. Although all of the TSOACs have been shown to be safe and effective for the treatment of DVT and PE, these medications have not been well studied in certain patient populations, including the elderly, those with cancer, as well as those with renal insufficiency. Conventional anticoagulation, such as warfarin or LMWH, likely will continue to be the anticoagulant of choice in these patient groups. **Fig. 2** summarizes a proposed algorithm for the treatment of VTE. Owing to the results of RCTs, many patients with VTE can be treated in the outpatient setting. Thrombolysis is generally reserved for patients with either impending limb gangrene or hemodynamic collapse. IVC filters should generally be avoided unless there is a contraindication to full-dose anticoagulation.

REFERENCES

1. Tagalakis V, Patenaude V, Kahn SR, et al. Incidence of and mortality from venous thromboembolism in a real-world population: the Q-VTE study cohort. Am J Med 2013;126(9):832.e13–21. http://dx.doi.org/10.1016/j.amjmed.2013.02.024.

2. Bates SM, Jaeschke R, Stevens SM, et al. Diagnosis of DVT: antithrombotic therapy and prevention of thrombosis, 9th ed: American College of Chest Physicians evidence-based clinical practice guidelines. Chest 2012;141(2 Suppl):e351S–418S. http://dx.doi.org/10.1378/chest.11-2299.

3. Carrier M, Le Gal G, Wells PS, et al. Systematic review: case-fatality rates of recurrent venous thromboembolism and major bleeding events among patients treated for venous thromboembolism. Ann Intern Med 2010;152(9):578–89. http://dx.doi.org/10.7326/0003-4819-152-9-201005040-00008.

4. Pengo V, Lensing AW, Prins MH, et al. Incidence of chronic thromboembolic pulmonary hypertension after pulmonary embolism. N Engl J Med 2004;350(22):2257–64. http://dx.doi.org/10.1056/NEJMoa032274.

5. Kahn SR, Ginsberg JS. Relationship between deep venous thrombosis and the postthrombotic syndrome. Arch Intern Med 2004;164(1):17–26. http://dx.doi.org/10.1001/archinte.164.1.17.

6. Kearon C, Akl EA, Comerota AJ, et al. Antithrombotic therapy for VTE disease: antithrombotic therapy and prevention of thrombosis, 9th ed: American College of Chest Physicians evidence-based clinical practice guidelines. Chest 2012;141(2 Suppl):e419S–94S. http://dx.doi.org/10.1378/chest.11-2301.

7. Othieno R, Abu Affan M, Okpo E. Home versus inpatient treatment for deep vein thrombosis. Cochrane Database Syst Rev 2007;(3):CD003076. http://dx.doi.org/10.1002/14651858.CD003076.pub2.

8. Aujesky D, Obrosky DS, Stone RA, et al. Derivation and validation of a prognostic model for pulmonary embolism. Am J Respir Crit Care Med 2005;172(8):1041–6. pii:200506-862OC.

9. Jimenez D, Aujesky D, Moores L, et al. Simplification of the pulmonary embolism severity index for prognostication in patients with acute symptomatic pulmonary embolism. Arch Intern Med 2010;170(15):1383–9. http://dx.doi.org/10.1001/archinternmed.2010.199.

10. Wicki J, Perrier A, Pornogor TV, et al. Predicting adverse outcome in patients with acute pulmonary embolism: a risk score. Thromb Haemost 2000;84(4):548–52. pii:00100548.

11. Otero R, Uresandi F, Jimenez D, et al. Home treatment in pulmonary embolism. Thromb Res 2010;126(1):e1–5. http://dx.doi.org/10.1016/j.thromres.2009.09.026.

12. Aujesky D, Roy PM, Verschuren F, et al. Outpatient versus inpatient treatment for patients with acute pulmonary embolism: an international, open-label, randomised, non-inferiority trial. Lancet 2011;378(9785):41–8. http://dx.doi.org/10.1016/S0140-6736(11)60824-6.

13. Squizzato A, Galli M, Dentali F, et al. Outpatient treatment and early discharge of symptomatic pulmonary embolism: a systematic review. Eur Respir J 2009;33(5):1148–55. http://dx.doi.org/10.1183/09031936.00133608.

14. Watson L, Broderick C, Armon MP. Thrombolysis for acute deep vein thrombosis. Cochrane Database Syst Rev 2014;(1):CD002783. http://dx.doi.org/10.1002/14651858.CD002783.pub3.

15. Jaff MR, McMurtry MS, Archer SL, et al. Management of massive and submassive pulmonary embolism, iliofemoral deep vein thrombosis, and chronic

thromboembolic pulmonary hypertension: a scientific statement from the American Heart Association. Circulation 2011;123(16):1788–830. http://dx.doi.org/10.1161/CIR.0b013e318214914f.

16. Konstantinides S, Geibel A, Heusel G, et al, Management Strategies and Prognosis of Pulmonary Embolism-3 Trial Investigators. Heparin plus alteplase compared with heparin alone in patients with submassive pulmonary embolism. N Engl J Med 2002;347(15):1143–50. http://dx.doi.org/10.1056/NEJMoa021274.

17. Meyer G, Vicaut E, Danays T, et al. Fibrinolysis for patients with intermediate-risk pulmonary embolism. N Engl J Med 2014;370(15):1402–11. http://dx.doi.org/10.1056/NEJMoa1302097.

18. Erkens PM, Prins MH. Fixed dose subcutaneous low molecular weight heparins versus adjusted dose unfractionated heparin for venous thromboembolism. Cochrane Database Syst Rev 2010;(9):CD001100. http://dx.doi.org/10.1002/14651858.CD001100.pub3.

19. van Dongen CJ, MacGillavry MR, Prins MH. Once versus twice daily LMWH for the initial treatment of venous thromboembolism. Cochrane Database Syst Rev 2005;(3):CD003074. http://dx.doi.org/10.1002/14651858.CD003074.pub2.

20. Prins MH, Lensing AW, Bauersachs R, et al. Oral rivaroxaban versus standard therapy for the treatment of symptomatic venous thromboembolism: a pooled analysis of the EINSTEIN-DVT and PE randomized studies. Thromb J 2013;11(1):21. http://dx.doi.org/10.1186/1477-9560-11-21.

21. Schulman S, Kakkar AK, Goldhaber SZ, et al. Treatment of acute venous thromboembolism with dabigatran or warfarin and pooled analysis. Circulation 2014;129(7):764–72. http://dx.doi.org/10.1161/CIRCULATIONAHA.113.004450.

22. Lega JC, Bertoletti L, Gremillet C, et al. Consistency of safety profile of new oral anticoagulants in patients with renal failure. J Thromb Haemost 2014;12(3):337–43. http://dx.doi.org/10.1111/jth.12486.

23. Uchino K, Hernandez AV. Dabigatran association with higher risk of acute coronary events: metaanalysis of noninferiority randomized controlled trials. Arch Intern Med 2012;172(5):397–402. http://dx.doi.org/10.1001/archinternmed.2011.1666.

24. Kahn SR, Shapiro S, Wells PS, et al. Compression stockings to prevent post-thrombotic syndrome: a randomised placebo-controlled trial. Lancet 2014;383(9920):880–8. http://dx.doi.org/10.1016/S0140-6736(13)61902-9.

25. Kahn SR, Shrier I, Kearon C. Physical activity in patients with deep venous thrombosis: a systematic review. Thromb Res 2008;122(6):763–73. pii:S0049-3848(07)00398-2.

26. Mahtani KR, Heneghan CJ, Nunan D, et al. Optimal loading dose of warfarin for the initiation of oral anticoagulation. Cochrane Database Syst Rev 2012;(12):CD008685. http://dx.doi.org/10.1002/14651858.CD008685.pub2.

27. Lijfering WM, Middeldorp S, Veeger NJ, et al. Risk of recurrent venous thrombosis in homozygous carriers and double heterozygous carriers of factor V Leiden and prothrombin G20210A. Circulation 2010;121(15):1706–12. http://dx.doi.org/10.1161/CIRCULATIONAHA.109.906347.

28. Christiansen SC, Cannegieter SC, Koster T, et al. Thrombophilia, clinical factors, and recurrent venous thrombotic events. JAMA 2005;293(19):2352–61. pii:293/19/2352.

29. Brouwer JL, Lijfering WM, Ten Kate MK, et al. High long-term absolute risk of recurrent venous thromboembolism in patients with hereditary deficiencies of protein S, protein C or antithrombin. Thromb Haemost 2009;101(1):93–9. pii:09010093.

30. Bruinstroop E, Klok FA, Van De Ree MA, et al. Elevated D-dimer levels predict recurrence in patients with idiopathic venous thromboembolism: a meta-analysis. J Thromb Haemost 2009;7(4):611–8. http://dx.doi.org/10.1111/j.1538-7836.2009.03293.x.

31. Douketis J, Tosetto A, Marcucci M, et al. Patient-level meta-analysis: effect of measurement timing, threshold, and patient age on ability of D-dimer testing to assess recurrence risk after unprovoked venous thromboembolism. Ann Intern Med 2010;153(8):523–31. http://dx.doi.org/10.7326/0003-4819-153-8-201010190-00009.

32. Verhovsek M, Douketis JD, Yi Q, et al. Systematic review: D-dimer to predict recurrent disease after stopping anticoagulant therapy for unprovoked venous thromboembolism. Ann Intern Med 2008;149(7):481–90. W94. pii:149/7/481.

33. Gomez-Outes A, Lecumberri R, Lafuente-Guijosa A, et al. Correlation between thrombus regression and recurrent venous thromboembolism. examining venographic and clinical effects of low-molecular-weight heparins: a meta-analysis. J Thromb Haemost 2004;2(9):1581–7. http://dx.doi.org/10.1111/j.1538-7836.2004.00862.x.

34. Carrier M, Rodger MA, Wells PS, et al. Residual vein obstruction to predict the risk of recurrent venous thromboembolism in patients with deep vein thrombosis: a systematic review and meta-analysis. J Thromb Haemost 2011;9(6):1119–25. http://dx.doi.org/10.1111/j.1538-7836.2011.04254.x.

35. Tan M, Mos IC, Klok FA, et al. Residual venous thrombosis as predictive factor for recurrent venous thromboembolism in patients with proximal deep vein thrombosis: a systematic review. Br J Haematol 2011;153(2):168–78. http://dx.doi.org/10.1111/j.1365-2141.2011.08578.x.

36. Becattini C, Agnelli G, Schenone A, et al. Aspirin for preventing the recurrence of venous thromboembolism. N Engl J Med 2012;366(21):1959–67. http://dx.doi.org/10.1056/NEJMoa1114238.

37. Brighton TA, Eikelboom JW, Mann K, et al. Low-dose aspirin for preventing recurrent venous thromboembolism. N Engl J Med 2012;367(21):1979–87. http://dx.doi.org/10.1056/NEJMoa1210384.

38. Castellucci LA, Cameron C, Le Gal G, et al. Efficacy and safety outcomes of oral anticoagulants and antiplatelet drugs in the secondary prevention of venous thromboembolism: systematic review and network meta-analysis. BMJ 2013;347:f5133. http://dx.doi.org/10.1136/bmj.f5133.

39. PREPIC Study Group. Eight-year follow-up of patients with permanent vena cava filters in the prevention of pulmonary embolism: the PREPIC (Prevention du Risque d'Embolie Pulmonaire par Interruption Cave) Randomized Study. Circulation 2005;112(3):416–22. http://dx.doi.org/10.1161/CIRCULATIONAHA.104.512834.

40. Kucher N, Rossi E, De Rosa M, et al. Massive pulmonary embolism. Circulation 2006;113(4):577–82. http://dx.doi.org/10.1161/CIRCULATIONAHA.105.592592.

41. Stein PD, Matta F, Keyes DC, et al. Impact of vena cava filters on in-hospital case fatality rate from pulmonary embolism. Am J Med 2012;125(5):478–84. http://dx.doi.org/10.1016/j.amjmed.2011.05.025.

42. Removing retrievable inferior vena cava filters: initial communication. Available at: http://www.fda.gov/MedicalDevices/Safety/AlertsandNotices/ucm221676.htm. Accessed November 12, 2011.

43. Ko SH, Reynolds BR, Nicholas DH, et al. Institutional protocol improves retrievable inferior vena cava filter recovery rate. Surgery 2009;146(4):809–14. http://dx.doi.org/10.1016/j.surg.2009.06.022 [discussion: 814–6].

Renal Artery Stenosis

Jose David Tafur-Soto, MD*, Christopher J. White, MD, FSCAI, FESC

KEYWORDS

- Renal artery stenting • Renal fractional flow reserve • Renovascular hypertension
- Ischemic nephropathy • Flash pulmonary edema • Chronic kidney disease • Renal atherosclerosis

KEY POINTS

- Screening for renal artery stenosis can be done with Doppler ultrasonography, CT angiography, and magnetic resonance angiography.
- Patients with medically controlled renovascular hypertension should not undergo renal stenting, because there is no added benefit of revascularization.
- Patients with (1) uncontrolled renovascular hypertension having failed 3 maximally tolerated antihypertensive medications (one of which is a diuretic), (2) ischemic nephropathy, and (3) cardiac destabilization syndromes with hemodynamically severe renal artery stenosis are likely to benefit from renal artery stenting.
- Physiologic measurements, including fractional flow reserve with hyperemic/resting translesional gradients, may be performed to select patients who should undergo renal artery revascularization.
- Patients should have routine 30-day, 3-month, 6-month, 12-month, and annual clinical, laboratory, and imaging follow-up for surveillance of in-stent restenosis.

INTRODUCTION

Renal artery stenosis (RAS), the single largest cause of secondary hypertension affecting 25% to 35% of the patients with secondary hypertension,[1,2] is associated with progressive renal insufficiency and causes cardiovascular complications such as refractory heart failure and flash pulmonary edema.[3–5] An understanding of the underlying pathophysiologic mechanisms, clinical manifestations, and medical and interventional treatment strategies is paramount in optimizing the care of patients with RAS. A critical issue is the appropriate patient selection for interventional procedures.

CAUSE AND PREVALENCE

RAS is caused by a heterogeneous group of conditions, including atherosclerosis, fibromuscular dysplasia (FMD), vasculitides, neurofibromatosis, congenital bands, and extrinsic compression of the renal artery. Atherosclerosis accounts for approximately 90% of the flow-limiting lesions of the renal arteries.[6]

ARAS typically involves the ostium and proximal portion of the renal artery and is frequently in continuity with atherosclerotic disease in the abdominal aorta. Patients with RAS frequently have associated atherosclerosis of multiple vascular beds, including coronaries, carotids, and peripheral vessels. Screening renal duplex ultrasonography (DUS) studies demonstrated RAS (>60% stenosis) in 6.8% of subjects in a "healthy" Medicare population with a mean age of 77 years.[7] There were almost twice as many men (9.1%) as women (5.5%, $P = .053$), and there were no racial differences (Caucasian = 6.9% and African American = 6.7%) in the prevalence of RAS.

An autopsy series found RAS (≥50% stenosis) in 27% of patients older than 50 years, and in 53% of

Disclosures: J.D. Tafur-Soto has nothing to disclose. Research participation and sponsorship from St. Jude (C.J. White).
Department of Cardiology, Ochsner Clinic Foundation, 1514 Jefferson Highway, New Orleans, LA 70121, USA
* Corresponding author.
E-mail addresses: jtafursoto@ochsner.org; jdtafur@gmail.com

0733-8651/15/$ – see front matter © 2015 Elsevier Inc. All rights reserved.

those with a history of diastolic hypertension (>100 mm Hg).[8] RAS is the cause of end-stage renal disease (ESRD) in 10% to 15% of patients starting dialysis[9]; approximately 25% of elderly patients with renal insufficiency (creatinine >2.0 mg/dL) have undiagnosed RAS.[5] RAS is present in 30% to 40% of patients with peripheral artery disease or abdominal aortic aneurysm.[10]

PATHOPHYSIOLOGY OF RENAL HYPOPERFUSION

Several processes contribute to the pathophysiologic process of RAS.[11] Renal hypoperfusion is a strong stimulus for renal neurohormonal activation, resulting in renin and subsequent angiotensin II release. Renin-angiotensin-aldosterone system (RAAS) activation occurs with both unilateral and bilateral (or solitary) renal hypoperfusion.[12]

In unilateral RAS, the ischemic kidney secretes renin, which leads to increased angiotensin formation and, hence, elevated blood pressure. As blood pressure rises, sodium excretion by the contralateral normal kidney increases; therefore, there is no sodium retention or subsequent volume overload. This mechanism for the hypertensive hyponatremia syndrome is seen in unilateral RAS.[13]

With bilateral (or solitary) RAS, the lack of compensation from a normal kidney in terms of sodium excretion leads to fluid retention, loss of kidney function, and congestive heart failure (CHF).[14] Angiotensin is also a potent stimulator of reactive oxygen species (ROS) generation. ROS are direct vasoconstrictors and produce multiple vasoactive and fibrogenic factors, which contribute to hypertension and renal dysfunction.[15] Apoptosis, possibly induced by ROS, may also contribute to loss of vascular cells by promoting inflammation and tissue injury.

In patients with moderate RAS, despite reduced renal blood flow (RBF), cortical and medullary oxygenation is preserved because of compensatory mechanisms that decrease oxygen consumption. However, compensation for impaired RBF is limited in patients with severe RAS, which results in significant decreases in cortical oxygenation.[16]

CLINICAL SYNDROMES ASSOCIATED WITH RENAL HYPOPERFUSION

The main clinical syndromes associated with hemodynamically significant RAS include renovascular hypertension, ischemic nephropathy, and cardiac destabilization syndromes.

Renovascular Hypertension

Resistant hypertension is defined as blood pressure higher than goal on 3 different classes of antihypertensive medications, ideally including a diuretic drug.[17,18] Patients with resistant hypertension should be evaluated for secondary causes of hypertension. Studies of refractory hypertension commonly reveal a high prevalence of previously unrecognized renovascular disease, particularly in older patient groups. In patients older than 50 years of age who were referred to a hypertension center, 13% had a secondary cause of hypertension, the most common of which was renovascular disease.[19]

RAS is a common finding in hypertensive patients undergoing cardiac catheterization to assess coronary artery disease. In a population of veterans with hypertension referred for coronary angiography, greater than 20% of patients were found to have hemodynamically significant atherosclerotic RAS (ARAS) (>70%).[20]

Ischemic Nephropathy

RAS is a potentially reversible form of renal insufficiency. However, if unrecognized, it can lead to ESRD. Some studies suggest that as much as 11% to 14% of ESRD is attributable to chronic ischemic nephropathy from ARAS.[21] Favorable predictors of improved success with intervention include a rapid recent increase in serum creatinine concentration, decrease in glomerular filtration rate (GFR) during angiotensin-converting-enzyme (ACE) inhibitor or angiotensin II receptor blockers (ARB) treatment, absence of glomerular or interstitial fibrosis on kidney biopsy, and kidney pole-to-pole length greater than 8.0 cm.[22] In 73 patients with chronic renal failure (creatinine clearance >50 mL/min) and clinical evidence of renal vascular disease and a mean follow-up of 2 years, renal function improved in 34 of 59 patients (57.6%). The most important predictor of improvement was the slope of the reciprocal serum creatinine plot before revascularization, suggesting that rapidly progressive renal failure is associated with a more favorable response on renal failure progression after revascularization in patients with vascular nephropathy and RAS.[23]

Cardiac Destabilization Syndromes

Exacerbations of coronary ischemia and CHF caused by increased vasoconstriction and/or volume overload can be attributed to RAS. The most widely recognized example of a cardiac destabilization syndrome is "flash" pulmonary or Pickering syndrome.[3,24] Renovascular disease may also complicate the treatment of patients with heart failure by preventing the administration of angiotensin antagonist therapy.

The importance of renal artery revascularization in the treatment of cardiac disturbance syndromes has been described in a series of patients presenting with either CHF or an acute coronary syndrome.[5] Successful renal stent placement resulted in a significant decrease in blood pressure and symptom improvement in 88% (42 of 48) of patients. For those patients who presented with unstable angina, renal artery stenting improved the Canadian Class Society symptoms at least by one regardless of concomitant coronary intervention. In patients presenting with heart failure, the New York Heart Association (NYHA) class of symptoms improved by at least one also independent of coronary revascularization (**Fig. 1**). Among 207 patients with decompensated heart failure, 19% had severe RAS and underwent renal artery stenting with decreased frequency of CHF admissions, flash pulmonary edema NYHA class symptoms, and tolerance to ACE inhibitors (**Table 1**).[4]

DIAGNOSTIC STRATEGIES
Doppler Ultrasound Evaluation

Renal artery Doppler ultrasound, or DUS, is a noninvasive examination useful for screening for RAS. It carries a sensitivity of 84%, specificity of 97%, and positive predictive value of 94% for the detection of significant RAS.[25] The success of this technology is highly dependent on technical skill in performing the examination.

A peak-systolic velocity (PSV) greater than 180 cm/s has a 95% sensitivity and 90% specificity significant to RAS. When the ratio of the PSV of the stenosed renal artery to the PSV in the aorta is greater than 3.5, DUS predicts greater than 60% RAS with a 92% sensitivity.[26,27] DUS also allows follow-up of stent patency in patients who have undergone renal artery stenting;

however, criteria for native RAS overestimate the degree of angiographic in-stent restenosis (ISR). Surveillance monitoring for renal stent patency should take into account that PSV and renal/aortic velocity ratio (RAR) obtained by DUS are higher for any given degree of arterial narrowing within the stent. PSV greater than 395 cm/s or RAR greater than 5.1 was the most predictive of angiographically significant ISR greater than 70%.[28]

DUS can be performed without risk to the patient because there is no iodinated contrast or ionizing radiation required. The main limitations for DUS include unsatisfactory examinations due to

Table 1
Results of patients undergoing renal artery stenting for control of recurrent hospitalizations for heart failure and flash pulmonary edema

	Renal Artery Stenting (n = 39)		
	Pre	Post	P Value
Mean blood pressure (mm Hg)	174/85	148/72	<.001
Mean number of BP medications	3	2.5	.006
Mean creatinine (mg/dL)	3.16	2.65	.06
ACE inhibitor use	15.40%	48.70%	.004
CHF hospitalizations per year	2.4	0.3	<.001
NYHA class symptoms	2.9	1.6	<.001

Data from Gray BH, Olin JW, Childs MB, et al. Clinical benefit of renal artery angioplasty with stenting for the control of recurrent and refractory congestive heart failure. Vasc Med 2002;7:275–9.

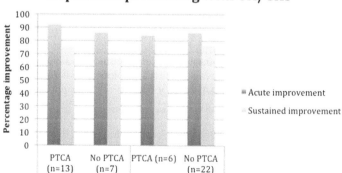

Symptoms after renal artery stenting in patients presenting with UA/CHF

- Acute improvement
- Sustained improvement

PTCA (n=13) / No PTCA (n=7) — Unstable angina (CCS)
PTCA (n=6) / No PTCA (n=22) — CHF (NYHA)

Fig. 1. Patients presenting with cardiac destabilization syndromes (acute coronary syndrome or CHF) and RAS benefited from renal artery revascularization independent of coronary intervention. CCS, Canadian Class Society; PTCA, percutaneous transluminal coronary angioplasty; UA, unstable angina. (*From* Khosla S, White CJ, Collins TJ, et al. Effects of renal artery stent implantation in patients with renovascular hypertension presenting with unstable angina or congestive heart failure. Am J Cardiol 1997;80:364; with permission.)

overlying bowel gas and large body habitus. There is a requirement for a capable sonographer who is allowed enough time to perform the examination.

The intrarenal resistive index (RI) is the ratio of the peak-systolic to end-diastolic velocity within the renal parenchyma at the level of the cortical blood vessels.[29] The RI is a representation of small-vessel glomerulosclerosis. There have been conflicting reports regarding the usefulness of RI to predict individual patient response to revascularization. One retrospective study demonstrated that an elevated resistance index greater than 0.80 predicted a lack of improvement in blood pressure and renal function after revascularization; however, it included balloon angioplasty without stent procedures, a strategy that is now recognized as less optimal compared with stenting (see later discussion).[30] A prospective study of renal stenting in 241 patients with an elevated RI (>0.70) showed improvement in blood pressure and renal function after intervention.[31] Patients with a higher RI (>0.8) actually benefitted more from revascularization than did those with milder elevations.

Computed Tomographic Angiography

CT angiography (CTA) can provide high-resolution cross-sectional imaging of RAS while supplying 3D angiographic images of the aorta, renal, and visceral arteries, which allows for localization and enumeration of the renal arteries, including accessory branches.[32] Sensitivity (59%–96%) and specificity (82%–99%) of CTA for detecting significant RAS compares well with invasive angiography.[33] CTA requires the administration of 100 to 150 mL of iodinated contrast and therefore carries the potential risk of contrast-induced nephropathy (CIN), especially in patients with estimated glomerular filtration rate (eGFR) less than 60 mL/1.73 m^2, diabetes mellitus, or anemia.[34,35] In addition, CTA requires the use of ionizing radiation. However, as CTA scanner technology advances, spatial resolution will improve, scanning time will decrease, the administered contrast load may be reduced, and the amount of radiation will be decreased.[36,37] In addition, iso-osmolar contrast media are now available with decreased potential for nephrotoxicity.[38] CTA allows for the detection of ISR in patients with prior stenting, which is an advantage over magnetic resonance angiography (MRA), in which metallic stents generate artifact.[33]

Magnetic Resonance Angiography

This imaging modality allows for localization and enumeration of the renal arteries and characterization of the stenosis. When compared with invasive angiography, it has sensitivity of 92% to 97% and specificity of 73% to 93% for the detection of RAS.[39,40] MRA does not require the use of ionizing radiation. Limitations for MRA include the association of gadolinium with nephrogenic systemic fibrosis when administered to patients with eGFR less than 30 mL/1.73 m^2 and that metal causes artifacts on MRA; therefore, it is not a useful test for patients with prior renal stents. Other patients who are not good candidates for MRA include those with claustrophobia or those with implanted medical devices (eg, artificial joints, permanent pacemakers).[41]

Captopril Renal Scans

Captopril renal scans (CRS) have been disappointing as screening tests. When evaluated in clinical practice, their sensitivity was 74% and specificity was 59%.[42] CRS are variable depending on the patient's medication use, hydration status, and underlying renal function. The American College of Cardiology/American Heart Association guidelines do not recommend the use of CRS for screening of RAS.[43] CRS may have a role in assessing the hemodynamic severity of a known stenosis, thereby providing physiologic information to guide revascularization decisions.

TREATMENT STRATEGIES
Medical Management of Renal Artery Stenosis

Medical management of atherosclerotic vascular disease involves blood pressure control, lipid-lowering therapy, an antiplatelet agent, and lifestyle advice, including dietary counseling, smoking cessation, and physical activity. Historically, the use of RAAS antagonists (ACE inhibitors or ARB) was contraindicated in this patient group owing to concerns of worsening renal function. Concerns with RAAS antagonists in this patient group are probably overstated, and observational studies have shown improved outcomes using this class of medication, perhaps because of interruption on many pathophysiologic processes described above. When used prospectively, RAAS antagonists were tolerated in 357 of 378 patients (92%), and this was even seen in 54 of 69 patients (78.3%) with bilateral RAS (>60%) or occlusion.[44] A subsequent observational study of 3750 patients with renovascular disease found that 53% were taking RAAS antagonists, and these patients had a significantly lower risk for the primary outcome (death, myocardial infarction, or stroke) (hazard ratio 0.70; 95% confidence interval [CI] 0.53–0.90).[45] The limitation of observational data is that it carries selection bias, and those able to tolerate RAAS antagonists may have less severe disease and could have better outcomes anyway. Patients who cannot tolerate medical therapy (MT) tend to have more extensive disease and are likely to benefit from revascularization.[46] Despite the lack of randomized trials, there is consensus that RAAS antagonists should be used in patients with RAS; however, they should be carefully monitored and introduced slowly.

Lipid-lowering therapy is widely accepted as one of the main treatments for all atherosclerotic vascular disease.[47] In a retrospective study, statin therapy was associated with a lower progression rate of renal insufficiency (7.4% vs 38.9%) and lower overall mortality (5.9% vs 36.1%; $P<.001$) for both with a mean follow-up of 11 years, suggesting the need for prospective, randomized controlled studies in renovascular disease patients to explore potential benefits of statins that may not be attributable solely to lipid lowering.[48]

The use of antiplatelet agents and smoking cessation in patients with RAS provide the same benefits that are seen in other forms of atherosclerotic disease, including peripheral and coronary artery disease. The recently published Cardiovascular Outcomes in Renal Atherosclerotic Lesions (CORAL) trial demonstrated the benefit of an initial strategy of MT versus MT plus renal artery stenting in patients with hypertension and RAS. All patients received, unless contraindicated, the angiotensin II type-1 receptor blocker, candesartan, with or without hydrochlorothiazide, and the combination agent, amlodipine–atorvastatin, with the dose adjusted on the basis of blood pressure and lipid status.[49]

Renal Artery Surgery

Surgical repair of RAS was the only available revascularization option before renal artery angioplasty. In an observational series of 500 patients with RAS and hypertension, managed with surgical revascularization and followed for up to 10 years, 12% of patients were cured of their hypertension and 73% were improved. Importantly, 30-day mortality ranged from 4.6% to 7.3%. Complications of surgery include surgical infections, such as surgery-related bleeding, urinary tract infection, and pseudomembranous colitis among others. Today, percutaneous, catheter-based therapy has largely replaced surgical renal revascularization for RAS because of the increased morbidity and mortality associated with surgery.[50,51]

Percutaneous Renal Artery Revascularization

Renal artery stenting is a reasonable option for patients with hemodynamically significant RAS (>70% angiographic diameter RAS or 50%–70% stenosis with a significant translesional gradient) and (1) resistant or uncontrolled hypertension and the failure of 3 antihypertensive drugs, one of which is a diuretic agent, or hypertension with intolerance to medication; (2) ischemic nephropathy; and (3) cardiac destabilization syndromes (**Table 2**).

Table 2
Management of patients with peripheral arterial disease

		Class	LOE
Asymptomatic stenosis	Solitary viable kidney with hemodynamically significant RAS	IIb	C
	Bilateral hemodynamically significant RAS	IIb	C
Hypertension	RAS and accelerated, resistant, or malignant hypertension	IIa	B
	RAS and hypertension with unilateral small kidney	IIa	B
	RAS and hypertension with medication intolerance	IIa	B
Preservation of renal function	Progressive CKD with bilateral RAS	IIa	B
	Progressive CKD with RAS to a solitary functioning kidney	IIa	B
	RAS and chronic renal insufficiency with unilateral RAS	IIb	C
CHF	RAS with recurrent, unexplained CHF or sudden, unexplained pulmonary edema	I	B
Unstable angina	Hemodynamically significant RAS and medically refractory unstable angina or recurrent heart failure	IIa	B

Abbreviation: LOE, level of evidence.

Data from Hirsch AT, Haskal ZJ, Hertzer NR, et al. ACC/AHA 2005 guidelines for the management of patients with peripheral arterial disease (lower extremity, renal, mesenteric, and abdominal aortic): executive summary a collaborative report from the American Association for Vascular Surgery/Society for Vascular Surgery, Society for Cardiovascular Angiography and Interventions, Society for Vascular Medicine and Biology, Society of Interventional Radiology, and the ACC/AHA Task Force on Practice Guidelines (Writing Committee to Develop Guidelines for the Management of Patients With Peripheral Arterial Disease) endorsed by the American Association of Cardiovascular and Pulmonary Rehabilitation; National Heart, Lung, and Blood Institute; Society for Vascular Nursing; TransAtlantic Inter-Society Consensus; and Vascular Disease Foundation. J Am Coll Cardiol 2006;47:1239–312.

Despite excellent angiographic outcomes achieved with renal stenting, there is a mismatch between angiographic (>97%) and clinical (~70%) success for controlling hypertension and renal dysfunction. Technically, renal artery stent placement is highly successful and safe. In a meta-analysis of 14 studies (678 patients) evaluating renal artery stenting for either hypertension or chronic kidney disease (CKD), the angiographic success rate was 98% (95% CI 95%–100%).[52] However, the clinical response rate for hypertension was only 69%, with a cure rate of 20%, and improvement in blood pressure in 49% (**Fig. 2**A). Renal function improved in 30% and stabilized in 38% of patients with an overall favorable response rate of 68% (see **Fig. 2**B).[52] The mismatch between angiographic success and clinical response may be explained by (1) the treatment of nonobstructive RAS lesions (visually overestimating the stenosis severity), or (2) symptoms (hypertension or CKD) that were not caused by RAS. The key to successful clinical outcomes is to identify which patients are likely to benefit from intervention.

Several recent randomized clinical trials have attempted to determine the clinical benefit of renal artery stenting. The STAR and ASTRAL trials have been flawed by poor design and the inability to assess RAS severity objectively. They have failed to select patients with hemodynamically significant RAS lesions that cause renal hypoperfusion and have failed to include operators with significant interventional experience.[53,54]

The recently published CORAL trial studied the optimal *initial* therapy for patients with 60% or more RAS and hypertension (systolic blood pressure >155 with ≥2 antihypertensive medications) or CKD (eGFR <60 mL/min/1.73 m^2). No hemodynamic measurements of lesion severity were performed. The CORAL study found that death from cardiovascular or renal causes, myocardial infarction, stroke, hospitalization for CHF, progressive renal insufficiency, or the need for dialysis in patients with ARAS (>60% diameter stenosis) and hypertension did not differ between groups treated with multifactorial MT alone compared with multifactorial MT plus renal stenting as an initial strategy.

The number of blood pressure medications in the group assigned to MT alone increased from baseline at 2.1 to 3.5 (similar to the stent group at 3.3), which demonstrated that these patients *did not* have resistant hypertension. Both groups had similar decreases in systolic blood pressure, 15.6 ± 25.8 mm Hg in the MT group and 16.6 ± 21.2 mm Hg in the stent group, which implies that patients had not actually failed 3-drug antihypertensive MT.[49] A major limitation of the CORAL study was the inability to identify hemodynamically severe RAS for treatment; this is particularly relevant for the moderate lesions (mean 67% diameter stenosis) studied in the CORAL study. Without measuring the hemodynamic severity of the RAS, one cannot discriminate between patients with true renovascular hypertension and those with RAS and essential hypertension.[55–57]

SELECTING PATIENTS LIKELY TO BENEFIT FROM REVASCULARIZATION

With a mismatch between technical and clinical response after renal revascularization, the question is how to select those patients who will most likely benefit from stenting. The "Achilles heel" of renal artery revascularization is that angiography is a very uncertain and unreliable best option for determining the hemodynamic severity of moderate RAS. When a single operator performed visual estimation of angiographic diameter stenosis in patients with moderate RAS (50%–90% diameter stenosis), the correlation was

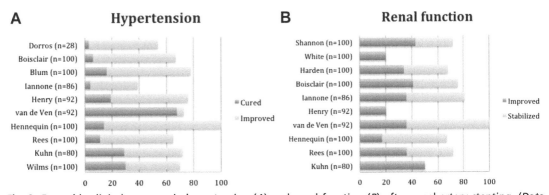

Fig. 2. Favorable clinical response in hypertension (*A*) and renal function (*B*) after renal artery stenting. (*Data from* Leertouwer TC, Gussenhoven EJ, Bosch JL, et al. Stent placement for renal arterial stenosis: where do we stand? A meta-analysis. Radiology 2000;216(1):78–85.)

poor between the angiographic diameter stenosis and resting mean translesional pressure gradient ($r = 0.43$; $P = .12$), hyperemic mean translesional pressure gradient ($r = 0.22$; $P = .44$), and renal fractional flow reserve (FFR) ($r = 0.18$; $P = .54$) (**Fig. 3**).[58] Therefore, physiologic assessment should always be performed in patients with moderate RAS lesions.

Translesional Pressure Gradients

A translesional systolic pressure gradient greater than 20 mm Hg, as well as a translesional resting pressure ratio of 0.90 (pressure distal to the stenosis/pressure proximal to the stenosis [P_d/P_a] less than 0.90), correlates with a significant increase in renin concentration in the ipsilateral renal vein.[59,60] Several series have shown improved blood pressure response when treating lesions with resting or hyperemic pressure gradients greater than 20 mm Hg.[56,57] Based on these observations, an expert consensus panel recommended that a peak-systolic gradient of at least 20 mm Hg, or a mean pressure gradient of 10 mm Hg, be used to confirm the severity of lesions less than or equal to 70% diameter stenosis in symptomatic patients with RAS.[61] Because the catheter itself can introduce an artificial gradient,[62] measurements should be done with either a 4-Fr or smaller catheter or a 0.014″ pressure wire.[63]

Renal Artery Fractional Flow Reserve

Another method to determine the severity of angiographic RAS is to quantify the FFR. This hemodynamic assessment of flow, which is widely used in the coronary circulation, is based on the principle that flow across a conduit artery is proportional to pressure across the vascular bed and is inversely proportional to the resistance of the vascular bed. Under conditions of maximum hyperemia, the flow through the conduit artery is maximal, while the resistance of the vascular bed is at a minimum and constant. Any reduction in flow under these conditions is caused by the stenosis and is proportional to the ratio of P_d and P_a.

FFR is measured after induction of maximum hyperemia. Renal hyperemia can be achieved with papaverine,[58,60] dopamine,[56] or acetylcholine (**Table 3**).[64] Translesional pressure gradients are measured, and FFR (P_d/P_a) is calculated using a 0.014-inch pressure guidewire. Renal artery FFR correlates well with other hemodynamic parameters of lesion severity[60,65] (**Fig. 4**) and in some series has been proven to be a better predictor of clinical response. In one study, renal FFR was measured after renal stent placement in 17 patients with refractory hypertension and moderate to severe (50%–90% stenosis), unilateral RAS. Ten patients had normal baseline renal FFR (FFR ≥ 0.80), whereas an abnormal baseline renal FFR (<0.80) was recorded in 7 patients. At 3 months after intervention, 86% of patients with an abnormal renal FFR experienced improvement in their blood pressure, compared with only 30% of those with normal renal FFR ($P = .04$) (**Fig. 5**). In this small series, baseline systolic, mean, or hyperemic translesional pressure gradients were not different between patients whose blood pressure improved and those in whom it did not.[55]

Renal Frame Count

In the coronary vasculature, the Thrombolysis in Myocardial Infarction (TIMI) frame count is a quantitative angiographic assessment of coronary blood flow that correlates with clinical outcomes.[66–69] The renal frame count (RFC) has been proposed as an alternative angiographic method to assess renal perfusion. RFC is the number of cine frames required for the contrast to reach the smallest visible distal branch in the renal parenchyma (**Fig. 6**). As in TIMI frame counting,

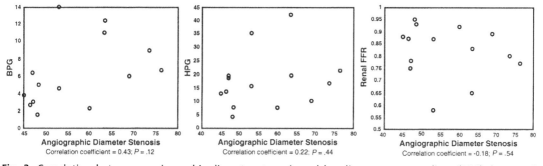

Fig. 3. Correlation between angiographic diameter stenosis and baseline pressure gradient (BPG), hyperemic pressure gradient (HPG), and renal FFR. (*From* Subramanian R, White CJ, Rosenfield K, et al. Renal fractional flow reserve: a hemodynamic evaluation of moderate renal artery stenoses. Catheter Cardiovasc Interv 2005;64:484; with permission.)

Table 3
Common agents used to induce renal hyperemia

Agent	Dose	Maximum Dose	Drug Considerations
Papaverine	32 mg	40 mg	Hypotension, crystallization with heparin
Acetylcholine	100 ug	1000 ug	Hypotension, tachyarrhythmias
Dopamine	50 ug/kg	—	Tachyarrhythmias

the first frame used for the RFC is the frame in which the contrast first fills the main renal artery. The last frame is when contrast enters the smallest visible branch of the distal renal parenchyma along the axis of the main renal artery. The measurements are done with angiography at 30 frames per second. RFC was initially described in patients with FMD of the renal arteries (15 kidneys), who were compared with subjects with normal renal arteries (50 kidneys) and had a significantly higher (prolonged) mean RFC (26.9 vs 20.4 $P = .0001$).[70] In a prospective series of 24 patients with uncontrolled hypertension who underwent renal artery stenting, reduction in RFC after stenting was associated with blood pressure reduction and greater than 4 RFC reduction after stenting predicted blood pressure reduction in 78% of subjects.[71]

Serum Biomarkers

Brain natriuretic peptide (BNP) is a neurohormone released from the ventricular myocardium in conditions that cause myocardial cell stretching, like CHF and pulmonary embolism.[72] BNP has been shown to directly correlate with pulmonary capillary wedge pressure.[73] In vitro studies have also shown that angiotensin II induces the synthesis and release of BNP, and in rats it has been found that BNP mRNA is upregulated 6 hours after clipping of the renal artery.[74]

In a series of 27 patients with significant RAS (>70% diameter stenosis) and uncontrolled hypertension, excluding patients with CHF, recent myocardial infarction, and chronic renal insufficiency (Cr $\geq$2), it was found that a baseline BNP greater than 80 and a BNP decreased by at least 30% had a significant correlation with clinical improvement in blood pressure. However, in the safety and efficacy of the RX HERCULink Elite renal Stent system trial, a single-arm, multicenter trial that included 202 patients with RAS and uncontrolled hypertension, BNP levels did not correlate with clinical improvement in blood pressure.[75] The usefulness of BNP as a predictor of good clinical outcome needs to be confirmed in a larger cohort of patients.

TECHNICAL ASPECTS OF REVASCULARIZATION

There are several important technical and procedural considerations to prevent complications during renal stenting. Selective renal angiography should be preceded by nonselective abdominal aortography. The catheter-in-catheter or no-touch techniques should be used to minimize contact with the aortic wall and injury to the renal

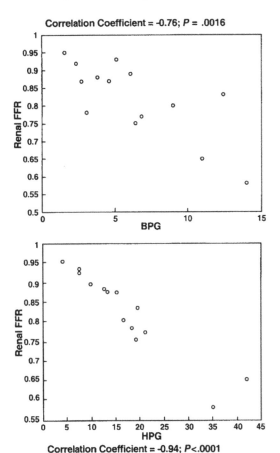

Fig. 4. Correlation between FFR and baseline pressure gradient (BPG) (*top*) and hyperemic pressure gradient (HPG) (*bottom*). (*From* Subramanian R, White CJ, Rosenfield K, et al. Renal fractional flow reserve: a hemodynamic evaluation of moderate renal artery stenoses. Catheter Cardiovasc Interv 2005;64:484; with permission.)

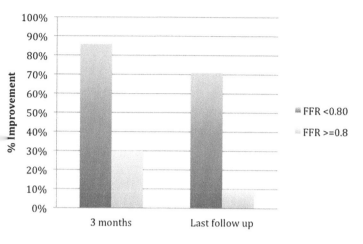

Fig. 5. Blood pressure improvement at follow-up stratified by baseline renal FFR (<0.8 vs ≥0.80). (*From* Mitchell JA, Subramanian R, White CJ, et al. Predicting blood pressure improvement in hypertensive patients after renal artery stent placement: renal fractional flow reserve. Catheter Cardiovasc Interv 2007;69:688; with permission.)

ostium during guiding catheter engagement (see later discussion). Aggressive hydration and limiting contrast volume are helpful to prevent the development of CIN.

Radial access, when compared with femoral access, is increasingly used to perform percutaneous diagnostic and interventional coronary procedures to reduce access site bleeding complications and improve postprocedural patient comfort. The Acute Candesartan Cilexetil Therapy in Stroke Survivors (ACCESS) study (n = 900) showed access site related bleeding complications of 2.3% in the brachial group, 2.3% in the femoral group, and 0% in the radial group (P = .035).[76]

The radial approach for renal stenting represents a valuable tool to reduce access site complications and to improve a patient's comfort. However, the operator needs specific technical skills as well as knowledge of device compatibility. Both radial arteries are suitable for renal intervention (**Fig. 7**). Depending on the configuration of the aortic arch, the left radial approach allows a shorter distance to the renal arteries. The right radial approach is more comfortable for the operator and there is less radiation exposure. The use of 125-cm-long catheters is appropriate for almost all patients, whereas the 100-cm-long catheters may not reach the renal arteries in taller patients or in patients with excessive aortic arch tortuosity.[77]

Embolic Protection Devices

Atheroembolism has been associated with an increase in morbidity and a dramatic reduction in 5-year survival compared with patients who had no evidence on biopsy of renal atheroembolization

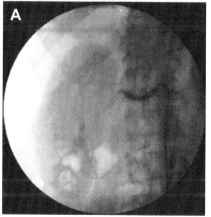
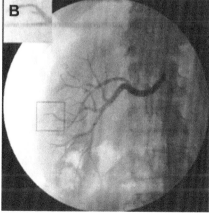

Fig. 6. (*A*) First frame, a column of contrast extending the entire width of the main renal artery with antegrade flow. (*B*) Last frame, contrast filling the smallest visible branch in the distal renal parenchyma. (*From* Mulumudi MS, White CJ. Renal frame count: a quantitative angiographic assessment of renal perfusion. Catheter Cardiovasc Interv 2005;65:184; with permission.)

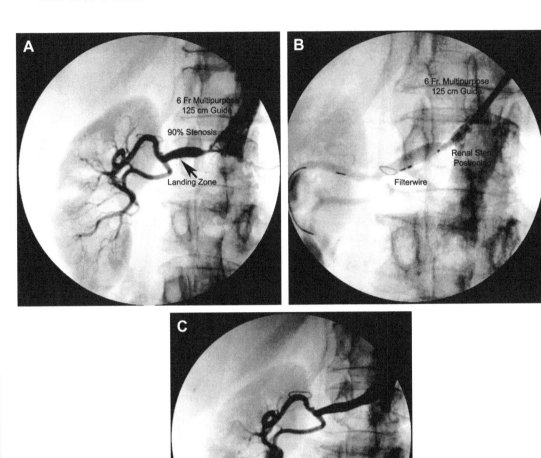

Fig. 7. (*A*) Right radial artery access using a 6-Fr multipurpose (125 cm) guide catheter. Note the landing zone before the bifurcation, suitable for a filter device (off-label use). (*B*) The filter device has been deployed, and the undeployed stent is being positioned across the lesion. (*C*) Final angiography after stent deployment and filter retrieval. (*From* White CJ. Optimizing outcomes for renal artery intervention. Circ Cardiovasc Interv 2010;3(2):189; with permission).

(54% vs 85%, $P = .011$).[78] Because atheroembolism is a potential complication of renal artery stenting, investigators have looked to embolic protection devices (EPD) to optimize outcomes after renal intervention. However, distal protection may be technically difficult if there is early bifurcation of the renal arteries. A randomized controlled study of 100 patients undergoing renal artery stenting was assigned to an open-label EPD or use of abciximab in a 2 × 2 factorial design. A positive interaction was observed between treatment with abciximab and embolic protection. Renal artery stenting alone, stenting with an EPD, and stenting with abciximab were associated with

similar and modest declines in eGFR at 1-month follow-up (-10, -12, -10 mL/min/1.73 m^2 eGFR change, respectively); however, the group treated with both EPD and abciximab was protected from a decline in eGFR and was superior to the other 3 groups ($+9$ mL/min/1.73 m^2 eGFR change, $P<.01$).[79]

In an uncontrolled, retrospective trial, RFC was measured in 66 patients undergoing renal artery intervention with and without EPD. EPD use was associated with improved RBF measured by RFC compared with the control group following RAS (mean reduction in RFC of 14.2 vs 6.7 $P = .03$).[80] EPDs may be effective in preventing renal atheroembolic injury, and a controlled trial measuring the impact of EPDs on RBF following RAS should be performed.

Stent Sizing with Intravascular Ultrasound

As described above, intravascular ultrasound (IVUS) can provide anatomic characterization of the atherosclerotic plaque. Twenty-two patients with ARAS were studied with IVUS after predilation and after angiographically successful stent deployment (diameter stenosis <10%). Modification based on IVUS, including selection of a larger balloon, additional dilation, and placement of a second stent, occurred in 5 patients after predilatation and in one patient after stent deployment. Mean blood pressure and amount of antihypertensive drugs decreased ($P<.05$); therefore, IVUS monitoring during renal artery stent placement resulted in additional lumen enlargement not considered necessary at angiography.[81] In a series of 363 renal artery interventions, follow-up angiography was available in 102 patients (34%) at an average of 303 days. Larger-diameter arteries were associated with a significantly lower incidence of angiographic restenosis. The restenosis rate was 36% for vessels with a reference diameter less than 4.5 mm compared with 16% in vessels with reference diameters of 4.5 to 6 mm ($P = .068$) and 6.5% in vessels with reference diameter greater than 6 mm ($P<.01$).[82] IVUS allows a more accurate way to measure vessel diameter than 2D angiography does, which allows the operator to safely maximize the stent size. Visual estimation tends to underestimate the size of the vessel, which can translate into higher rates of ISR.

Drug-eluting Stent Versus Bare Metal Stent

Restenosis after stent angioplasty of ARAS is a limitation, especially in small-diameter renal arteries. Two meta-analyses of renal artery intervention with bare metal stent (BMS) have demonstrated average restenosis rates after stent placement of 16% and 17%.[52,83] More recent reports suggest that with optimal deployment techniques, restenosis rates of less than 11% can be achieved when followed for to 60 months.[84,85]

The Palmaz Genesis Peripheral Stainless Steel Balloon Expandable Stent, comparing a Sirolimus Coated with an Uncoated Stent in REnal Artery Treatment (GREAT), study[86] was a prospective, multicenter study of angiographic patency of renal artery stents placed in 105 patients with ARAS. The restenosis rate was determined as binary restenosis with a cutoff point at 50% diameter stenosis. The binary restenosis rate was

6.7% with sirolimus-eluting stents (SES) versus 14.6% with BMS ($P = .30$). After 6 months and 1 year, target lesion revascularization (TLR) rates were 7.7% and 11.5%, respectively, in the BMS group versus 1.9% at both time points in the SES group ($P = .21$). This rate remained stable up to 2 years of follow-up but did not reach significance because of the small sample size. TLR was performed in 8% of the patients in the BMS group and in 2% of the drug-eluting stent (DES) group. At 1-year follow-up, the clinical patency was 88.5% in the BMS group and 98.1% in the DES group ($P = .21$). In one study of renal artery stenting, vessels with a diameter less than 4.5 mm had a restenosis rate of 36%, compared with a 6.5% rate of restenosis in vessels with diameters greater than 6 mm.[82]

The use of covered stents in the renal arteries has been reported in the management of complications, including perforation.[87] Polytetrafluoroethylene-covered stents may offer a way to treat recurrent RAS. In case reports, the covered stents remained free of any significant neointimal tissue or obstruction after used for recurrent ISR management.[88,89] Their safety is currently being evaluated in clinical trials.

Restenotic Lesions

The durability of renal artery interventions is limited by the development of ISR and the need for secondary or tertiary renal interventions. Two meta-analyses of renal artery intervention have demonstrated mean restenosis rates after stent placement of 16% and 17% at 2- and 5-years follow-up, respectively.[52,83] Renal stents have excellent long-term patency rates, with cumulative primary patency of 79% to 85% and a secondary patency of 92% to 98% at 5 years.[84,85] A larger reference vessel diameter (RVD) and larger acute gain (poststent minimal lumen diameter) after stent deployment are associated with a lower incidence of restenosis. The restenosis rate for smaller renal arteries (RVD $\leq$4.5 mm) was 36% compared with a restenosis rate of 6.5% for larger renal arteries (RVD >6.0 mm).[82]

The optimal treatment of renal artery ISR is uncertain. An initial report including 20 renal arteries in 15 patients found that, at a mean follow-up of 11 months, the restenosis rate for percutaneous transluminal angioplasty treatment of ISR was 25%. Renal function remained stable or improved in 80%, and hypertension was classified as improved or cured in 47%.[90] There are no reports of efficacy in treating ISR with cutting balloons[88,91] or brachytherapy.[92]

FOLLOW-UP AND NATURAL HISTORY

Patients should be followed clinically in terms of blood pressure control with laboratory results to monitor renal function, and surveillance DUS imaging is recommended to evaluate stent patency. DUS is the recommended imaging technique to screen for ISR. DUS surveillance monitoring for renal stent patency should take into account that a stented artery is less compliant than a native artery and that PSV and RAR obtained by DUS are higher for any given degree of arterial narrowing within the stent[28]; therefore, obtaining a postprocedure DUS is reasonable to establish a new baseline PSV. Patients should have routine 30-day, 3-month, 6-month, 12-month, and annual clinical, laboratory, and DUS follow-up for surveillance of ISR.[93]

CURRENT INDICATIONS FOR RENAL ARTERY STENTING
Renovascular Hypertension

Percutaneous revascularization is reasonable for patients with hemodynamically significant RAS and accelerated hypertension, resistant hypertension, malignant hypertension, hypertension with an unexplained unilateral small kidney, and hypertension with intolerance to medication (Class IIa Level of Evidence: B).[43]

Ischemic nephropathy
a. Percutaneous revascularization is reasonable for patients with RAS and progressive CKD with bilateral RAS or a RAS to a solitary functioning kidney (Class IIa Level of Evidence: B).
b. Percutaneous revascularization may be considered for patients with RAS and chronic renal insufficiency with unilateral RAS (Class IIb Level of Evidence: C).

Cardiac destabilization syndromes
c. Percutaneous revascularization is indicated for patients with hemodynamically significant RAS and recurrent, unexplained CHF or sudden, unexplained pulmonary edema (Class I Level of Evidence: B).
d. Percutaneous revascularization is reasonable for patients with hemodynamically significant RAS and unstable angina (Class IIa Level of Evidence: B).

REFERENCES

1. Benjamin MM, Fazel P, Filardo G, et al. Prevalence of and risk factors of renal artery stenosis in patients with resistant hypertension. Am J Cardiol 2014; 113:687–90.

2. Crowley JJ, Santos RM, Peter RH, et al. Progression of renal artery stenosis in patients undergoing cardiac catheterization. Am Heart J 1998;136:913–8.

3. Messerli FH, Bangalore S, Makani H, et al. Flash pulmonary oedema and bilateral renal artery stenosis: the Pickering syndrome. Eur Heart J 2011;32:2231–5.

4. Gray BH, Olin JW, Childs MB, et al. Clinical benefit of renal artery angioplasty with stenting for the control of recurrent and refractory congestive heart failure. Vasc Med 2002;7:275–9.

5. Khosla S, White CJ, Collins TJ, et al. Effects of renal artery stent implantation in patients with renovascular hypertension presenting with unstable angina or congestive heart failure. Am J Cardiol 1997;80: 363–6.

6. Tynes WV 2nd. Unusual renovascular disorders. Urol Clin North Am 1984;11:529–42.

7. Hansen KJ, Edwards MS, Craven TE, et al. Prevalence of renovascular disease in the elderly: a population-based study. J Vasc Surg 2002;36:443–51.

8. Holley KE, Hunt JC, Brown AL Jr, et al. Renal artery stenosis. A clinical-pathologic study in normotensive and hypertensive patients. Am J Med 1964;37:14–22.

9. Guo H, Kalra PA, Gilbertson DT, et al. Atherosclerotic renovascular disease in older US patients starting dialysis, 1996 to 2001. Circulation 2007;115:50–8.

10. Olin JW, Melia M, Young JR, et al. Prevalence of atherosclerotic renal artery stenosis in patients with atherosclerosis elsewhere. Am J Med 1990;88: 46N–51N.

11. Eirin A, Lerman LO. Darkness at the end of the tunnel: poststenotic kidney injury. Physiology (Bethesda) 2013;28:245–53.

12. Agarwal M, Lynn KL, Richards AM, et al. Hyponatremic-hypertensive syndrome with renal ischemia: an underrecognized disorder. Hypertension 1999;33: 1020–4.

13. Pickering TG. Renovascular hypertension: etiology and pathophysiology. Semin Nucl Med 1989;19: 79–88.

14. Textor SC, Lerman L. Renovascular hypertension and ischemic nephropathy. Am J Hypertens 2010; 23:1159–69.

15. Zhu XY, Chade AR, Rodriguez-Porcel M, et al. Cortical microvascular remodeling in the stenotic kidney: role of increased oxidative stress. Arterioscler Thromb Vasc Biol 2004;24:1854–9.

16. Gloviczki ML, Glockner JF, Lerman LO, et al. Preserved oxygenation despite reduced blood flow in poststenotic kidneys in human atherosclerotic renal artery stenosis. Hypertension 2010;55:961–6.

17. Pimenta E, Calhoun DA. Resistant hypertension: incidence, prevalence, and prognosis. Circulation 2012;125:1594–6.

18. Calhoun DA, Jones D, Textor S, et al. Resistant hypertension: diagnosis, evaluation, and treatment: a scientific statement from the American Heart

Association Professional Education Committee of the Council for High Blood Pressure Research. Circulation 2008;117:e510–26.

19. Anderson GH Jr, Blakeman N, Streeten DH. The effect of age on prevalence of secondary forms of hypertension in 4429 consecutively referred patients. J Hypertens 1994;12:609–15.

20. Aqel RA, Zoghbi GJ, Baldwin SA, et al. Prevalence of renal artery stenosis in high-risk veterans referred to cardiac catheterization. J Hypertens 2003;21:1157–62.

21. Preston RA, Epstein M. Ischemic renal disease: an emerging cause of chronic renal failure and end-stage renal disease. J Hypertens 1997;15:1365–77.

22. Garovic VD, Textor SC. Renovascular hypertension and ischemic nephropathy. Circulation 2005;112:1362–74.

23. Muray S, Martin M, Amoedo ML, et al. Rapid decline in renal function reflects reversibility and predicts the outcome after angioplasty in renal artery stenosis. Am J Kidney Dis 2002;39:60–6.

24. Messerli FH, Bangalore S. The Pickering Syndrome–a pebble in the mosaic of the cardiorenal syndrome. Blood Press 2011;20:1–2.

25. Taylor DC, Kettler MD, Moneta GL, et al. Duplex ultrasound scanning in the diagnosis of renal artery stenosis: a prospective evaluation. J Vasc Surg 1988;7:363–9.

26. Strandness DE Jr. Duplex imaging for the detection of renal artery stenosis. Am J Kidney Dis 1994;24:674–8.

27. Olin JW, Piedmonte MR, Young JR, et al. The utility of duplex ultrasound scanning of the renal arteries for diagnosing significant renal artery stenosis. Ann Intern Med 1995;122:833–8.

28. Chi YW, White CJ, Thornton S, et al. Ultrasound velocity criteria for renal in-stent restenosis. J Vasc Surg 2009;50:119–23.

29. Radermacher J. Ultrasonography of the kidney and renal vessels. I. Normal findings, inherited and parenchymal diseases. Urologe A 2005;44:1351–63 [quiz: 1364]. [in German].

30. Radermacher J, Chavan A, Bleck J, et al. Use of Doppler ultrasonography to predict the outcome of therapy for renal-artery stenosis. N Engl J Med 2001;344:410–7.

31. Zeller T, Muller C, Frank U, et al. Stent angioplasty of severe atherosclerotic ostial renal artery stenosis in patients with diabetes mellitus and nephrosclerosis. Catheter Cardiovasc Interv 2003;58:510–5.

32. Kawashima A, Sandler CM, Ernst RD, et al. CT evaluation of renovascular disease. Radiographics 2000;20:1321–40.

33. Kim TS, Chung JW, Park JH, et al. Renal artery evaluation: comparison of spiral CT angiography to intra-arterial DSA. J Vasc Interv Radiol 1998;9:553–9.

34. McCullough PA, Adam A, Becker CR, et al. Risk prediction of contrast-induced nephropathy. Am J Cardiol 2006;98:27K–36K.

35. McCullough PA, Adam A, Becker CR, et al. Epidemiology and prognostic implications of contrast-induced nephropathy. Am J Cardiol 2006;98:5K–13K.

36. Cho ES, Yu JS, Ahn JH, et al. CT angiography of the renal arteries: comparison of lower-tube-voltage CTA with moderate-concentration iodinated contrast material and conventional CTA. AJR Am J Roentgenol 2012;199:96–102.

37. Lufft V, Hoogestraat-Lufft L, Fels LM, et al. Contrast media nephropathy: intravenous CT angiography versus intraarterial digital subtraction angiography in renal artery stenosis: a prospective randomized trial. Am J Kidney Dis 2002;40:236–42.

38. Davenport MS, Khalatbari S, Cohan RH, et al. Contrast material-induced nephrotoxicity and intravenous low-osmolality iodinated contrast material: risk stratification by using estimated glomerular filtration rate. Radiology 2013;268:719–28.

39. Turgutalp K, Kiykim A, Ozhan O, et al. Comparison of diagnostic accuracy of Doppler USG and contrast-enhanced magnetic resonance angiography and selective renal arteriography in patients with atherosclerotic renal artery stenosis. Med Sci Monit 2013;19:475–82.

40. Tan KT, van Beek EJ, Brown PW, et al. Magnetic resonance angiography for the diagnosis of renal artery stenosis: a meta-analysis. Clin Radiol 2002;57:617–24.

41. Dellegrottaglie S, Sanz J, Rajagopalan S. Technology insight: clinical role of magnetic resonance angiography in the diagnosis and management of renal artery stenosis. Nat Clin Pract Cardiovasc Med 2006;3:329–38.

42. Huot SJ, Hansson JH, Dey H, et al. Utility of captopril renal scans for detecting renal artery stenosis. Arch Intern Med 2002;162:1981–4.

43. Hirsch AT, Haskal ZJ, Hertzer NR, et al. ACC/AHA guidelines for the management of patients with peripheral arterial disease (lower extremity, renal, mesenteric, and abdominal aortic): a collaborative report from the American Associations for Vascular Surgery/Society for Vascular Surgery, Society for Cardiovascular Angiography and Interventions, Society for Vascular Medicine and Biology, Society of Interventional Radiology, and the ACC/AHA Task Force on Practice Guidelines (writing committee to develop guidelines for the management of patients with peripheral arterial disease)–summary of recommendations. J Vasc Interv Radiol 2006;17:1383–97 [quiz: 1398].

44. Chrysochou C, Foley RN, Young JF, et al. Dispelling the myth: the use of renin-angiotensin blockade in atheromatous renovascular disease. Nephrol Dial Transplant 2012;27:1403–9.

45. Hackam DG, Duong-Hua ML, Mamdani M, et al. Angiotensin inhibition in renovascular disease: a population-based cohort study. Am Heart J 2008; 156:549–55.

46. Hirsch AT, Haskal ZJ, Hertzer NR, et al. ACC/AHA 2005 guidelines for the management of patients with peripheral arterial disease (lower extremity, renal, mesenteric, and abdominal aortic): executive summary a collaborative report from the American Association for Vascular Surgery/Society for Vascular Surgery, Society for Cardiovascular Angiography and Interventions, Society for Vascular Medicine and Biology, Society of Interventional Radiology, and the ACC/AHA Task Force on Practice Guidelines (Writing Committee to Develop Guidelines for the Management of Patients with Peripheral Arterial Disease) endorsed by the American Association of Cardiovascular and Pulmonary Rehabilitation; National Heart, Lung, and Blood Institute; Society for Vascular Nursing; TransAtlantic Inter-Society Consensus; and Vascular Disease Foundation. J Am Coll Cardiol 2006;47:1239–312.

47. Stone NJ, Robinson JG, Lichtenstein AH, et al. 2013 ACC/AHA guideline on the treatment of blood cholesterol to reduce atherosclerotic cardiovascular risk in adults: a report of the American College of Cardiology/American Heart Association Task Force on Practice Guidelines. Circulation 2014;129:S1–45.

48. Silva VS, Martin LC, Franco RJ, et al. Pleiotropic effects of statins may improve outcomes in atherosclerotic renovascular disease. Am J Hypertens 2008; 21:1163–8.

49. Cooper CJ, Murphy TP, Cutlip DE, et al. Stenting and medical therapy for atherosclerotic renal-artery stenosis. N Engl J Med 2014;370:13–22.

50. Libertino JA, Beckmann CF. Surgery and percutaneous angioplasty in the management of renovascular hypertension. Urol Clin North Am 1994;21: 235–43.

51. Zinman LN, Libertino JA. Surgery of the renal artery: hepato and spleno renal bypass. J Mal Vasc 1994; 19(Suppl A):96–101.

52. Leertouwer TC, Gussenhoven EJ, Bosch JL, et al. Stent placement for renal arterial stenosis: where do we stand? A meta-analysis. Radiology 2000;216:78–85.

53. Investigators A, Wheatley K, Ives N, et al. Revascularization versus medical therapy for renal-artery stenosis. N Engl J Med 2009;361:1953–62.

54. Bax L, Woittiez AJ, Kouwenberg HJ, et al. Stent placement in patients with atherosclerotic renal artery stenosis and impaired renal function: a randomized trial. Ann Intern Med 2009;150:840–8. W150–1.

55. Mitchell JA, Subramanian R, White CJ, et al. Predicting blood pressure improvement in hypertensive patients after renal artery stent placement: renal fractional flow reserve. Catheter Cardiovasc Interv 2007;69:685–9.

56. Mangiacapra F, Trana C, Sarno G, et al. Translesional pressure gradients to predict blood pressure response after renal artery stenting in patients with renovascular hypertension. Circ Cardiovasc Interv 2010;3:537–42.

57. Leesar MA, Varma J, Shapira A, et al. Prediction of hypertension improvement after stenting of renal artery stenosis: comparative accuracy of translesional pressure gradients, intravascular ultrasound, and angiography. J Am Coll Cardiol 2009;53:2363–71.

58. Subramanian R, White CJ, Rosenfield K, et al. Renal fractional flow reserve: a hemodynamic evaluation of moderate renal artery stenoses. Catheter Cardiovasc Interv 2005;64:480–6.

59. De Bruyne B, Manoharan G, Pijls NH, et al. Assessment of renal artery stenosis severity by pressure gradient measurements. J Am Coll Cardiol 2006; 48:1851–5.

60. Kapoor N, Fahsah I, Karim R, et al. Physiological assessment of renal artery stenosis: comparisons of resting with hyperemic renal pressure measurements. Catheter Cardiovasc Interv 2010;76:726–32.

61. Rundback JH, Sacks D, Kent KC, et al. Guidelines for the reporting of renal artery revascularization in clinical trials. American Heart Association. Circulation 2002;106:1572–85.

62. Nahman NS Jr, Maniam P, Hernandez RA Jr, et al. Renal artery pressure gradients in patients with angiographic evidence of atherosclerotic renal artery stenosis. Am J Kidney Dis 1994;24:695–9.

63. Colyer WR Jr, Cooper CJ, Burket MW, et al. Utility of a 0.014″ pressure-sensing guidewire to assess renal artery translesional systolic pressure gradients. Catheter Cardiovasc Interv 2003;59:372–7.

64. Jones NJ, Bates ER, Chetcuti SJ, et al. Usefulness of translesional pressure gradient and pharmacological provocation for the assessment of intermediate renal artery disease. Catheter Cardiovasc Interv 2006;68:429–34.

65. White CJ, Olin JW. Diagnosis and management of atherosclerotic renal artery stenosis: improving patient selection and outcomes. Nat Clin Pract Cardiovasc Med 2009;6:176–90.

66. Kunadian V, Harrigan C, Zorkun C, et al. Use of the TIMI frame count in the assessment of coronary artery blood flow and microvascular function over the past 15 years. J Thromb Thrombolysis 2009;27: 316–28.

67. Gibson CM, Cannon CP, Murphy SA, et al. Relationship of the TIMI myocardial perfusion grades, flow grades, frame count, and percutaneous coronary intervention to long-term outcomes after thrombolytic administration in acute myocardial infarction. Circulation 2002;105:1909–13.

68. Gibson CM, Murphy SA, Rizzo MJ, et al. Relationship between TIMI frame count and clinical outcomes after thrombolytic administration. Thrombolysis in

Myocardial Infarction (TIMI) Study Group. Circulation 1999;99:1945–50.

69. Gibson CM, Cannon CP, Daley WL, et al. TIMI frame count: a quantitative method of assessing coronary artery flow. Circulation 1996;93:879–88.

70. Mulumudi MS, White CJ. Renal frame count: a quantitative angiographic assessment of renal perfusion. Catheter Cardiovasc Interv 2005;65:183–6.

71. Mahmud E, Smith TW, Palakodeti V, et al. Renal frame count and renal blush grade: quantitative measures that predict the success of renal stenting in hypertensive patients with renal artery stenosis. JACC Cardiovasc Interv 2008;1:286–92.

72. Morrison LK, Harrison A, Krishnaswamy P, et al. Utility of a rapid B-natriuretic peptide assay in differentiating congestive heart failure from lung disease in patients presenting with dyspnea. J Am Coll Cardiol 2002;39:202–9.

73. Troughton RW, Prior DL, Pereira JJ, et al. Plasma B-type natriuretic peptide levels in systolic heart failure: importance of left ventricular diastolic function and right ventricular systolic function. J Am Coll Cardiol 2004;43:416–22.

74. Wolf K, Kurtz A, Pfeifer M, et al. Different regulation of left ventricular ANP, BNP and adrenomedullin mRNA in the two-kidney, one-clip model of renovascular hypertension. Pflugers Arch 2001;442:212–7.

75. Jaff MR, Bates M, Sullivan T, et al. Significant reduction in systolic blood pressure following renal artery stenting in patients with uncontrolled hypertension: results from the HERCULES trial. Catheter Cardiovasc Interv 2012;80:343–50.

76. Kiemeneij F, Laarman GJ, Odekerken D, et al. A randomized comparison of percutaneous transluminal coronary angioplasty by the radial, brachial and femoral approaches: the access study. J Am Coll Cardiol 1997;29:1269–75.

77. Trani C, Tommasino A, Burzotta F. Transradial renal stenting: why and how. Catheter Cardiovasc Interv 2009;74:951–6.

78. Olin JW. Atheroembolic renal disease: underdiagnosed and misunderstood. Catheter Cardiovasc Interv 2007;70:789–90.

79. Cooper CJ, Haller ST, Colyer W, et al. Embolic protection and platelet inhibition during renal artery stenting. Circulation 2008;117:2752–60.

80. Paul TK, Lee JH, White CJ. Renal embolic protection devices improve blood flow after stenting for atherosclerotic renal artery stenosis. Catheter Cardiovasc Interv 2012;80:1019–22.

81. Leertouwer TC, Gussenhoven EJ, van Overhagen H, et al. Stent placement for treatment of renal artery stenosis guided by intravascular ultrasound. J Vasc Interv Radiol 1998;9:945–52.

82. Lederman RJ, Mendelsohn FO, Santos R, et al. Primary renal artery stenting: characteristics and outcomes after 363 procedures. Am Heart J 2001;142:314–23.

83. Isles CG, Robertson S, Hill D. Management of renovascular disease: a review of renal artery stenting in ten studies. QJM 1999;92:159–67.

84. Blum U, Krumme B, Flugel P, et al. Treatment of ostial renal-artery stenoses with vascular endoprostheses after unsuccessful balloon angioplasty. N Engl J Med 1997;336:459–65.

85. Henry M, Amor M, Henry I, et al. Stents in the treatment of renal artery stenosis: long-term follow-up. J Endovasc Surg 1999;6:42–51.

86. Zahringer M, Sapoval M, Pattynama PM, et al. Sirolimus-eluting versus bare-metal low-profile stent for renal artery treatment (GREAT Trial): angiographic follow-up after 6 months and clinical outcome up to 2 years. J Endovasc Ther 2007;14:460–8.

87. Rasmus M, Huegli R, Jacob AL, et al. Extensive iatrogenic aortic dissection during renal angioplasty: successful treatment with a covered stent-graft. Cardiovasc Intervent Radiol 2007;30:497–500.

88. Patel PM, Eisenberg J, Islam MA, et al. Percutaneous revascularization of persistent renal artery in-stent restenosis. Vasc Med 2009;14:259–64.

89. Zeller T, Sixt S, Rastan A, et al. Treatment of reoccurring instent restenosis following reintervention after stent-supported renal artery angioplasty. Catheter Cardiovasc Interv 2007;70:296–300.

90. Bax L, Mali WP, Van De Ven PJ, et al. Repeated intervention for in-stent restenosis of the renal arteries. J Vasc Interv Radiol 2002;13:1219–24.

91. Munneke GJ, Engelke C, Morgan RA, et al. Cutting balloon angioplasty for resistant renal artery in-stent restenosis. J Vasc Interv Radiol 2002;13:327–31.

92. Spratt JC, Leslie SJ, Verin V. A case of renal artery brachytherapy for in-stent restenosis: four-year follow-up. J Invasive Cardiol 2004;16:287–8.

93. American College of Cardiology Foundation (ACCF), American College of Radiology (ACR), American Institute of Ultrasound in Medicine (AIUM), et al. ACCF/ACR/AIUM/ASE/ASN/ICAVL/SCAI/SCCT/SIR/SVM/SVS/SVU [corrected] 2012 appropriate use criteria for peripheral vascular ultrasound and physiological testing part I: arterial ultrasound and physiological testing: a report of the American College of Cardiology Foundation appropriate use criteria task force, American College of Radiology, American Institute of Ultrasound in Medicine, American Society of Echocardiography, American Society of Nephrology, Intersocietal Commission for the Accreditation of Vascular Laboratories, Society for Cardiovascular Angiography and Interventions, Society of Cardiovascular Computed Tomography, Society for Interventional Radiology, Society for Vascular Medicine, Society for Vascular Surgery, [corrected] and Society for Vascular Ultrasound. [corrected]. J Am Coll Cardiol 2012;60:242–76.

Resistant Hypertension
Medical Management and Alternative Therapies

Hossein Ghofrani, MD[a], Fred A. Weaver, MD, MMM[b],
Mitra K. Nadim, MD[c],*

KEYWORDS

- Hypertension • Joint National Committee • Resistant hypertension • Secondary hypertension
- Device

KEY POINTS

- Resistant hypertension (HTN) is failure to achieve goal blood pressure (BP) in spite of using a minimum of 3 antihypertensive drugs of different classes, at maximal tolerated doses, one of which must be a diuretic.
- In patients with resistant HTN, causes of pseudoresistance (both patient- and provider-related factors), and secondary HTN should be ruled out.
- Treatment of resistant HTN focuses on lifestyle modification and pharmacologic management. The basic principle for intervention is to ensure that all possible mechanisms for BP elevation are blocked.
- In general, most patients with resistant HTN should be on a renin angiotensin system blocker along with a calcium antagonist and a diuretic. Further medications can be added on an individual basis.
- Device-based therapies for resistant HTN should be reserved for those in whom available pharmacologic agents failed to control BP.

INTRODUCTION

Hypertension (HTN) is a major public health problem that affects approximately 1 billion people worldwide.[1] In the United States, 1 in 3 adults ($\approx$73 million) has high blood pressure (BP).[2] Several studies, including meta-analyses, have demonstrated a linear relationship between BP level and the risk for cardiovascular events, such as stroke, myocardial infarction, congestive heart failure, and chronic kidney disease (CKD), with the risk of cardiovascular mortality doubles with every 20/10 mm Hg increase in systolic and diastolic BP.[3] In the United States, the total cost of treating HTN in 2010 was estimated to be $76 billion.[2] Persistent, suboptimal BP control is consequently the most common attributable risk for death worldwide, being responsible for 62% of cerebrovascular disease and 49% of ischemic heart disease as well as the progression of CKD, and an estimated 7 million deaths and 64 million disability-adjusted life years annually.[4,5] Analyses of the National Health and Nutrition Examination Survey (NHANES) have demonstrated that not

F.A. Weaver is a consultant and on the advisory board for CRVx Inc; M.K. Nadim is a consultant for CVRx Inc.
[a] Division of Nephrology, Department of Medicine, Keck School of Medicine, University of Southern California, 2020 Zonal Avenue, IRD 806, Los Angeles, CA 90033, USA; [b] Division of Vascular Surgery & Endovascular Therapy, Department of Surgery, Keck School of Medicine, University of Southern California, 1520 San Pablo Street, Suite 4300, Los Angeles, CA 90033, USA; [c] Division of Nephrology, Department of Medicine, Keck School of Medicine, University of Southern California, 1520 San Pablo Street, Suite 4300, Los Angeles, CA 90033, USA
* Corresponding author.
E-mail address: mitra.nadim@med.usc.edu

Cardiol Clin 33 (2015) 75–87
http://dx.doi.org/10.1016/j.ccl.2014.09.003
0733-8651/15/$ – see front matter © 2015 Elsevier Inc. All rights reserved.

only is HTN awareness poor, but approximately 50% of hypertensive patients are not adequately treated to their goal BP of less than 140/90 mm Hg, with worse control rates in participants greater than 60 years of age, CKD and diabetes mellitus (DM).[6] Several, large HTN outcome trials also demonstrate a failure to achieve BP goals despite protocol-defined treatment regimens; 20% to 35% of participants were unable to achieve BP control despite receiving 3 antihypertensive medications or more.[7–9] These patients, by definition, are referred to as having refractory or resistant HTN.

Evaluation and treatment of patients with resistant HTN should be focused on identifying and removal of contributing factors, correct diagnosis and management of secondary causes, and use of effective multidrug regimens. Management of these patients often necessitates consultation with an HTN specialist.

DEFINITION OF RESISTANT HYPERTENSION

The Seventh Joint National Committee Report on Prevention, Detection, Evaluation, and Treatment of High Blood Pressure (JNC-7) defined resistant HTN as failure to achieve goal BP less than 140/90 mm Hg or less than 130/80 mm Hg in patients with DM or CKD in patients with HTN who are on maximum doses of an appropriate antihypertensive drug regimen consisting of 3 or more agents of different classes, including a diuretic.[10] The American Heart Association, however, defined resistant HTN as uncontrolled HTN despite at least 3 antihypertensive drugs or controlled HTN with at least 4 medications.[11] Although resistant HTN was not specifically addressed in the JNC-8 2014 Hypertension Guidelines, recommended goal BP was raised to less than 150/90 mm Hg in adults aged 60 years or older, and less than 140/90 mm Hg in patients less than 60 years old, including those with CKD, DM, or both.[12] Resistant HTN is not synonymous with uncontrolled HTN (**Box 1**). The latter includes all hypertensive patients who lack BP control under treatment, namely those receiving an inadequate treatment regimen, those with poor compliance, those who have elevated BP in the office but normal at home (white coat HTN) and those with undetected secondary HTN, as well as those with true treatment resistance.

PREVALENCE OF RESISTANT HYPERTENSION

Several clinical trials and epidemiologic data have estimated the prevalence of resistant HTN to be 20% to 30%,[7–9,13–15] although the exact

---

Box 1
Definitions of various forms of hypertension

Resistant hypertension

Failure to achieve goal BP using a minimum of 3 antihypertensive drugs at maximal tolerated doses, 1 of which must be a diuretic.

Controlled resistant hypertension[11]

Patients who meet the definition of resistant hypertension but whose BP is controlled on maximal tolerated doses of 4 or more antihypertensive medications.

Refractory hypertension

Patients who meet the definition of resistant hypertension but whose BP is not controlled on maximal tolerated doses of 4 or more antihypertensive medications.

Pseudoresistance

Lack of BP control with appropriate treatment in a patient who does not have resistant hypertension.

White-Coat hypertension

Patients who have clinic/office BP readings above goal on at least 3 separate visits with 2 measurements taken at each visit, and at least 2 BP readings at or below goal taken outside the clinic/office, and show no evidence of end-organ damage.

Masked hypertension

Patients who have normal clinic but high ambulatory BPs (opposite of white-coat hypertension).

Abbreviation: BP, blood pressure.

---

prevalence has been difficult to determine owing to the lack of large, prospective cohort studies of patients with true resistant HTN. Individuals with resistant HTN are more likely to be older than age 55, male, non-Hispanic black, have a high body mass index, with a history of DM, renal dysfunction, and cardiovascular disease, including coronary heart disease, heart failure, and stroke.[6] A 2012 estimation by the American Heart Association based on NHANES 2005–2008 data showed that only 54% of hypertensive participants had a well-controlled BP on medications and that the prevalence of uncontrolled HTN despite being on 3 medications has almost doubled from 16% in 1998 through 2004 to 28% in 2005 through 2008.[16] In patients with controlled as well as uncontrolled HTN, the number of medications taken has increased with time.[6] NHANES data from 2005 through 2008 has shown that

28% of uncontrolled hypertensive patients are on at least 3 medications and 7.3% of controlled patients are on at least 4 BP medications. Based on the JNC-7 recommended BP goals for patients with CKD and DM, only 37% of patients with CKD[17] and 25% of those with diabetes were controlled to the recommended level.[18–20] One should keep in mind that many of these studies had limitations owing to the lack of control over medication adherence, use of suboptimal dosages and inappropriate drug combinations, lack of workup for patients with possible white coat HTN or secondary causes of HTN and therefore may have overestimated the prevalence of resistant HTN. Regardless, given the trend of a more obese and older population with increased numbers of comorbidities, such as DM and CKD, the prevalence of resistant HTN will most likely increase over the next decade.

PROGNOSIS

Evidence suggests that the prognosis of individuals with long-standing, poorly controlled, resistant HTN is unfavorable. Major cohort studies have shown that the extent of BP elevation directly increases the relative risk of stroke, myocardial infarction, kidney failure, and congestive heart failure in patients with HTN.[21–25] Ambulatory BP monitoring has played a special role in the diagnosis of resistant HTN, in differentiation with pseudoresistance, and in the assessment of cardiovascular risk and prognosis. Large cohort, cross-sectional studies have confirmed that individuals whose resistant HTN was diagnosed on the basis of ambulatory BP monitoring had a higher number of comorbidities, more target-organ damage (including left ventricular hypertrophy, impaired renal function, and microalbuminuria), and higher rates of cardiovascular morbidity and mortality, even after adjustment for different cardiovascular risk factors.[26–30] A nondipping, nocturnal BP pattern and the ambulatory arterial stiffness index are other variables that have been independently associated with increased cardiovascular events in patients with resistant HTN.[28,29] However, the extent to which the excess cardiovascular morbidity and mortality related to resistant HTN is reduced by adequate BP control remains unknown.

DIAGNOSIS, EVALUATION, AND MONITORING

Evaluation of patients with resistant HTN should focus on identifying patients who meet the definition criteria for resistant HTN, confirming true treatment resistance, identification of causes contributing to treatment resistance (including secondary causes of HTN), and documentation of target-organ damage. In most cases, treatment resistance is multifactorial in etiology, and factors such as lifestyle, medications, associated conditions, and identifiable causes contribute to the difficulty in achieving BP control in patients with resistant HTN (**Box 2**).

Pseudoresistant Hypertension

Pseudoresistance refers to lack of BP control with appropriate treatment in a patient who does not actually have resistant HTN. Various factors, such as suboptimal BP measurement, white coat effect, poor compliance with prescribed therapy, heavily calcified, sclerotic, and noncompressible

---

Box 2
Patient characteristics associated with treatment-resistant hypertension

Older age

High baseline blood pressure

Obesity

Smoking

Excessive dietary salt intake

Chronic kidney disease

Diabetes

Left ventricular hypertrophy

Black race

Female sex

Heavy alcohol intake (>3 drinks/d)

Medications

  Nonnarcotic analgesics

    Nonsteroidal antiinflammatory agents, including aspirin

    Selective cyclooxygenase-2 inhibitors

  Sympathomimetic agents (decongestants, diet pills, cocaine)

  Stimulants (amphetamine, methamphetamine)

  Corticosteroids

  Oral contraceptives

  Cyclosporine and tacrolimus

  Erythropoietin

  Natural licorice

  Herbal compounds (ginseng, ephedra, yohimbine, or ma huang)

arteries, and inappropriate medication combination or dosing can result in elevated BP readings and produce the misconception of resistant HTN (**Box 3**). Careful evaluation to exclude these factors should be performed on all patients who present with resistant HTN.

White coat HTN is a cause of pseudoresistance and refers to patients with elevated BP in the clinical setting while having significantly lower or normal blood pressures at home. The white coat effect is not uncommon and as many as 25% of patients referred for resistant HTN have been shown to be at goal BP control when ambulatory measurements are performed.[31,32] These patients have less target-organ damage compared with truly resistant hypertensive patients; however, their prognosis is worse than that of the general normotensive population.[25,33,34] In patients with white coat HTN, continued home BP or repeated ambulatory BP monitoring within 3 to 6 months is recommended because 20% to 25% of these patients may go on to develop true resistant HTN.[35]

Poor compliance is another common cause of apparent resistant HTN. Studies have shown that up to 50% of newly diagnosed hypertensive patients stop taking their medications during the first year, and only 40% of the remaining patients continue to take their medications over the next 5 to 10 years.[36–39] Single-point measurement of drug concentration in urine samples or therapeutic drug monitoring in serum samples in patients with resistant HTN have shown that 50% to 60% of patients had medication noncompliance.[40] This problem might be less common (about 16%) among patients followed by HTN specialists.[41] Once medication nonadherence is established, efforts should be made to identify the barriers to adherence. Factors that improve medication compliance include use of agents with a low side effect profile, avoidance of complicated dosing schedules, use of pill boxes, patient education regarding importance of BP management, and use of medications with lower out-of-pocket costs.[42,43] Electronic monitoring systems to assess drug adherence have demonstrated that one third of hypertensive patients who are poorly controlled on an adequately dosed triple therapy actually normalized their BP when drug adherence was monitored.[21,39,44]

Physician-related factors contributing to resistant HTN include inappropriate selection and dosing of medication, as well as "clinical inertia," defined as the conscious decision by a clinician to not adequately treat a condition despite knowing that it is present.[45] Clinical inertia, which is not uncommon among physicians, may be owing to lack of training and experience in the proper use of antihypertensive agents.[46] An open survey among primary care physicians in 1596 centers from 16 countries in four different continents showed that the main reasons for not intensifying antihypertensive treatment when BP remained above goal were the assumption that the time after starting the new drug was too short to attain its full effect, the satisfaction with a clear improvement of BP or with a BP nearing the goal, and the acceptance of good self-measurements.[47]

Secondary Causes of Hypertension

Secondary causes of HTN are thought to occur in fewer than 10% of hypertensive individuals (**Box 4**). Correct diagnosis and treatment can help with achieving goal BP and in some cases, can lead to potential cure. Patients with known or suspected secondary HTN should be referred to an HTN specialist for workup and management.

Primary aldosteronism is the most common cause of resistant HTN, with a prevalence of 10% to 30%.[48–50] Hypokalemia may not be present early in the stage of the disease and is thought to be a late manifestation of this disorder.[50] A plasma aldosterone level/plasma renin

---

Box 3
Causes of pseudoresistant hypertension

Improper technique

  Wrong cuff size

  One reading only

  Patient not sitting quietly for 3–5 minutes before measurement

White coat hypertension

Recent smoking or caffeine intake before measurement

Noncompressable calcified or atherosclerotic arteries in elderly

Poor patient compliance

  Medication side effects

  Medication cost

  Complicated drug dosing

  Lack of patient education

Physician-related factors

  Inadequate/incorrect regimen

  Physician inertia to add or modify drug regimen

Box 4
Causes of secondary hypertension

Primary aldosteronism

Renovascular disease

- Atherosclerotic renal artery stenosis
- Fibromuscular dysplasia

Obstructive sleep apnea

Chronic kidney disease

Hypothyroidism/hyperthyroidism

Cushing syndrome

Pheochromocytoma

Coarctation of the aorta

Hyperparathyroidism

---

adrenal hyperplasia. Patients with unilateral adenoma should undergo surgical removal, which has been shown to cure HTN in 50% to 60% of patients.[51]

Renovascular disease is a common finding in hypertensive patients occurring in approximately 20% of patients undergoing cardiac catheterization.[52] More than 90% of cases are atherosclerotic in origin, with a higher likelihood occurring in older patients with a history of smoking, known atherosclerotic disease, especially peripheral artery disease, DM, and sudden loss of renal function after the initiation of an angiotensin-converting enzyme inhibitor or angiotensin receptor blocker (ARB). Even though several, prospective, randomized trials over the past decade have failed to demonstrate clinical advantages to revascularization compared with medical therapy (**Table 1**), management of patients with renovascular disease remains controversial.[34,53–58] Many criticized that these trials were subject to selection bias by excluding patients with severe cases of stenosis or HTN and progressive renal disease, and including patients with minor renovascular disease; therefore, the outcomes of these studies cannot be generalized to all patients. In addition, observational studies support the concept that BP control, improvement in kidney function, and reversal of progressive kidney injury can be improved in some patients after revascularization. Medical therapy should be the first line of treatment in patients with presumed renovascular HTN. For patients who fail medical therapy or

ratio of greater than 20 in the setting of a plasma aldosterone concentration greater than 15 ng/dL is highly suggestive of primary hyperaldosteronism. However, confirmatory assessment with an intravenous or oral salt suppression test is required to confirm the diagnosis. Adrenal vein sampling is the gold standard for localizing aldosterone-producing adenomas in patients with primary hyperaldosteronism. Medical management with a mineralocorticoid receptor antagonist, such as spironolactone or eplerenone, has been shown to control BP in patients with primary aldosteronism, especially those with bilateral

---

Table 1
Summary of trials of renal artery stenting versus medical therapy in the management of atherosclerotic renal artery stenosis

Study	Year	Country	Patient Population	Follow-up (mo)	Outcomes
ASTRAL[55]	2009	UK, Australia, New Zealand	806 patients with refractory HTN or CKD, 54% with bilateral RAS	34	No difference in BP, renal function or mortality between the groups
STAR[54]	2009	The Netherlands, France	138 patients with CKD; 48% with bilateral RAS	24	No difference in renal function; significant complication with the procedures
CORAL[53]	2013	US	947 patients with HTN or CKD, 20% with bilateral RAS	43	No difference in incidence of renal or cardiovascular events, or all-cause mortality; modest difference in systolic BP (−2 mm Hg) in stent group

Abbreviations: BP, blood pressure; CKD, chronic kidney disease; HTN, hypertension; RAS, renal artery stenosis.

develop progressive loss of renal function, renal revascularization offers therapeutic benefit. In patients less than 50 years of age, especially women, fibromuscular dysplasia should be considered.

CKD is both a common cause and a complication of long-standing, poorly controlled HTN. In the antihypertensive and Lipid-lowering Treatment to Prevent Heart Attack Trial (ALLHAT) study, CKD, as indicated by a serum creatinine of greater than 1.5 mg/dL, was a strong predictor of failure to achieve goal BP.[7] Increased sodium and fluid retention, and consequently an expansion of intravascular volume, is the main factor leading to treatment resistance in patients with CKD.[59]

Obstructive sleep apnea (OSA) is very common in patients with resistant HTN, with prevalence rates of up to 83% based on an apnea–hypopnea index greater than 10 events per hour in patients with unsuspected sleep apnea.[60–65] OSA is both more common and more severe in men. A history of snoring and daytime sleepiness, especially in the presence of obesity, should prompt one to suspect OSA. Both nocturnal and daytime BP are increased with a lack of nocturnal dipping. The more severe the sleep apnea, the less likely BP is controlled despite the use of an increasing number of medications.[62,65] However, results of several clinical trials have shown only modest BP reductions (3–5 mm Hg) after treatment of OSA with continuous positive airway pressure.[63,64,66]

Pheochromocytoma is very rare, with a prevalence in a general hypertensive population of only 0.1% to 0.6%.[67] The diagnosis should be considered in a hypertensive patient with a combination of headaches, palpitations, and sweating, typically occurring in an episodic fashion. The best screening test for pheochromocytoma is plasma free metanephrines (normetanephrine and metanephrine), which carries a 99% sensitivity and an 89% specificity. Surgical resection of the tumor is the treatment of choice for this group of patients.

TREATMENT
Lifestyle Modification

All patients with HTN should be counseled about lifestyle modification. Although not specifically evaluated in patients with resistant HTN, lifestyle modifications, such as weight loss, dietary salt reduction, diet rich in fruit and vegetables and low in saturated fats (ie, the Dietary Approaches to Stop Hypertension [DASH] diet), increased physical activity, limiting daily alcohol consumption to no more than 2 drinks for men and 1 drink for women, and ingestion of a high-fiber, low-fat diet, have clear benefit in terms of reducing

BP.[68–71] In the United States, the average sodium consumption is approximately 8.5 g/d. High sodium intake is among the major contributing factors to resistant HTN and a sodium restriction to 1.7 g/d is associated with a reduction in BP with a more pronounced effects in patients with resistant HTN.[23]

Pharmacologic Treatment

Inappropriate antihypertensive drug combinations or suboptimal dosing are the most common causes of resistant HTN. In a retrospective cohort study in a large population with resistant HTN, only 3% and 5.9% of patients were on chlorthalidone or a mineralocorticoid receptor antagonist, respectively, both of which are evidence-based recommended antihypertensive agents.[72]

The basic principle for intervention in resistant HTN is to ensure that all possible mechanisms for BP elevation, including volume expansion, renin–angiotensin–aldosterone system activation, and peripheral vascular resistance, are blocked. Moreover, there are few fixed-dose combination antihypertensive agents that have been approved by the Food and Drug Administration for use as first-line therapy. These have been especially useful for patients with resistant HTN who have compliance problems.[73] In general, most patients with resistant HTN should be on a renin–angiotensin–aldosterone system blocker along with a calcium antagonist and a diuretic, all of which are preferred to be prescribed in full dosages and for appropriate time intervals.

An appropriate diuretic to decrease volume overload remains a cornerstone of therapy and can help about 60% of patients achieve BP goals.[13,14,41,74] Chlorthalidone, a thiazidelike diuretic, has been shown to provide greater BP reduction, longer duration of action, and better cardiovascular risk profile compared with hydrochlorothiazide 50 mg/d,[75,76] and was the only diuretic recommended by the American Heart Association position statement in 2008.[11] In patients with CKD stage 4 or 5 (glomerular filtration rate of <30 mL/min), loop diuretics should be used for effective volume and BP control.[11] Furosemide or bumetanide must be given twice or even thrice daily, because the once-daily use is associated with intermittent natriuresis and consequent reactive sodium retention caused by increases in renin–angiotensin–aldosterone system activity. Torsemide has a longer duration of action; therefore, once or twice daily dosing may be sufficient.

Aldosterone blockade by adding spironolactone or eplerenone to a 3-medication regimen may be beneficial in reducing BP in patients with or without primary hyperaldosteronism, especially in certain settings, such as obesity or sleep apnea.[77–83] However, results of several randomized and non-randomized studies on the BP-lowering effect of aldosterone antagonists has been inconclusive.[84–86] A meta-analysis of 13 studies (3 randomized and 10 observational) in 2640 patients, that evaluated the antihypertensive benefit of aldosterone antagonists as an add-on therapy in patients with resistant HTN, showed an average systolic BP reduction between 16 and 20 mm Hg in patients treated with aldosterone antagonists.[83] Reduction in BP was more pronounced in patients with a baseline systolic BP greater than 150 mm Hg; however, a mild but significant increase in serum potassium and creatinine was also present in treated patients. Amiloride is an inhibitor of the aldosterone-regulated epithelial sodium channel in the distal nephron, and in a prospective, randomized, placebo-controlled, double-blind study of African-American patients, it was shown to provide a reduction in BP comparable to spironolactone.[87]

β-Blockers should be used as fifth-line drug therapy unless there are compelling indications, such as congestive heart failure or prior myocardial infarction, to initiate them earlier. Large clinical trials have shown inferior cardiovascular protection with the combination of β-blockers and thiazide diuretics in comparison with combinations of calcium channel blockers plus an angiotensin-converting enzyme inhibitor or an angiotensin II receptor blocker plus thiazide diuretic.[8]

Device Therapies for Resistant Hypertension

Despite lifestyle modification and the various pharmacologic agents available, there remains a subset of patients who are unable to reach goal BP. Over the last decade, 2 new approaches to treat resistant HTN have been developed that mainly target the sympathetic nervous system: catheter-based renal denervation (RDN) ablation therapy and carotid sinus baroreflex activation therapy (BAT; **Table 2**). Increased sympathetic tone increases peripheral vascular resistance, which leads to increased renin secretion, reduced renal blood flow, and increased sodium retention. Stimulation of carotid baroreceptors via BAT or ablation of the renal nerve via RDN, leads to sustained reduction in arterial pressure and heart rate by suppressing sympathetic activity.

Carotid Baroreflex Activation Therapy

BAT uses a carotid sinus baroreceptor stimulator that is surgically implanted by means of open carotid exposure and activates the receptors with variable and programmable amounts of energy.

Similar to a pacemaker, the generator is implanted in a pocket in the infraclavicular space. Electrical stimulation of the carotid baroreceptors has been shown to cause a depressor response through sympathetic inhibition. Both the Rheos system (CVRx, Minneapolis, MN, USA) and the newer generation BAT, Barostim neo (CVRx), have been shown to reduce BP in patients with resistant HTN.[88–93] The efficacy and safety of Rheos system was investigated in the phase II, multicenter, nonrandomized Device Based Therapy of Hypertension Trial (DEBuT-HT) in 45 patients with drug-resistant HTN. After 1 year of therapy, patients demonstrated a mean decrease of 30 ± 6 mm Hg for systolic BP, which was maintained for 2 years.[93] Shortly thereafter, a double-blind, randomized, prospective, multicenter, placebo-controlled trial in the United States of 265 subjects with resistant HTN, demonstrated a reduction of systolic BP by greater than 30 mm Hg with 55% of patients achieved goal BP with BAT,[90] which persisted for up to 53 months.[91] However, this trial did not meet the acute efficacy endpoint for the proportion of patients with at least a 10 mm Hg-drop in systolic BP with a superiority margin of 20% between the 2 groups at 6 months. In addition, the implant procedure safety did not meet the pre-specified 82% event-free objective performance criterion; however, the adverse event profile compared favorably with results from endarterectomy trials, which were more like the dissection for the Rheos procedure in the carotid region.

Owing to the higher than expected device-related complications with the Rheos system in the pivotal trial, a second-generation system for delivering BAT, the Barostim neo system, was developed which involves unilateral lead placement (instead of bilateral with the Rheos system), a much smaller implantable device, and a safety profile comparable with that of a pacemaker. In a single-arm, open-label study of 30 patients with resistant HTN (including patients with prior RDN), a systolic BP reduction of 26 mm Hg after 6 months was demonstrated in patients with baseline systolic BP of 172 mm Hg, which is comparable to the results seen with the Rheos system, with minor procedure-related complications.[92] Currently, a randomized BP efficacy trial has started in the United States with the Barostim neo system. The Barostim neo is approved for sale in Europe; however, the indication is restricted to patients with therapy-resistant HTN or heart failure. However, it is registered as an investigational device and limited to investigational use by the US law.

In addition to BP control, BAT may provide additional cardiovascular benefit. In early stage

Table 2
Trials on device-based approaches to management of resistant hypertension

Study	Year	Study Type	No. of Patients	Mean SBP	No. of Antihypertensive Medications	Outcome Summary
Carotid baroreceptor activation therapy						
DEBuT-HT[93]	2010	Single arm, Open label	45	179	5.0	Reduction in systolic BP of 30 mm Hg at 1, 2 and 3 y; 67% of patients with systolic BP <140 mm Hg at 3 y
Rheos Pivotal[90]	2011	2:1 randomized (active: control)	265	168 ± 26	5.2 ± 1.6	Reduction in systolic BP by 26 mm Hg at 6 mo and 35 mm Hg at 12 mo; 63% of patients achieved SBP <140 mm Hg at 1 y
Barostim neo[92]	2012	Single arm, open label	30	172 ± 20	6.1 ± 2.7	Reduction in systolic BP by 26 mm Hg at 6 mo; reduction in systolic BP by 22 mm Hg in subset of patients with prior RDN therapy
Renal denervation						
Symplicity HTN-1[95]	2009	Single arm, Open label	45	177 ± 19	4.7 ± 1.4	Reduction in systolic BP by 22 mm Hg at 6 and 27 mm Hg at 12 mo
Symplicity HTN-2[96]	2010	1:1 Randomized	106	178 ± 18	5.2 ± 1.5	Reductions in systolic BP by 32 mm Hg at 6 mo in patients treated with RDN; no difference in 24-h ambulatory BP
Symplicity HTN-3[97]	2014	2:1 Randomized (active: control)	535	180 ± 16	5.1 ± 1.4	No difference in systolic BP between the groups at 6 mo (14 mm Hg SBP reduction in RDN group, 12 mm Hg SBP reduction in control group)

Abbreviations: BP, blood pressure; RDN, renal denervation; SBP, systolic BP.

heart failure patients with resistant HTN, BAT lowered BP and effectively reversed cardiac remodeling with a significant reduction in left ventricular mass index and concentric hypertrophy.[94] In another analysis, 3 months of BAT reduced left ventricular mass index similarly to a 12-month course of ARB therapy, and a 12-month therapy with BAT provided twice the effect of reducing left ventricular mass index as did 12 months of ARB therapy.

Renal Denervation Therapy

RDN therapy using a radiofrequency ablation catheter that directly targets the sympathetic nerves adjacent to the renal artery is a recently proposed, minimally invasive procedure to control BP.[95–97] The Symplicity Renal Denervation System involves an endovascular energy delivery catheter and an automated generator. Once in place within the renal artery, the tip of the catheter is placed against the arterial wall in several places where it delivers radiofrequency energy to the surrounding sympathetic nerves. Typical procedure comprises 4 to 6 treatments for each renal artery.[95]

The Symplicity -1 study was the first clinical trial that enrolled 50 patients with resistant HTN (on 4.7 ± 1.4 medications at the beginning of the study) and an estimated glomerular filtration rate of greater than 45 mL/min/1.73 m^2, at 5 Australian and European centers.[95] In this cohort study, RDN lowered office systolic BP by 14 mm Hg at 1 month and by 27 mm Hg at 12 months; 85% of the patients responded to therapy with a reduction of office systolic BP exceeding 10 mm Hg. RDN successfully restored nocturnal dipping in 50% of previously nondipping or reverse-dipping patients.[95] However, the study did not include a control group. In a subsequent multicenter, prospective, randomized study, Symplicity HTN-2, patients with resistant HTN were randomly assigned to undergo RDN with medical therapy (n = 52) or to medical therapy alone (control group; n = 54).[96] Similar to the Symplicity HTN-1 trial, patients with type 1 diabetes and a glomerular filtration rate of less than 45 mL/min/1.73 m^2 were excluded. Six-month office-based BP measurements were significantly lower in the RDN group (32/12 mm Hg reduction compared with 0/1 mm Hg change in control group, both from a baseline of 178/96 mm Hg). However, home BP and 24-hour ambulatory BP were similar in the two groups.[96] Symplicity HTN-3, a large, US, randomized, controlled trial included 535 patients with resistant HTN who were assigned in a 2:1 ratio to RDN or a sham procedure. However, this study showed no difference in the office BP or 24-hour ambulatory BP in the RDN group compared with the sham procedure group treated with medical therapy alone.[97,98]

Although reported procedure-related complications of RDN in all 3 Symplicity-HTN trials were low, recent reports suggest that diffuse renal artery constriction owing to vasospasm and local tissue damage at the ablation site with endothelial edema and thrombus formation may occur after RDN.[99,100]

SUMMARY

Treating resistant HTN, particularly in patients who are already prescribed 4 or more drugs, is a true challenge. Entertaining correct diagnosis, ruling out secondary causes of HTN, dealing with patients' noncompliance and proper medication dosing, and selecting appropriate additional BP-lowering agents are issues that commonly need attention. Choice of medication should be based not only on the antihypertensive efficacy but also on the incremental cost, the adverse effect profile, and its potential cardiovascular benefits. Ongoing investigation and research on development of new fixed-dose combination medications and innovative medical, minimally invasive or invasive methods of BP management are arenas never to be left abandoned.

REFERENCES

1. Wolf-Maier K, Cooper R, Banegas J, et al. Hypertension prevalence and blood pressure levels in 6 European countries, Canada, and the United States. JAMA 2003;289:2363–9.
2. Lloyd-Jones D, Adams R, Carnethon M, et al. Heart disease and stroke statistics–2009 update: a report from the American Heart Association Statistics Committee and Stroke Statistics Subcommittee. Circulation 2009;119(3):e21–181.
3. Turnbull F, Neal B, Ninomiya T, et al. Effects of different regimens to lower blood pressure on major cardiovascular events in older and younger adults: meta-analysis of randomized trials. BMJ 2008;336:1121–3.
4. Mancia G, DeBacker G, Dominiczak A, et al. ESH-ESC Practice guidelines for the management of arterial hypertension: ESH-ESC Task Force on the Management of Arterial Hypertension. J Hypertens 2007;25(9):1751–62.
5. Perkovic V, Huxley R, Wu Y, et al. The burden of blood pressure-related disease: a neglected priority for global health. Hypertension 2007;50: 991–7.
6. Egan B, Zhao Y, Axon R, et al. Uncontrolled and apparent treatment resistant hypertension in the United States, 1988 to 2008. Circulation 2011; 124:1046–58.
7. ALLHAT Officers and Coordinators for the ALLHAT Collaborative Research Group. The Antihypertensive and Lipid-Lowering Treatment to Prevent Heart Attack Trial. Major outcomes in high-risk hypertensive patients randomized to angiotensin-converting enzyme inhibitor or calcium channel blocker vs diuretic: the Antihypertensive and Lipid-Lowering Treatment to Prevent Heart Attack Trial (ALLHAT). JAMA 2002;288(23):2981–97.
8. Dahlof B, Devereux R, Kjeldsen S, et al. Cardiovascular morbidity and mortality in the Losartan Intervention for Endpoint Reduction in Hypertension

Study (LIFE): a randomized trial against atenolol. Lancet 2002;359:995–1003.

9. Pepine C, Handberg E, Cooper-DeHoff R, et al. A calcium antagonist vs a non-calcium antagonist hypertension treatment strategy for patients with coronary artery disease. The International Verapamil-Trandolapril Study (INVEST): a randomized controlled trial. JAMA 2003;290:2805–16.

10. Chobanian A, Bakris G, Black H. Seventh report of the Joint National Committee on Prevention, Detection, Evaluation, and Treatment of High Blood Pressure. Hypertension 2003;42:1206–52.

11. Calhoun D, Jones D, Textor S, et al. Resistant hypertension: diagnosis, evaluation, and treatment. A scientific statement from the American Heart Association Professional Education Committee of the Council for High Blood Pressure Research. Hypertension 2008;51:1403–19.

12. James P, Oparil S, Carter B. 2014 evidence-based guideline for the management of high blood pressure in adults: report from the panel members appointed to the Eighth Joint National Committee (JNC 8). JAMA 2014;311(5):507–20.

13. Black H, Elliott W, Grandits G, et al. Principal results of the controlled onset verapamil investigation of cardiovascular end points (CONVINCE) trial. JAMA 2003;289(16):2073–82.

14. Jamerson K, Weber M, Bakris G, et al. Benazepril plus amlodipine or hydrochlorothiazide for hypertension in high-risk patients. Avoiding cardiovascular events through combination therapy in patients living with systolic hypertension (ACCOMPLISH) trial. N Engl J Med 2008;359(23):2417–28.

15. Sarafidis P, Bakris G. State of hypertension management in the United States: confluence of risk factors and the prevalence of resistant hypertension. J Clin Hypertens (Greenwich) 2008;10:130–9.

16. Roger V, Go A, Lloyd-Jones D, et al. Heart disease and stroke statistics 2012 update: a report from the American Heart Association. Circulation 2012; 125(1):e2–220.

17. Peralta C, Hicks L, Chertow G, et al. Control of hypertension in adults with chronic kidney disease in the United States. Hypertension 2005;45:1119–24.

18. Hajjar I, Kotchen T. Trends in prevalence, awareness, treatment, and control of hypertension in the United States, 1988–2000. JAMA 2003;290: 199–206.

19. Ong K, Cheung B, Man Y, et al. Prevalence, awareness, treatment, and control of hypertension among United States adults 1999–2004. Hypertension 2007;49:69–75.

20. Sarafidis P, Li S, Chen S, et al. Hypertension awareness, treatment, and control in chronic kidney disease. Am J Med 2008;121(4):332–40.

21. McAdam-Marx C, Ye X, Sung JC, et al. Results of a retrospective, observational pilot study using electronic medical records to assess the prevalence and characteristics of patients with resistant hypertension in an ambulatory care setting. Clin Ther 2009;31:1116–23.

22. Daugherty S, Powers J, Magid D, et al. Incidence and prognosis of resistant hypertension in hypertensive patients. Circulation 2012;125(13): 1635–42.

23. Gupta A, Nasothimiou E, Chang C, et al. Baseline predictors of resistant hypertension in the Anglo-Scandinavian Cardiac Outcome Trial (ASCOT): a risk score to identify those at high-risk. J Hypertens 2011;29(10):2004–13.

24. Persell S. Prevalence of resistant hypertension in the United States, 2003–2008. Hypertension 2011;57(6):1076–80.

25. Pierdomenico S, Lapenna D, Bucci A, et al. Cardiovascular outcome in treated hypertensive patients with responder, masked, false resistant, and true resistant hypertension. Am J Hypertens 2005;18: 1422–8.

26. de-la-Sierra A, Banegas J, Oliveras A, et al. Clinical differences between resistant hypertensives and patients treated and controlled with three or less drugs. J Hypertens 2012;30(6):1211–6.

27. de-la-Sierra A, Segura J, Banegas J, et al. Clinical features of 8295 patients with resistant hypertension classified on the basis of ambulatory blood pressure monitoring. Hypertension 2011; 57:898–902.

28. Muxfeldt E, Cardoso C, Dias V, et al. Prognostic impact of the ambulatory arterial stiffness index in resistant hypertension. J Hypertens 2010;28: 1547–53.

29. Muxfeldt E, Cardoso C, Salles G. Prognostic value of nocturnal blood pressure reduction in resistant hypertension. Arch Intern Med 2009;169:874–80.

30. Salles G, Cardoso C, Muxfeldt E. Prognostic influence of office and ambulatory blood pressures in resistant hypertension. Arch Intern Med 2008;168: 2340–6.

31. Brown M, Buddle M, Martin A. Is resistant hypertension really resistant? Am J Hypertens 2001;14: 1263–9.

32. Hermida R, Ayala D, Calvo C, et al. Effects of time of day of treatment on ambulatory blood pressure pattern of patients with resistant hypertension. Hypertension 2005;46:1053–9.

33. Muxfeldt E, Bloch K, Nogueira A, et al. Twenty-four hour ambulatory blood pressure monitoring pattern of resistant hypertension. Blood Press Monit 2003; 8:181–5.

34. Textor SC, Lerman LO. Renal artery stenosis: medical versus interventional therapy. Curr Cardiol Rep 2013;15(10):409.

35. Muxfeldt E, Fiszman R, deSouza F, et al. Appropriate time interval to repeat ambulatory blood

pressure monitoring in patients with white-coat resistant hypertension. Hypertension 2012;59: 384–9.

36. Daugherty S, Powers J, Magid D, et al. The association between medication adherence and treatment intensification with blood pressure control in resistant hypertension. Hypertension 2012;60: 303–9.

37. Mazzaglia G, Mantovani L, Sturkenboom M, et al. Patterns of persistence with antihypertensive medications in newly diagnosed hypertensive patients in Italy: a retrospective cohort study in primary care. J Hypertens 2005;23:2093–100.

38. VanWijk B, Klungel O, Heerdink E, et al. Rate and determinants of 10-year persistence with antihypertensive drugs. J Hypertens 2005;23:2101–7.

39. Vrijens B, Vincze G, Kristanto P, et al. Adherence to prescribed antihypertensive drug treatments: longitudinal study of electronically compiled dosing histories. BMJ 2008;336:1114–7.

40. Jung O, Gechter JL, Wunder C, et al. Resistant hypertension? Assessment of adherence by toxicological urine analysis. Journal of hypertension 2013;31(4):766–74.

41. Garg J, Elliot W, Folker A, et al. Resistant hypertension revisited: a comparison of two university-based cohorts (RUSH Hypertensive Service). Am J Hypertens 2005;18(5 Pt 1):619–26.

42. Haynes R, Yao X, Degani A, et al. Interventions to enhance medication adherence. Cochrane Database Syst Rev 2005;(4):CD000011.

43. Takiya L, Peterson A, Finley R. Meta-analysis of interventions for medication adherence to antihypertensives. Ann Pharmacother 2004;38:1617–24.

44. Burnier M, Schneider MP, Chiolero A, et al. Electronic compliance monitoring in resistant hypertension: the basis for rational therapeutic decisions. Journal of Hypertension 2001;19(2):335–41.

45. Phillips L, Branch W, Cook C, et al. Clinical inertia. Ann Intern Med 2001;135:825–34.

46. Oliveria S, Lapuerta P, McCarthy B, et al. Physician-related barriers to the effective management of uncontrolled hypertension. Arch Intern Med 2002;162:413–20.

47. Ferrari P. Reasons for therapeutic inertia when managing hypertension in clinical practice in non-Western countries. J Hum Hypertens 2009; 23(3):151–9.

48. Aronova A, Fahey T, Zarnegar R. Management of hypertension in primary aldosteronism. World J Cardiol 2014;6(5):227–33.

49. Calhoun D, Nishizaka M, Zaman M, et al. Hyperaldosteronism among black and white subjects with resistant hypertension. Hypertension 2002;40: 892–6.

50. Fardella C, Mosso L, Gómez-Sánchez C, et al. Primary hyperaldosteronism in essential hypertensives: prevalence, biochemical profile, and molecular biology. J Clin Endocrinol Metab 2008;85:1863–7.

51. Rossi GP, Cesari M, Cuspidi C, et al. Response to effectiveness of adrenalectomy and aldosterone antagonists for long-term treatment of primary aldosteronism. Hypertension 2013;62(4):e14.

52. Aqel RA, Zoghbi GJ, Baldwin SA, et al. Prevalence of renal artery stenosis in high-risk veterans referred to cardiac catheterization. J Hypertens 2003;21(6):1157–62.

53. Cooper C, Murphy T, Cutlip D, et al, For The CORAL Investigators. Stenting and medical therapy for atherosclerotic renal artery stenosis. N Engl J Med 2014;370(1):13–22.

54. Bax L, Woittiez A, Kouwenberg H, et al. Stent placement in patients with atherosclerotic renal artery stenosis and impaired renal function: a randomized trial. Ann Intern Med 2009;150:840–8.

55. Wheatley K, Ives N, et al, For The ASTRAL Investigators. Revascularization versus medical therapy for renal-artery stenosis. N Engl J Med 2009; 361(20):1953–62.

56. Watson P, Hadjipetrou P, Cox S, et al. Effect of renal artery stenting on renal function and size in patients with atherosclerotic renovascular disease. Circulation 2000;102:1671–7.

57. Chrysochou C, Kalra PA. Current management of atherosclerotic renovascular disease–what have we learned from ASTRAL? Nephron Clin Pract 2010;115(1):73–81.

58. Burket M, Cooper C, Kennedy D, et al. Renal artery angioplasty and stent placement: predictors of a favorable outcome. Am Heart J 2000;139:64–71.

59. Campese VM, Mitra N, Sandee D. Hypertension in renal parenchymal disease: why is it so resistant to treatment? Kidney Int 2006;69(6):967–73.

60. Logan A, Perlikowski S, Mente A, et al. High prevalence of unrecognized sleep apnoea in drug-resistant hypertension. J Hypertens 2001;19:2271–7.

61. Nieto F, Young T, Lind B, et al. Association of sleep-disordered breathing, sleep apnea, and hypertension in a large community-based study. Sleep Heart Health Study. JAMA 2000;283:1829–36.

62. Lavie P, Hoffstein V. Sleep apnea syndrome: a possible contributing factor to resistant. Sleep 2001;24(6):721–5.

63. Lozano L, Tovar JL, Sampol G, et al. Continuous positive airway pressure treatment in sleep apnea patients with resistant hypertension: a randomized, controlled trial. Journal of hypertension 2010; 28(10):2161–8.

64. Martinez-Garcia MA, Capote F, Campos-Rodriguez F, et al. Effect of CPAP on blood pressure in patients with obstructive sleep apnea and resistant hypertension: the HIPARCO randomized clinical trial. JAMA 2013;310(22):2407–15.

65. Grote L, Hedner J, Peter J. Sleep-related breathing disorder is an independent risk factor for uncontrolled hypertension. J Hypertens 2000;18:679–85.

66. Duchna H, Orth M, Schultze-Werninghaus G. Long-term effects of nasal continuous positive airway pressure on vasodilatory endothelial function in obstructive sleep apnea syndrome. Sleep Breath 2005;9:97–103.

67. Hodin R, Lubitz C, Phitayakorn R, et al. Diagnosis and management of pheochromocytoma. Curr Probl Surg 2014;51(4):151–87.

68. Aucott L, Poobalan A, Smith W, et al. Effects of weight loss in overweight/obese individuals and long-term hypertension outcomes: a systematic review. Hypertension 2005;45:1035–41.

69. Vollmer W, Sacks F, Ard J, et al, DASH Sodium Trial Collaborative Research Group. Effects of diet and sodium intake on blood pressure: subgroup analysis of the DASH-sodium trial. Ann Intern Med 2001;135:1019–28.

70. Whelton S, Chin A, Xin X, et al. Effect of aerobic exercise on blood pressure: a meta-analysis of randomized, controlled trials. Ann Intern Med 2002; 136:493–503.

71. Dimeo F, Pagonas N, Seibert F, et al. Aerobic exercise reduces blood pressure in resistant hypertension. Hypertension 2012;60:653–8.

72. Zhang X, Eirin A, Li ZL, et al. Angiotensin receptor blockade has protective effects on the poststenotic porcine kidney. Kidney Int 2013;84(4): 767–75.

73. Khanna A, Lefkowitz L, White W. Evaluation of recent fixed-dose combination therapies in the management of hypertension. Curr Opin Nephrol Hypertens 2008;17:477–83.

74. White WB, Calhoun DA, Samuel R. Improving blood pressure control: increase the dose of diuretic or switch to a fixed-dose angiotensin receptor blocker/diuretic? the valsartan hydrochlorothiazide diuretic for initial control and titration to achieve optimal therapeutic effect (Val-DICTATE) trial. Journal of clinical hypertension 2008;10(6):450–8.

75. Ernst M, Carter B, Goerdt C, et al. Comparative antihypertensive effects of hydrochlorothiazide and chlorthalidone on ambulatory and office blood pressure. Hypertension 2006;47:352–8.

76. Khosla N, Chua D, Elliott W, et al. Are chlorthalidone and hydrochlorothiazide equivalent bloodpressure-lowering medications? J Clin Hypertens (Greenwich) 2005;7:354–6.

77. Nishizaka M, Zaman M, Calhoun D. Efficacy of lowdose spironolactone in subjects with resistant hypertension. Am J Hypertens 2003;16:925–30.

78. Pratt-Ubunama M, Nishizaka M, Boedefeld R, et al. Plasma aldosterone is related to severity of obstructive sleep apnea in subjects with resistant hypertension. Chest 2007;131:453–9.

79. Cheung CM, Chrysochou C, Shurrab AE, et al. Effects of renal volume and single-kidney glomerular filtration rate on renal functional outcome in atherosclerotic renal artery stenosis. Nephrol Dial Transplant 2010;25(4):1133–40.

80. Alvarez-Alvarez B, Abad-Cardiel M, Fernandez-Cruz A, et al. Management of resistant arterial hypertension: role of spironolactone versus double blockade of the renin-angiotensin-aldosterone system. Journal of Hypertension 2010;28(11): 2329–35.

81. Calhoun D, Nishizaka M, Zaman M, et al. Aldosterone excretion among subjects with resistant hypertension and symptoms of sleep apnea. Chest 2004;125:112–7.

82. Calhoun DA, White WB. Effectiveness of the selective aldosterone blocker, eplerenone, in patients with resistant hypertension. Journal of the American Society of Hypertension JASH 2008;2(6): 462–8.

83. Liu G, Zheng XX, Xu YL, et al. Effect of aldosterone antagonists on blood pressure in patients with resistant hypertension: a meta-analysis. Journal of Human Hypertension 2014.

84. Hanselin MR, Saseen JJ, Allen RR, et al. Description of antihypertensive use in patients with resistant hypertension prescribed four or more agents. Hypertension 2011;58(6):1008–13.

85. Saha C, Eckert GJ, Ambrosius WT, et al. Improvement in blood pressure with inhibition of the epithelial sodium channel in blacks with hypertension. Hypertension 2005;46(3):481–7.

86. Cefalu WT, Boulton AJ, Tamborlane WV, et al. Status of Diabetes Care: "It just doesn't get any better... or does it?". Diabetes Care 2014;37(7): 1782–5.

87. Lane DA, Beevers DG. Amiloride 10 mg is less effective than spironolactone 25 mg in patients with hypertension resistant to a multidrug regime including an angiotensin-blocking agent. Journal of Hypertension 2007;25(12):2515–6.

88. Bisognano J, Sloand J, Papademetriou V, et al. An implantable carotid sinus baroreflex activating system for drug-resistant hypertension: interim chronic efficacy results from the multicenter Rheos Feasibility Trial. Circulation 2006;114(Suppl 18):II575.

89. Illig K, Levy M, Sanchez L, et al. An implantable carotid sinus stimulator for drug-resistant hypertension: surgical technique and short-term outcome from the multicenter phase II Rheos Feasibility Trial. J Vasc Surg 2006;44(6):1213–8.

90. Bisognano J, Bakris G, Nadim M, et al. Baroreflex activation therapy lowers blood pressure in patients with resistant hypertension: results from the double-blind, randomized, placebo-controlled Rheos Pivotal Trial. J Am Coll Cardiol 2011;58: 765–73.

91. Bakris G, Nadim M, Haller H, et al. Baroreflex activation therapy provides durable benefit in patients with resistant hypertension: results of long-term follow-up in the Rheos Pivotal Trial. J Am Soc Hypertens 2012;6:152–8.

92. Hoppe U, Brandt M, Wachter R, et al. Minimally invasive system for baroreflex activation therapy chronically lowers blood pressure with pacemaker-like safety profile: results from the Barostim neo trial. J Am Soc Hypertens 2012;6:270–6.

93. Scheffers IJ, Kroon AA, Schmidli J, et al. Novel baroreflex activation therapy in resistant hypertension: results of a European multi-center feasibility study. Journal of the American College of Cardiology 2010;56(15):1254–8.

94. Bisognano J, Kaufman C, Bach D, et al, DEBuT-HT, Rheos Feasibility Trial Investigators. Improved cardiac structure and function with chronic treatment using an implantable device in resistant hypertension: results from European and United States trials of the Rheos system. J Am Coll Cardiol 2011;57: 1787–8.

95. Krum H, Schlaich M, Whitbourn R, et al. Catheter-based renal sympathetic denervation for resistant hypertension: a multicentre safety and proof-of-principle cohort study. Lancet 2009;373:1275–81.

96. SYMPLICITY-HTN-2-Investigators. Renal sympathetic denervation in patients with treatment-resistant hypertension (The SYMPLICITY HTN-2 Trial): a randomized controlled trial. Lancet 2010; 376(9756):1903–9.

97. Bhatt DL, Kandzari DE, O'Neill WW, et al. A controlled trial of renal denervation for resistant hypertension. The New England Journal of Medicine 2014;370(15):1393–401.

98. Bakris GL, Townsend RR, Liu M, et al. Impact of Renal Denervation on 24-hour Ambulatory Blood Pressure: Results from SYMPLICITY HTN-3. Journal of the American College of Cardiology 2014. May 17.

99. Stabile E, Ambrosini V, Squarcia R, et al. Percutaneous sympathectomy of the renal arteries: the OneShot Renal Denervation System is not associated with significant vessel wall injury. EuroIntervention 2013;9(6):694–9.

100. Templin C, Jaguszewski M, Ghadri JR, et al. Vascular lesions induced by renal nerve ablation as assessed by optical coherence tomography: pre- and post-procedural comparison with the Simplicity catheter system and the EnligHTN multi-electrode renal denervation catheter. Eur Heart J 2013;34(28):2141–8, 2148b.

Advances in Peripheral Arterial Disease Endovascular Revascularization

 CrossMark

Ambrose Panico, DO[a], Asif Jafferani, MD[a], Falak Shah, MD[a],
Robert S. Dieter, MD, RVT[b],*

KEYWORDS

- Peripheral arterial disease • Chronic total occlusion • Atherectomy • Complication • Outcome

KEY POINTS

- Peripheral arterial disease (PAD) has increasingly become a worldwide problem; in the United States PAD affects 8-12 million Americans.
- Significant advances have been made in the endovascular treatment of lower extremity arterial occlusive disease.
- Since the last update in 2011, new technologies have been developed, predominantly in reentry devices and treatment of chronic total occlusion lesions.

HISTORY OF PERIPHERAL ARTERIAL DISEASE INTERVENTION

Peripheral arterial disease (PAD) has increasingly become a worldwide problem; in the United States, PAD has a prevalence of 12% in the general population, affecting 8-12 million Americans.[1,2] The prevalence of PAD increases with age and is as high as 20% in Americans older than 65, affecting as many as 7.6 million people (prevalence becomes exponentially higher with the presence additional risk factors for vascular disease).[1,2] PAD of the lower extremities encompasses a wide clinical spectrum that ranges from asymptomatic disease to critical limb ischemia. Left untreated, advanced PAD can lead to significant morbidity,[2] and is the most common cause of lower extremity amputation when not revascularized.[3] Limb preservation can lead to significantly decreased mortality (2-year mortality in patients undergoing amputation is nearly 40%[3]).

Over the last decade, the number of endovascular procedures for critical limb ischemia has increased by nearly 4-fold, which has coincided with a significant decrease in amputation rates.[4]

Lower extremity PAD presents unique clinical and therapeutic challenges. The management of lower extremity PAD can be extremely difficult given the diffuse atherosclerotic burden, chronic total occlusion (CTO), presence of critical limb ischemia, and lack of quality distal run-off. These unique features limit the success of traditional, angioplasty-based (endovascular) therapies/interventions and contribute to the disappointing results observed with balloon angioplasty for management of these complex lesions.[5] These clinical and technical challenges have led to the development of a myriad of new technologies aimed to enhance the safety and improve the effectiveness of percutaneous revascularization strategies in the management of PAD.

The authors have nothing to disclose.
[a] Loyola University Medical Center, Maywood, IL 60153, USA; [b] Stritch School of Medicine, Loyola University Medical Center, Maywood, IL 60153, USA
* Corresponding author. 2160 S First Ave, Maywood, IL 60153.
E-mail address: RDIETER@LUMC.EDU

Cardiol Clin 33 (2015) 89–98
http://dx.doi.org/10.1016/j.ccl.2014.09.002
0733-8651/15/$ – see front matter Published by Elsevier Inc.

cardiology.theclinics.com

This review builds on the recent advances in the endovascular management of PAD as discussed in 2011.[6] Therefore, for relevancy, it focuses on the technologies related to atherectomy, advances in nitinol self-expanding balloon stents, and advances in device technology for the treatment of CTO. Available drug-eluting technologies are reviewed elsewhere in this issue of *Cardiology Clinics*. For other interventions, please refer to the 2011 update.[6]

ADVANCES IN PLAQUE REMOVAL AND DEBULKING
Atherectomy

Excimer laser
Early attempts at laser-based endovascular devices used continuous-wave, heat-tipped laser technology. These early attempts were quickly abandoned in the late 1980s owing to high complication rates from thermal damage to the surrounding vascular tissues, leading to high restenosis rates.[7] The advent of the excimer laser-assisted system (Spectranetics Corporation, Colorado Springs, CO) allowed for the use of flexible fiberoptic catheters capable of directing ultraviolet light to penetrate into the fibrous cap/plaque. The 308-nm laser a has short penetration depth of 50 μm, which allows for direct ablation of the plaque on contact alone, without a subsequent rise in surrounding temperature delivered to the surrounding tissue. These catheters showed promising initial success rates of 90.5% with primary and secondary patency rates of 33% and 75.9%, respectively, as reported by Scheinert and colleagues.[8] These results were echoed in the Peripheral Excimer Laser Angioplasty (PELA) Trial with primary patency rates determined by ultrasound of 48% in the laser arm and 58% in the angioplasty arm.[9]

The design of the TURBO-Booster catheter (Spectranetics Corporation) aimed to create a channel larger than the diameter of the catheter itself, utilizing a custom guide catheter that allowed for the laser to directionally ablate tissue, thus creating a larger lumen. Utilizing these catheters, the Clirpath Excimer Laser System to Enlarge Lumen Openings (CELLO) study demonstrated patency rates (percent stenosis <50%) of 59% and 54% at 6 and 12 months, respectively, with target lesion revascularization (TLR) required in 23.1% of study participants.[10]

Excisional and orbital atherectomy
Since the 2011 update,[6] there have been only a few significant trials comparing directional atherectomy devices to primary balloon angioplasty

(PBA). In a prospective, 2-center, randomized trial, the SilverHawk atherectomy catheter (Covidien, Plymouth, CO) with adjunctive PBA was compared with PBA alone for treatment of infrainguinal disease.[11] Fifty-eight patients were randomized (36 vessels in the atherectomy arm and 48 vessels in PBA arm) and followed for the primary endpoint of TLR at 1 year, secondary outcomes rate of "bailout" stent placement, and the rate of target vessel revascularization. Results of the study showed no difference in TLR at 1 year (16.7% vs 11.1%) or target vessel revascularization (21.4% vs 11.1%). There was, however, a significant difference in the need for bailout stent placement (27.6% in the atherectomy arm vs 62.1% in the PBA arm; $P = .017$).

Major adverse outcomes were similar between groups; however, there was a significant difference in distal microembolization (64.7% [n = 17] vs 0% [n = 10]) when an embolic filter was used.[11] The prospective, multicenter, single-arm DEFINITIVE Ca^{++} study aimed at evaluating the effectiveness and safety of the SilverHawk and TurboHawk (Covidien, Plymouth, CO) catheters when used with a distal embolic protection device.[12] The 30-day freedom from major adverse events was 93.1%, with a primary effectiveness endpoint ($\leq$50% residual diameter stenosis) of 92%. Technical success showed a residual diameter stenosis of 33.3% (further reduced to 24.1% with adjunctive therapy). The clinical improvement to asymptomatic status (Rutherford–Becker Class = 0) at 30 days increased from 0% to 52.3%; 88.5% of patients experienced a symptomatic improvement of at least 1 Rutherford–Becker Class categories.

Jetstream
Jetstream systems (Bayer Health System, Leverkusen, Germany) offer both expandable and single-cutter options. The expandable system achieves graded atherectomy using 2 sets of rotating stainless steel blades. The first set of blades sits within a fenestrated metal housing situated at the tip of the catheter, which allows cutting in a diameter just over 3 mm when rotated clockwise. The second set of 5 blades are hinged and mounted just proximal from the distal housing, also allowing for cutting to a diameter of 3 mm when rotated counterclockwise. The single-cutter catheter system has a longer working shaft, which allows for it to be utilized for the revascularization of more distal lesions and is available in sizes ranging from 1.6 to 1.85 mm. Both systems work via differential cutting, which allows for fibrous and calcified tissue/plaque to be preferentially cut sparing the normal more compliant tissue.

Before approval, the Jetstream device was studied by Zeller and colleagues[13] in the Pathway PVD trial. Lesion crossing and debulking success rate was 99%, minor embolic events were observed in 10% of cases, and perforations were seen in 2% (n = 4). Patients were followed for major adverse events, which occurred in 19% of patients; most of these events were TLR at a rate of 15% and 26%, at 6 and 12 months, respectively.

Distal embolism among the more common concerns when atherectomy is pursued, especially in the setting of single vessel run-off. Shrikhande and colleagues[14] reviewed available prospective registry data to examine the incidence of distal embolization during the treatment of 2137 lesions in 1029 patients undergoing atherectomy using 4 different atherectomy devices. Significantly, they found an overall embolization rate of 1.6% (review based on pre and post run-off angiograms) with higher rates of embolization seen in both more complex lesions and CTO compared with de novo lesions (3.2% vs 2.4% vs 0.9%, respectively; P = .01), as well as with specific devices (**Fig. 1**).

RECENT ADVANCES IN NITINOL STENT TECHNOLOGIES

Among the non–drug-eluting, self-expanding stents, the SUPERA peripheral stent system (Abbott Vascular, Santa Clara, CA) is among the newer technologies that has recently been made available.

SUPERA

Self-expanding nitinol stents have improved the patency rates of conventional percutaneous transluminal angioplasty with provisional stenting. However, restenosis and stent fracture rates,

particularly in anatomically vulnerable positions like the superficial femoral artery (SFA) or popliteal lesions, remain a concern. The SUPERA stent aims to improve on these rates through a novel design. The SUPERA stent is an interwoven nitinol stent constructed from 6 pairs of nitinol wires forming closed loops at both ends (**Fig. 2**). The biomechanics of this helical stent imparts greater radial compression resistance and flexibility without unwanted chronic outward force or barotrauma against the artery, theoretically allowing this stent to be ideal for revascularization of SFA and popliteal lesions. Accumulated clinical experience seems to support this hypothesis. Registry data from Leipzig, Germany, have shown significant success in SFA (137 stents) and popliteal lesions (125 stents) with primary patency at 12 months reported at 84.7% ± 3.6% and 87.7 ± 3.7%, respectively.[15,16] No stent fractures were reported in both studies, with clinically significant improvements in the Ankle–Brachial Index and Rutherford–Becker class scores. Similarly, experience from the United States has indicated that the primary patency rate with the use of the SUPERA stent (39 stent cases) is 79.2% at 1 year in the popliteal artery.[17] No stent fractures were reported.

These results have been reproduced in another registry that reported a patency rate of 78.6% for 96 stent cases.[18] Similarly, George and colleagues[19] also reported primary patency rates of 85.8% at 1 year in 08 limbo with SUPERA stents. These studies have not reported any stent fractures. This clinical success has prompted the SUPERB trial. Preliminary data from SUPERB suggests that in 266 lesions treated with SUPERA stents, primary patency rates remained at 86% with the freedom from TLR reported to be 90% at 1 year.[20] No stent fractures were observed.

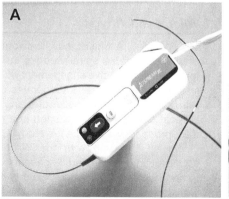 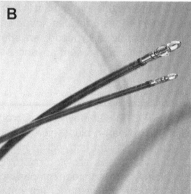

Fig. 1. JETSTREAM atherectomy system. (*A*) Ergonomic design allows for single or dual operator options. (*B*) Catheters available in both single and eXpandable cutting design. (*Courtesy of* Bayer HealthCare LLC, Whippany, NJ; with permission. JETSTREAM is a required trademark of Bayer HealthCare LLC.)

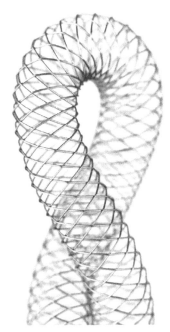

Fig. 2. The SUPERA stent is an interwoven nitinol stent constructed from 6 pairs of nitinol wires forming closed loops at both ends. This helical stent imparts greater radial compression resistance and flexibility without unwanted chronic outward force or barotrauma against the artery. Theoretically, this stent is ideal for revascularization of SFA and popliteal lesions. Illustration is artist rendition. Not drawn to scale. (*Courtesy of* Abbott Vascular. © 2014 Abbott. All Rights Reserved.)

RECENT ADVANCES IN ENDOVASCULAR TREATMENT OF CHRONIC TOTAL OCCLUSION

Endovascular treatment of CTO presents a special set of challenges to the interventionalist. Fortunately, many devices and techniques are available to tackle this issue. This section reviews devices that allow cap penetration, lesion crossing, and entry into the true lumen with improvement in technical success. Some of these devices have been reviewed in the 2011 update[6]; hence, an effort has been made to limit this to recent advances in CTO devices (**Table 1**).

FrontRunner

The FrontRunner XP CTO catheter (J & J Cordis, New Brunswick, NJ) relies on blunt microdissection. The catheter has a blunt end with a hinged jaw, which opens and closes allowing microdissection of the plaque and consequent passage of the guidewire through the lesion for adjunctive angioplasty.

A number of studies have reported good success with the use of the FrontRunner device,[21–23]

with complications of minor perforations or distal extensions of dissections reported. Recently, Shetty and colleagues[24] reported a 95.5% procedural success rate with the use of FrontRunner XP device in 26 SFA and popliteal Trans-Atlantic Inter-Society Class D (TASC D) CTOs. No procedural complications were reported. Additionally, the FrontRunner XP device has been successful in the recanalization of CTO of other peripheral arteries, such as the subclavian and celiomesenteric arteries.[25,26]

Crosser Device

The Crosser CTO Recanalization system (Flow-Cardia, Sunnyvale, CA) utilizes high-frequency (20 kHz), low-amplitude, vibrational energy to break the CTO cap. The system consists of a generator, a transducer, and a disposable, monorail, hydrophilic catheter with irrigation ports at the hub. The catheter is placed in direct contact with the fibroatheromatous plaque cap of the CTO, and transmits vibration energy, allowing recanalization of the CTO and passage of the guidewire. Preliminary experience in small case series reported a greater than 70% success rate with the use of the Crosser catheter.[27,28] However, Khalid and colleagues[29] reported a series of 25 patients with 27 CTOs, in which the Crosser catheter was used as the primary CTO crossing device. The success rate was only 41%. Only 1 complication of a small, local perforation at the lesion site was directly attributed to the Crosser catheter. A study by Staniloae and colleagues[30] reported a technical success rate of 77% in 73 CTOs that underwent recanalization using the Crosser device with no direct catheter related complications noted. Preliminary findings from the Peripheral Approach To Recanalization In Occluded Totals (PATRIOT) study show a success rate 81% for revascularization of CTOs.[31]

Wildcat and Kittycat

The Wildcat (Avinger, Inc, Redwood City, CA) employs rotatable spiral wedges in its distal tip for active and passive engagement with the plaque lesion. The Kittycat device operates on the same principle, but with a smaller crossing profile. The Wildcat catheter was evaluated in a nonrandomized, prospective, multicenter study, Chronic Total Occlusion Crossing with the Wildcat Catheter (CONNECT) that enrolled 88 patients with a single femoropopliteal CTO lesion.[32] Eighty-four patients were treated per protocol with the Wildcat catheter after conventional guidewire failure, with 89% technical success as well as secondary endpoints, which included device, lesion, and procedural

Table 1
Summary of devices used in the treatment of chronic total occlusions

Devices	Study	Patients (n)	Mean Lesion Length (cm)	Success Rate, % (Level)	Clinically Significant Complications (n)
FrontRunner XP (J & J Cordis, New Brunswick, NJ)	Mossop et al,[22] 2006	36 patients (44 lesions)	9.275	91 (II)	0
	Charalambous et al,[23] 2010	26	17.6	65.38 (I)	2
	Shetty et al,[24] 2013	22	18	95.5 (I)	NR
CROSSER (FlowCardia, Sunnyvale, CA)	Khalid et al,[29] 2010	25 patients (27 lesions)	11.7	41 (I)	2
	Staniloae et al,[30] 2011	56 patients (73 lesions)	NR	76.7 (I)	0
	PATRIOT,[31] 2007	85	14	81.2 (I)	0
Wildcat (Avinger, Inc, Redwood City, CA)	CONNECT,[32] 2012	84	17.4	89 (I)	4
Vibrational Angioplasty	Kapralos et al,[35] 2014	27 patients (28 lesions)	5.6	89.3 (II)	0
Ocelot System (Avinger, Inc, Redwood City, CA)	Schwindt et al,[36] 2013	33	20.5	94 (I)	0
	CONNECT II,[37] 2013	100	16.6	97 (I)	2
TruePath Catheter (Boston Scientific, Natick, MA)	ReOpen,[38] 2014	85	16.7	80 (I)	1
	Banerjee et al,[39] 2014	13	17	77 (I), 100 (II)[a]	0
Excimer laser angioplasty	Steinkamp et al,[40] 2000	94	17.5	80.9 (II)	8
	Boccalandro et al,[42] 2004	25	18	84 (II)	1
Outback LTD (Cordis Corp., Bridgewater, NJ)	Smith et al,[46] 2011	15	18.5	87 (II)	0
	Bausback et al,[48] 2011	113 patients (118 lesions)	19.5	91.5 (I), 90.7 (II)	2
	Aslam et al,[47] 2013	51	23	96 (II)	1
	Gandini et al,[49] 2013	52 patients (26 with interventions)[b]	24.75	100 (I)	0
Pioneer (Medtronic Vascular, Santa Rosa, CA)	Al-Ameri et al,[51] 2009	21	10.7	95 (II)	1
	Smith et al,[46] 2011	8	24.8	100 (II)	0
Bridgepoint system	Banerjee et al,[54] 2014	15 patients (17 lesions)	18.3	88 (I), 100 (II)[a]	0
Viance and Enteer System	PFAST-CTO,[55] 2012	66	19.5	84 (I)	3

Smaller case series have not been included. Clinically significant complications include device-related complications that required further interventions.

Success rates have been defined as follows: (I) technical success, which is achieving successful lesion crossing; or (II) procedural success, which is the successful recanalization of the target lesion.

Abbreviation: NR, not reported.

[a] Does not include lesions that employed the use of a reentry device additionally in technical success rates.

[b] Randomized, controlled trial of 52 patients equally divided into intervention and control arms.

success. Complications included a 4.8% rate of perforations (measured per protocol). Per the authors, this rate is comparable with the efficacy and safety rates reported for other devices.

Vibrational Angioplasty

Vibrational angioplasty is a technique in which a conventional guidewire is connected to a device that imparts mechanical vibration to the guidewire. This is used to break the cap of the CTO to allow access and further navigation along the path of least resistance for successful crossing of the CTO. Smaller separate series in the literature have reported technical success rates of 100% in 6 cases of femoropopliteal lesions,[33] and of 92% in 13 infrapopliteal cases with 1 arterial perforation without sequelae.[34] More recently, however, Kapralos and colleagues[35] reported a series of 28 CTO cases in 27 patients with a technical success rate of 89% and no complications reported. Failure to cross was attributed to the inability to penetrate the calcified cap in 2 cases and the inability to cross the obstruction intraluminally after successful cap penetration.

Ocelot Catheter

The Ocelot system (Avinger, Inc.) has a distal tip with spiral wedges allowing clockwise and counterclockwise rotation to advance the catheter through the occlusion. It is additionally connected to an optical coherence tomography lightbox that allows real-time visualization of the catheter and the ability to discriminate between healthy tissue and plaque. The catheter was evaluated in a European trial of 33 CTOs with a technical success rate of 94% and no adverse events reported.[36] As part of the study, interventionalists using the Ocelot system were asked to rate the catheter as well as the optical coherence tomography system across different performance categories. The average experience was rated from excellent to good.

The Chronic Total Occlusion Crossing with the Ocelot System II (CONNECT II) trial was designed as a nonrandomized, single-arm, multicenter, prospective study to evaluate the safety and efficacy of the Ocelot catheter.[37] One hundred patients were enrolled and the device achieved technical success in 97% of the cases. Two patients experienced vessel perforations as adverse events. The clinical endpoint of improvement in Ankle–Brachial Index to greater than 0.95 was achieved in 88% at discharge, and in 94% at 30 days' follow-up, with significant improvement ($P < .001$) in Rutherford–Becker class.

TruePath Catheter

The TruePath catheter (Boston Scientific Corporation, Natick, MA) is an intraluminal crossing device that uses a distal, diamond coated, radiopaque tip revolving at 13,000 rpm to create a pathway through the CTO. The device is facilitated by a 1:1 torquer and the distal tip is able to bend by 15° to avoid side branches or subintimal passage

of the needle. The ReOpen study was a prospective, nonrandomized, single-arm study to evaluate the TruePath catheter in CTOs of the lower extremity.[38] Technical success in crossing the CTO was achieved in 80% of patients with successful guidewire placement in 76%. Only 1 clinically significant perforation was noted requiring intervention.

In the Excellence in Peripheral Arterial Disease (XLPAD) registry, 13 patients underwent CTO crossing via TruePath.[39] Procedural success was achieved in all cases; however, in 3 cases the guidewire passed into the subintimal space and required the use of a reentry device. The only adverse event noted was a small hematoma (<5 cm) at the entry site in 1 case.

Excimer Laser Angioplasty

Excimer laser angioplasty, as the name suggests, uses an excimer laser to photochemically ablate a path through the atherosclerotic plaque to allow crossing of the CTO. This system is very similar to excimer laser atherectomy, although here only an intraluminal path is sought for the guidewire to cross the CTO. The most widely used system consists of the CVX-300 Excimer Laser System (Spectranetics Corporation) and the Turbo Elite catheter (Spectranetics Corporation), which transmits the laser from the generation system to the tissue. It is frequently used in a step-by-step technique with gradual ablation of the occlusion and attempts made to pass the guidewire repeated in multiple steps until lesion crossing is successful. The procedural success rate has been reported to be greater than 80% in multiple studies,[40–42] with major complications being reported as local perforation of the vessel, acute reocclusion, and distal thromboembolism.

Reentry devices

Subintimal angioplasty (SIA) is a popular technique used to cross a CTO. The technique, first described by Bolia and colleagues[43] in 1990, is successful in about 80% of the cases for successful crossing of the CTO.[44,45] However, the most common reason for the failure of this technique is the inability to regain access to the true vascular lumen. Accordingly, devices have been developed that aim to increase the success rate of this specialized technique for reentry into the true vascular lumen.

Outback Catheter

The Outback Catheter (Cordis Corp., Bridgewater, NJ) utilizes a hollow, 22-G distal needle that allows controlled entry via fluoroscopy. With the help of

2 fluoroscopic markers at the catheter, the device is positioned appropriately allowing the needle to pierce the subintimal space accessing the true lumen. A number of smaller studies have evaluated the device and reported high technical success rates.[46,47] More recently, however, larger studies and experiences with the device have been reported. Bausback and colleagues,[48] in their center's retrospective review of 118 cases, reported a successful reentry in 91.5% of cases, with revascularization completed in 90.7%. Device-related complications included minor hematomas (4.2%) and 2 cases of failure to withdraw the needle into the catheter. Interestingly, Outback is also the only device evaluated for CTOs that has been subjected to a randomized, controlled trial.

Gandini and colleagues[49] recently reported on 52 patients comparing the Outback catheter with manual reentry. Technical success was achieved in all cases; however, the use of the Outback catheter improved on successful in-target reentry rates (defined as reentry within 5 cm of the dissection). The Outback catheter was 100% successful, whereas the manual method was successful in only 42% of the cases. Use of the Outback catheter was also significantly associated with reduced mean procedural and mean fluoroscopy time (36.0 ± 9.4 and 29.8 ± 8.9 min compared with 55.4 ± 14.2 min and 39.6 ± 13.9 min, respectively). No device-related complications were reported.

Furthermore, another study has looked at factors influencing failure of the Outback device in allowing successful reentry after SIA.[50] Moderate to severe calcification remained the only significant predictor of failure with the Outback device (odds ratio, 6.3; 95% CI, 1.45–24.48).

Pioneer Catheter

The Pioneer catheter (Medtronic Vascular, Santa Rosa, CA) is another reentry device that utilizes intravascular ultrasound technology to gain successful reentry into the vascular lumen. Intravascular ultrasonography allows imaging of the true lumen distal to the CTO, allowing the catheter to be positioned appropriately for a needle deployment, which gains access to the true lumen, through which a guidewire can be passed and conventional angioplasty can proceed. The Pioneer catheter has also reported a high success rate in several small case series. A series by Al-Ameri and colleagues[51] reported the successful use of the device in 21 CTOs, which had failed reentry via conventional guidewire techniques. Pioneer was successful in 95% of the cases. No complications related to the reentry device were reported. Similarly, Smith and colleagues[46] in

their experience with both of the reentry devices reported a 100% success rate with the use of the Pioneer catheter in 8 patients, with no complications.

Bridgepoint System

Of the reviewed devices, which aim for direct cap penetration and crossing of the CTO while remaining in the true lumen, cases of entry into the subintimal space invariably do occur, requiring the use of either the conventional Bolia technique for subintimal angioplasty or the use of reentry devices. The Bridgepoint system is unique in that it contains a catheter for intraluminal passage of CTOs—the CrossBoss catheter, which has a rotating tip that rotates along a torque device allowing penetration of the CTO cap and passage of the guidewire. Also present are the Stingray Balloon catheter and Stingray Guidewire. These are useful in instances when the CrossBoss is unable to be advanced and SIA needs to be attempted, with the Stingray system allowing reentry into the true lumen. The Stingray balloon catheter is a self-orienting, flat-topped balloon that allows entry of the guidewire through a port adjacent to the true vascular lumen. Although this system is designed for use in the coronary vasculature, case reports have described the successful use of this device in peripheral CTOs.[52,53] Banerjee and colleagues,[54] however, demonstrated 100% success with the use of the CrossBoss catheter in 17 infrainguinal CTOs, with 15 not requiring the use of a reentry device. Two patients with minor access site hematomas were the only complications experienced.

Another similar device system, comprising the Viance crossing catheter and the Enteer reentry catheter (Covidien, Mansfield, MA) were investigated in the Peripheral Facilitated Antegrade Steering Technique in Chronic Total Occlusions (PFAST-CTO) trial.[55] In this study, 66 patients with CTOs were treated first with the Viance catheter and then had SIA attempted with the help of the Enteer catheter to regain true lumen reentry. Of the 45 patients with only the Viance catheter used, technical success was reported at 84%, whereas the success rate was 86% in the 21 patients requiring reentry with the Enteer catheter. The overall technical success rate remained at 85% with rates of major adverse events at 3% in the observed 30-day period.

SUMMARY

Significant advances have been made in the endovascular treatment of lower extremity arterial occlusive disease. Since the last update in 2011, new technologies have been developed, predominantly in reentry devices and treatment of CTO lesions. These advances have allowed for the revascularization of complex vascular lesions in terms of procedural success rates. Although this technical success is encouraging, these technologies must ultimately prove to provide measurable long-term clinical success at a reasonable cost to the health care system. In the ever-changing field of health care where increasingly more importance is placed on cost-conscious practices, more and more scrutiny will be placed on these endovascular procedures. More large, randomized, controlled trials need to be designed to focus on clinical outcomes and success rates for treatment of lower extremity arterial occlusive disease. These trials are required to compare the various options available for treating lower extremity vascular lesions. These trials cannot only evaluate important and meaningful clinical endpoints, but also compare costs among the newer devices. These future studies will serve as the guide by which clinicians can provide the most successful clinical and cost effect care in treating patients with lower-extremity PAD.

REFERENCES

1. Go AS, Mozaffarian D, Roger VL, et al. Heart disease and stroke statistics–2014 update: a report from the American Heart Association. Circulation 2014;129:e28–292.
2. Hirsch AT, Criqui MH, Treat-Jacobson D, et al. Peripheral arterial disease detection, awareness, and treatment in primary care. JAMA 2001;286:1317–24.
3. Norgren L, Hiatt WR, Dormandy JA, et al. Inter-society consensus for the management of peripheral arterial disease (TASC II). J Vasc Surg 2007; 45(Suppl S):S5–67.
4. Egorova NN, Guillerme S, Gelijns A, et al. An analysis of the outcomes of a decade of experience with lower extremity revascularization including limb salvage, lengths of stay, and safety. J Vasc Surg 2010;51:878–85, 885.e1.
5. Rogers JH, Laird JR. Overview of new technologies for lower extremity revascularization. Circulation 2007;116:2072–85.
6. Gandhi S, Sakhuja R, Slovut DP. Recent advances in percutaneous management of iliofemoral and superficial femoral artery disease. Cardiol Clin 2011;29: 381–94.
7. Wollenek G, Laufer G. Comparative study of different laser systems with special regard to angioplasty. Thorac Cardiovasc Surg 1988;36(Suppl 2): 126–32.
8. Scheinert D, Laird JR Jr, Schroder M, et al. Excimer laser-assisted recanalization of long, chronic superficial femoral artery occlusions. J Endovasc Ther 2001;8:156–66.
9. Laird J. Peripheral excimer laser angioplasty (PELA) Trial results. Paper presented at: 14th Annual Scientific Symposium Transcatheter Cardiovascular Therapeutics. Washington, DC, September 24–28, 2002.
10. Dave RM, Patlola R, Kollmeyer K, et al. Excimer laser recanalization of femoropopliteal lesions and 1-year patency: results of the CELLO registry. J Endovasc Ther 2009;16:665–75.
11. Shammas NW, Coiner D, Shammas GA, et al. Percutaneous lower-extremity arterial interventions with primary balloon angioplasty versus Silverhawk atherectomy and adjunctive balloon angioplasty: randomized trial. J Vasc Interv Radiol 2011;22:1223–8.
12. Roberts D, Niazi K, Miller W, et al. Effective endovascular treatment of calcified femoropopliteal disease with directional atherectomy and distal embolic protection: final results of the DEFINITIVE Ca(++) trial. Catheter Cardiovasc Interv 2014;84:236–44.
13. Zeller T, Krankenberg H, Steinkamp H, et al. One-year outcome of percutaneous rotational atherectomy with aspiration in infrainguinal peripheral arterial occlusive disease: the multicenter pathway PVD trial. J Endovasc Ther 2009;16:653–62.
14. Shrikhande GV, Khan SZ, Hussain HG, et al. Lesion types and device characteristics that predict distal embolization during percutaneous lower extremity interventions. J Vasc Surg 2011;53:347–52.
15. Scheinert D, Grummt L, Piorkowski M, et al. A novel self-expanding interwoven nitinol stent for complex femoropopliteal lesions: 24-month results of the SUPERA SFA registry. J Endovasc Ther 2011;18: 745–52.
16. Scheinert D, Werner M, Scheinert S, et al. Treatment of complex atherosclerotic popliteal artery disease with a new self-expanding interwoven nitinol stent: 12-month results of the Leipzig SUPERA popliteal artery stent registry. JACC Cardiovasc Interv 2013;6:65–71.
17. Leon LR Jr, Dieter RS, Gadd CL, et al. Preliminary results of the initial United States experience with the Supera woven nitinol stent in the popliteal artery. J Vasc Surg 2013;57:1014–22.
18. Chan YC, Cheng SW, Ting AC, et al. Primary stenting of femoropopliteal atherosclerotic lesions using new helical interwoven nitinol stents. J Vasc Surg 2014;59:384–91.
19. George JC, Rosen ES, Nachtigall J, et al. SUPERA interwoven nitinol stent outcomes in above-knee interventions (SAKE) study. J Vasc Interv Radiol 2014;25:954–61.
20. Rosenfield K. Comparison of the Supera peripheral system to a performance goal derived from balloon angioplasty clinical trials in the superficial femoral artery Paper presented at: Vascular InterVentional Advances (VIVA). Las Vegas, October 9–12, 2012.

21. Mossop P, Cincotta M, Whitbourn R. First case reports of controlled blunt microdissection for percutaneous transluminal angioplasty of chronic total occlusions in peripheral arteries. Catheter Cardiovasc Interv 2003;59:255–8.

22. Mossop PJ, Amukotuwa SA, Whitbourn RJ. Controlled blunt microdissection for percutaneous recanalization of lower limb arterial chronic total occlusions: a single center experience. Catheter Cardiovasc Interv 2006;68:304–10.

23. Charalambous N, Schafer PJ, Trentmann J, et al. Percutaneous intraluminal recanalization of long, chronic superficial femoral and popliteal occlusions using the Frontrunner XP CTO device: a single-center experience. Cardiovasc Intervent Radiol 2010;33:25–33.

24. Shetty R, Vivek G, Thakkar A, et al. Safety and efficacy of the frontrunner XP catheter for recanalization of chronic total occlusion of the femoropopliteal arteries. J Invasive Cardiol 2013;25:344–7.

25. Michael TT, Banerjee S, Brilakis ES. Use of the frontrunner catheter to cross a chronic total occlusion of the left subclavian artery. Hellenic J Cardiol 2011;52: 86–90.

26. Ayers NP, Zacharias SJ, Abu-Fadel MS, et al. Successful use of blunt microdissection catheter in a chronic total occlusion of a celiomesenteric artery. Catheter Cardiovasc Interv 2007;69:546–9.

27. Al-Ameri H, Mayeda GS, Shavelle DM. Use of high-frequency vibrational energy in the treatment of peripheral chronic total occlusions. Catheter Cardiovasc Interv 2000;74:1110–5.

28. Gandini R, Volpi T, Pipitone V, et al. Intraluminal recanalization of long infrainguinal chronic total occlusions using the Crosser system. J Endovasc Ther 2009;16:23–7.

29. Khalid MR, Khalid FR, Farooqui FA, et al. A novel catheter in patients with peripheral chronic total occlusions: a single center experience. Catheter Cardiovasc Interv 2010;76:735–9.

30. Staniloae CS, Mody KP, Yadav SS, et al. Endoluminal treatment of peripheral chronic total occlusions using the Crosser(R) recanalization catheter. J Invasive Cardiol 2011;23:359–62.

31. Joye J. The PATRIOT (Peripheral approach to recanalization in occluded totals) study results. Paper presented at: 19th Annual Symposium Transcatheter Cardiovascular Therapeutics. Washington, DC, October 20–25, 2007.

32. Pigott JP, Raja ML, Davis T, Connect Trial Investigators. A multicenter experience evaluating chronic total occlusion crossing with the Wildcat catheter (the CONNECT study). J Vasc Surg 2012;56:1615–21.

33. Michalis LK, Tsetis DK, Katsamouris AN, et al. Vibrational angioplasty in the treatment of chronic femoropopliteal arterial occlusions: preliminary experience. J Endovasc Ther 2001;8:615–21.

34. Tsetis DK, Michalis LK, Rees MR, et al. Vibrational angioplasty in the treatment of chronic infrapopliteal arterial occlusions: preliminary experience. J Endovasc Ther 2002;9:889–95.

35. Kapralos I, Kehagias E, Ioannou C, et al. Vibrational angioplasty in recanalization of chronic femoropopliteal arterial occlusions: single center experience. Eur J Radiol 2014;83:155–62.

36. Schwindt A, Reimers B, Scheinert D, et al. Crossing chronic total occlusions with the Ocelot system: the initial European experience. EuroIntervention 2013; 9:854–62.

37. Selmon MR, Schwindt AG, Cawich IM, et al. Final results of the chronic total occlusion crossing with the ocelot system II (CONNECT II) study. J Endovasc Ther 2013;20:770–81.

38. Bosiers M, Diaz-Cartelle J, Scheinert D, et al. Revascularization of lower extremity chronic total occlusions with a novel intraluminal recanalization device: results of the ReOpen study. J Endovasc Ther 2014;21:61–70.

39. Banerjee S, Sarode K, Das T, et al. Endovascular treatment of infrainguinal chronic total occlusions using the TruePath device: features, handling, and 6-month outcomes. J Endovasc Ther 2014; 21:281–8.

40. Steinkamp HJ, Werk M, Haufe M, et al. Laser angioplasty of peripheral arteries after unsuccessful recanalization of the superficial femoral artery. Int J Cardiovasc Intervent 2000;3:153–60.

41. Steinkamp HJ, Rademaker J, Wissgott C, et al. Percutaneous transluminal laser angioplasty versus balloon dilation for treatment of popliteal artery occlusions. J Endovasc Ther 2002;9:882–8.

42. Boccalandro F, Muench A, Sdringola S, et al. Wireless laser-assisted angioplasty of the superficial femoral artery in patients with critical limb ischemia who have failed conventional percutaneous revascularization. Catheter Cardiovasc Interv 2004;63:7–12.

43. Bolia A, Miles KA, Brennan J, et al. Percutaneous transluminal angioplasty of occlusions of the femoral and popliteal arteries by subintimal dissection. Cardiovasc Intervent Radiol 1990;13:357–63.

44. Klimach SG, Gollop ND, Ellis J, et al. How does subintimal angioplasty compare to transluminal angioplasty for the treatment of femoral occlusive disease? Int J Surg 2014;12:361–4.

45. London NJ, Srinivasan R, Naylor AR, et al. Reprinted article "Subintimal angioplasty of femoropopliteal artery occlusions: the long-term results". Eur J Vasc Endovasc Surg 2011;42(Suppl 1):S9–15.

46. Smith M, Pappy R, Hennebry TA. Re-entry devices in the treatment of peripheral chronic occlusions. Tex Heart Inst J 2011;38:392–7.

47. Aslam MS, Allaqaband S, Haddadian B, et al. Subintimal angioplasty with a true reentry device for treatment of chronic total occlusion of the arteries

of the lower extremity. Catheter Cardiovasc Interv 2013;82:701–6.

48. Bausback Y, Botsios S, Flux J, et al. Outback catheter for femoropopliteal occlusions: immediate and long-term results. J Endovasc Ther 2011;18: 13–21.

49. Gandini R, Fabiano S, Spano S, et al. Randomized control study of the outback LTD reentry catheter versus manual reentry for the treatment of chronic total occlusions in the superficial femoral artery. Catheter Cardiovasc Interv 2013;82:485–92.

50. Shin SH, Baril D, Chaer R, et al. Limitations of the Outback LTD re-entry device in femoropopliteal chronic total occlusions. J Vasc Surg 2011;53: 1260–4.

51. Al-Ameri H, Shin V, Mayeda GS, et al. Peripheral chronic total occlusions treated with subintimal angioplasty and a true lumen re-entry device. J Invasive Cardiol 2009;21:468–72.

52. Casserly IP, Rogers RK. Use of Stingray re-entry system in treatment of complex tibial artery occlusive disease. Catheter Cardiovasc Interv 2010;76:584–8.

53. Jessup DB, Lombardi W. Re-canalization of peripheral chronic total occlusions using the BridgePoint Stingray re-entry device. J Interv Cardiol 2011;24: 569–73.

54. Banerjee S, Hadidi O, Mohammad A, et al. Blunt microdissection for endovascular treatment of infrainguinal chronic total occlusions. J Endovasc Ther 2014;21:71–8.

55. Gray WA. Peripheral facilitated antegrade steering technique in chronic total occlusions. Paper presented at: Vascular InterVentional Advances (VIVA). Las Vegas, October 9–12, 2012.

Reperfusion Therapy in the Acute Management of Ischemic Stroke

Michelle P. Lin, MD, MPH[a], Nerses Sanossian, MD[a,b],*

KEYWORDS

- Acute ischemic stroke • Stroke system of care
- Intravenous recombinant tissue plasminogen activator (IV-tPA) • Mechanical thrombectomy
- Thrombolysis in cerebral infarction (TICI score) • American Heart Association
- American Stroke Association

KEY POINTS

- Reperfusion, or restoration of blood flow, is an effective means of reducing disability in the setting of acute stroke.
- Rapid evaluation of stroke begins with community education to recognize signs and symptoms of stroke, an organized system of care by the emergency medical services (EMS) and the emergency department (ED), timely evaluation by the stroke team, and critical care capability.
- Stroke is the fourth leading cause of death after ischemic heart disease, lung cancer, and chronic lower respiratory disease and a leading cause of disability and societal cost in the United States.

INTRODUCTION

An estimated 6.8 million Americans greater than or equal to 20 years of age have had a stroke, and there are approximately 795,000 new or recurrent cases per year with an annual direct and indirect cost of $36.5 billion in 2010.[1,2] Stroke is the fourth leading cause of death after ischemic heart disease, lung cancer, and chronic lower respiratory disease[3] and a leading cause of disability and societal cost in the United States.[3]

This review provides an overview of the acute evaluation and treatment of ischemic stroke, focusing on the role of reperfusion therapy. The discussion is framed around the most recent American Heart Association/American Stroke Association guidelines.[4] Rapid evaluation of stroke begins with community education to recognize signs and symptoms of stroke, an organized system of care by the EMS and the ED, timely evaluation by the stroke team, and critical care capability. Intravenous (IV) thrombolysis with a recombinant tissue plasminogen activator (IV-tPA) within the first 3 hours of stroke symptom onset is the only therapy approved by the US Food and Drug Administration (FDA) for acute ischemic stroke.[5] Recanalization rates for IV-tPA are limited, however, in large-vessel occlusions, which led to the exploration of endovascular therapy.[6] Landmark trials in IV-tPA, endovascular perfusion therapy, and acute medical treatments, including

The authors have nothing to disclose.

[a] Department of Neurology, University of Southern California, Los Angeles, CA 90033, USA; [b] Department of Neurology, Roxanna Todd Hodges Comprehensive Stroke Clinic, University of Southern California, 1520 San Pablo Street, Suite 3000, Los Angeles, CA 90026, USA
* Corresponding author. Roxanna Todd Hodges Comprehensive Stroke Clinic, University of Southern California, 1520 San Pablo Street, Suite 3000, Los Angeles, CA 90026.
E-mail address: sanossia@yahoo.com

Cardiol Clin 33 (2015) 99–109
http://dx.doi.org/10.1016/j.ccl.2014.09.009
0733-8651/15/$ – see front matter © 2015 Elsevier Inc. All rights reserved.

blood pressure (BP) management, aspirin, statin, and anticoagulation, have shaped current understanding of acute stroke care.

EVALUATION OF ACUTE REPERFUSION THERAPY

Rapid recognition of stroke is critical for stroke outcome. The National Institutes of Neurological Disorders and Stroke (NINDS) has established target timeframes in the evaluation of stroke suspects, dubbed "stroke chain of survival" (**Table 1**). A fairly standardized algorithm for evaluating and treating acute ischemic stroke. The first step is to recognize traditional stroke symptoms, including acute facial paresis, arm drift, or abnormal speech, for instance. Analogous to atypical angina, many patients, in particular women, may present with nontraditional stroke symptoms, such as generalized weakness, fatigue, and cognitive changes that can make rapid diagnosis challenging.[7,8] There are major campaigns aimed at the public to improve stroke system recognition, including the face, arm, speech, and time (FAST) educational program. Emergency dispatch operators and paramedics are also trained in stroke recognition using tools, such as the Los Angeles Prehospital Stroke Screen. Routing of patients with suspected stroke to specialized centers bypassing the nearest hospital is increasing throughout the United States.

After arrival in the ED, door-to-noncontrast CT head initiation ought to be done in less than or equal to 25 minutes, and door-to-CT head interpretation in less than or equal to 45 minutes. CT head is useful in differentiating ischemic stroke from hemorrhage stroke, because the treatment pathways of these 2 entities is different. MRI head with diffusion-weighted images is helpful in distinguishing true stroke from stroke mimics, although a vast majority of centers in the US use CT only in the ED. Common stroke mimics include seizure, migraine, hypertensive encephalopathy, space-occupying lesions, toxic/septic/metabolic conditions, or psychogenic.[9] Key blood work to obtain includes complete blood cell count, international normalized ratio/partial thromboplastin time, blood glucose, creatinine, toxicology screen, and troponin. Clinical assessment (history, general examination, and neurologic examination) remains the cornerstone of the evaluation. Stroke scales, such as the National Institutes of Health Stroke Scale (NIHSS), provide important information about the severity of stroke and prognostic information and influence decisions about the acute treatment.

INTRAVENOUS THROMBOLYSIS (INTRAVENOUS THROMBOLYSIS WITH A RECOMBINANT TISSUE PLASMINOGEN ACTIVATOR)

In 1996, the FDA approved the use of IV-tPA for the treatment of acute ischemic stroke within 3 hours of symptom onset, based on the results of the NINDS tPA stroke trial.[5] The trial showed that patients treated with tPA were 30% more likely to have minimal or no functional disability at 3 months (defined as a modified Rankin Scale score [mRS] of 0 or 1)].[4] Later, the European Cooperative Acute Stroke Study III further demonstrated global favorable outcomes when IV-tPA was administered 3 to 4.5 hours after symptom onset (52% vs 45%; OR 1.28; 95% CI, 1.0–1.6), although the effect was less pronounced than in those who received IV-tPA from 0 to 3 hours in the NINDS study (odds ratio [OR] 1.9; 95% CI, 1.2–2.9).[10] Approximately 4.5 patients need to be treated within 1.5 hours, 9 from 1.5 to 3 hours, and 14.1 from 3 to 4.5 hours to have 1 additional patient with no disability at 90 days.[11] The primary complication of treating patients with IV-tPA for acute ischemic stroke is brain hemorrhage. In a pooled analysis, large intracranial hemorrhage (ICH) occurred in 5.2% of patients in the IV-tPA group versus 1.0% of controls (OR 5.37; 95% CI, 3.22–8.95).[11]

Similar to recanalization of occluded coronary vessels, recanalization of intracranial vessels is clearly associated with improved clinical outcome. Zangerle and colleagues[12] reported that 58.3% of patients with recanalization had favorable 90-day mRS scores compared with 5.6% of patients without recanalization (P<.001). In a meta-analysis, Rha and Saver[6] showed that recanalization significantly improved 90-day clinical

Table 1
Emergency department–based care: stroke chain of survival

Action	Time
Door-to-physician	≤10 min
Door-to-stroke team	≤15 min
Door-to-CT scan initiation	≤25 min
Door-to-CT scan interpretation	≤45 min
Door-to-drug (≥80% compliance)	≤60 min
Door-to-stroke unit admission	≤3 h

From Jauch EC, Saver JL, Adams HP, et al. Guidelines for the early management of patients with acute ischemic stroke: a guideline for healthcare professionals from the American Heart Association/American Stroke Association. Stroke 2013;44:870–947; with permission.

outcome (OR 4.43; 95% CI, 3.32–5.91) and mortality (OR 0.24; 95% CI, 0.7–17.4). Clinical efficacy of IV-tPA and its ability to achieve successful recanalization, however, are limited in patients presenting with acute stroke due to large-vessel occlusion, in particular proximally located clots. Sillanpää and colleagues[13] found that greater than 80% of stroke patients treated with IV-tPA with a more distally located clot had good neurologic outcome at 3 months. Proximal middle cerebral artery (MCA) occlusion was associated with only a 22% chance of good outcome, and none of the patients with occlusion located in the most distal segment of the internal carotid artery (ICA) experienced good recovery.[13]

ENDOVASCULAR INTERVENTIONS

Endovascular procedures are often performed in individuals who have received IV-tPA but who have severe strokes with large vessel occlusion and high clot burden. These individuals are thought to respond poorly to IV-tPA, and most ongoing clinical trials with the newer devices are aimed at demonstrating a benefit of a combined IV and intra-arterial (IA) approach versus IV alone.[14] The second group in whom endovascular therapy is potentially beneficial is those ineligible for IV-tPA (eg, time of onset beyond 3–4.5 hours, coagulopathy, recent major surgery within 14 days, or on anticoagulation). Although clinical trials have focused on intervention within a 6-hour window for thrombolytic- and an 8-hour window for device-based therapy, there are situations in which procedures can be performed outside of these time windows, such as in the setting of basilar artery occlusion.

Revascularization Grading Systems

Thrombolysis in Myocardial Infarction (TIMI) and Thrombolysis in Cerebral Infarction (TICI) are 2 of the most commonly used angiographic scores for revascularization/reperfusion in neurointervention for acute ischemic stroke.[15] The TIMI grading system was originally developed to assess the degree of cardiac reperfusion during interventions for acute myocardial infarction. Its prognostic value categorizes a patient's risk of death and ischemic events and provides a basis for therapeutic decision making; it was subsequently applied to neurointerventions.[16] The TICI grading system is a modification of the TIMI scale developed specifically for the intracranial circulation.[17] Grades in both systems range from 0 (no recanalization/reperfusion) to 3 (complete recanalization/reperfusion), but TICI allows a more detailed description of partial recanalization and a greater reperfusion range: none to minimal limited to the parent artery (TICI grade 0 or 1), partial reperfusion beyond the occlusion site (TICI grade 2a), near-complete or greater than 50% reperfusion beyond the occlusion site (TICI grade 2b), or complete (TICI grade 3). **Fig. 1** provides examples of cerebral angiographic runs that correspond to different degrees of the TICI scale.

Intra-arterial Fibrinolysis

As with IV fibrinolysis therapy, reduced time from symptom onset to reperfusion with IA therapies is highly correlated with better clinical outcomes. The Prolyse in Acute Cerebral Thromboembolism (PROACT) II trial evaluated IA thrombolysis with recombinant prourokinase (r-proUK) in patients with NIHSS score greater than or equal to 4 and

| TICI 0 | TICI 1 | TICI 2a | TICI 2b | TICI 3 |

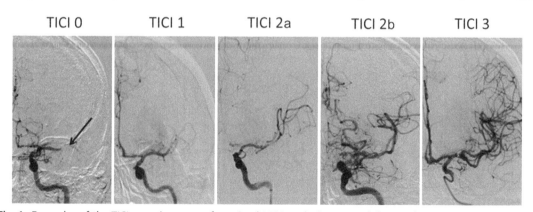

Fig. 1. Examples of the TICI score in a case of proximal MCA occlusion. From left to right: TICI 0 shows no recanalization/reperfusion of the primary occluded vessel (*arrow*). TICI 1 shows partial reperfusion beyond the initial occlusion but no filling of distal MCA branches. TICI 2a and TICI 2b correspond to partial (<50%) and near-complete (>50% but less than full) reperfusion beyond the occlusion site, respectively. TICI 3 indicates complete reperfusion of the entire MCA territory. (*From* Mokin M, Khalessi A, Mocco J, et al. Endovascular treatment of acute ischemic stroke: the end or just the beginning? Neurosurg Focus 2014;36:E5; with permission.)

suspected of having MCA occlusion.[18] Among the 180 randomized patients, 40% of the 121 patients treated with IA thrombolysis (IV r-proUK + IV heparin) and 25% of the 59 control (IV heparin) patients had an mRS score of 0 to 2 at 90 days (P = .04). MCA recanalization was achieved in 66% of the r-proUK arm and in 18% of the control group (P = .001). Symptomatic ICH occurred in 10% of patients treated with r-proUK and in 2% of the control group (P = .06).[18] Mortality rates were similar between the 2 groups.

Mechanical Thrombectomy

The number of options for endovascular treatment of ischemic stroke has increased substantially over the past decade to include IA fibrinolysis, mechanical clot retrieval, mechanical aspiration, and acute angioplasty and stenting. There are currently 4 devices cleared by the FDA for recanalization of arterial occlusion in patients with ischemic stroke. **Fig. 2**A shows the Mechanical Embolus Removal in Cerebral Ischemia (MERCI) clot retrieval system (Stryker Neurovascular, Fremont, California). **Fig. 2**C shows the mechanical clot aspiration with the Penumbra system (Penumbra Inc, Alameda, California). **Fig. 2**B, D shows the stent retrieval systems, Solitaire (ev3 Neurovascular, Irvine, California) and Trevo (Stryker Neurovascular).

Table 2 summarizes the key randomized controlled trials done on endovascular therapy for acute ischemic stroke. Two randomized trials—Solitaire With the Intention for Thrombectomy (SWIFT) and Trevo versus MERCI retrievers for thrombectomy revascularization of large vessel occlusions in acute ischemic stroke (TREVO2)—that compared the MERCI clot-retriever to Solitaire or Trevo stent retrievers in patients treated

within 8 hours of symptom onset demonstrated higher revascularization rates of greater than 80%.[19,20] In the SWIFT trial, a remarkable 58% of patients achieved good neurologic outcome at 3 months, compared with only 33% of patients in the MERCI group.[19] At the same time, mortality rates were lower in the Solitaire group than in the MERCI group (17% vs 38%, respectively). Solitaire FR and Trevo were both approved by FDA for treatment of stroke due to large-vessel occlusion. The relative effectiveness of the Penumbra system versus stent retrievers is not yet characterized.

Angioplasty/Stenting Versus Intravenous Thrombolysis with Recombinant Tissue Plasminogen Activator Trials

Three randomized controlled trials, Interventional Management of Stroke (IMS) III, Mechanical Retrieval and Recanalization of Stroke Clots Using Embolectomy (MR RESCUE), and SYNTHESIS-Expansion,[21–23] aimed to compare the efficacy of endovascular treatment to IV-tPA. The design and key outcomes of the trials are summarized in **Table 2**.

The IMS III trial randomized eligible patients who had received IV alteplase within 3 hours after symptom onset to receive additional endovascular treatment or no additional treatment, in a 2:1 ratio.[21] The primary outcome measure was an mRS score of less than or equal to 2 at 90 days (see **Table 2**). The proportion of participants with the desired primary outcome at 90 days was not statistically significant among patients treated with endovascular treatment and those treated with IV-tPA (40.8% vs 38.7%; P .25). The proportion of patients with symptomatic ICH within

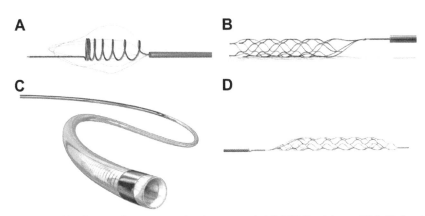

Fig. 2. Devices approved by the FDA for acute stroke clot removal: (A) MERCI retriever, (B) Solitaire stent retriever, (C) Penumbra aspiration system, and (D) TREVO2 stent retriever (ev3 Neurovascular, Irvine, California). (From Khatri P. Evaluation and management of acute ischemic stroke. Continuum (Minneap Minn) 2014;20:283–95; with permission.)

30 hours after initiation of IV-tPA was similar between the 2 groups (6.2% vs 5.9%; $P = .8$).[21]

In the MR RESCUE trial, patients were randomized to mechanical embolectomy (MERCI retriever or Penumbra system) with optional IA thrombolysis or IV-tPA.[22] Patients were further stratified by the presence of a favorable penumbral pattern (substantial salvageable tissue and small infarct core) or not, prior to randomization on pretreatment CT or MRI of the brain. The mean scores on the mRS at 3 months did not differ between embolectomy and standard care (3.9 vs 3.9; $P = .99$). Symptomatic ICH was seen in 3 of 64 and in 2 of 54 patients randomized to embolectomy or standard care, respectively. Patients with penumbral pattern had smaller infarct volumes and lower mRS at 90 days regardless of the treatment modality.[22]

The SYNTHESIS-Expansion trial randomized 362 patients to endovascular treatment, which was predominantly IA thrombolysis and the option of mechanical thrombectomy or IV-tPA The primary outcome was defined by an mRS of 0 or 1 at 3 months.[23] The primary outcome was seen in 30.4% of the patients treated with endovascular treatment and in 34.8% of those treated with IV alteplase at 3 months.[23] The adjusted odds of primary outcome were not statistically significant (OR 0.71; 95% CI, 0.44–1.14; $P = .16$). Symptomatic ICH within 7 days occurred in 6% of patients from each group.[23]

Overall, the 3 trials did not demonstrate superiority of endovascular treatment and the safety parameters were comparable. However, it is possible that endovascualr treatment may benefit selected subgroups such as in those with severe deficits (NIHSS>20), in patients with large proximal arterial occlusion. In addition, the effectiveness of newer retriever devices have not been thoroughly studied.[24,25]

Coronary Versus Cerebral Artery Reperfusion Therapy

Endovascular reperfusion therapies for myocardial infarction and ischemic stroke have evolved in similar patterns: first was IV fibrinolysis, followed by IA fibrinolysis, and then mechanical thrombectomy. Patel and Saver[26] performed a systematic, comparative analysis of recanalization/reperfusion outcomes of these 2 distinctive circulatory beds: 37 trials of coronary reperfusion that enrolled 10,908 patients from 1983 to 2009 and 10 trials of cerebral reperfusion that enrolled 1064 patients from 1992 to 2009 were compared.[26] In both circulatory beds, endovascular treatments were more efficacious at achieving reperfusion than

peripherally administered fibrinolytics. In the coronary bed, rates of achieved reperfusion began at high levels in the 1980s and improved modestly over the subsequent 3 decades. In the cerebral bed, reperfusion rates began at modest levels in the early 1990s and increased more slowly (Fig. 3).[26] With an anchor added for spontaneous reperfusion rates in the reperfusion therapy era, analysis of complete reperfusion rates showed a rapid rise to plateau of 80% to 90% for coronary reperfusion versus a slow rise to plateau of 20% to 25% for cerebral reperfusion (see Fig. 3).[26]

STANDARD MEDICAL THERAPY

Postreperfusion therapy care is essential because approximately 25% of patients may have neurologic worsening during the first 24 to 48 hours after stroke and it is difficult to predict which patients will deteriorate.[27] A dedicated stroke unit with nursing expertise is pivotal in the management of acute stroke patients. Key components of medical therapy for acute stroke beyond IV-tPA include BP modulation, antiplatelet and neuroprotective agents (statins), cardiac monitoring, respiratory support, normothermia, and normoglycemia.[4,27]

Blood Pressure

Elevated BP is common during the acute phase of ischemic stroke, but, owing to a lack of data, BP goal in this setting is controversial and is based on expert opinion. Due to the concern regarding reducing perfusion to an already ischemic brain, "permissive hypertension" is recommended to a goal of less than 220/120 mm Hg among those who did not receive tPA or less than 185/110 mm Hg over the first 24 hours. In cases where systemic hypotension has produced neurologic sequelae, vasopressors may be used to improve cerebral blood flow.[4] Several recent trials have found that lowering BP in the acute setting may be associated with worse clinical outcomes.

First, one analysis found that low-normal systolic BP (SBP) was associated with a higher risk of early recurrence by 2 weeks and poor functional outcome at 6 months compared with high-normal SBP.[28] Second, results of a randomized trial in patients with acute stroke and raised BP levels (SBP $\geq$140 mm Hg) suggested a trend toward greater risk of poor functional outcome at 180 days after BP-lowering treatment was initiated within 30 hours of the index stroke.[29] Third, the recent China Antihypertensive Trial in Acute Ischemic Stroke showed that immediate BP reduction by 10% to 25% within 24 hours of acute ischemic stroke, or achievement of BP less than 140/90 mm Hg within 7 days of acute ischemic stroke,

Table 2
Characteristics of the included randomized controlled trials on endovascular therapy for acute ischemic stroke

Author	Intervention vs Control	No. of Patients (% Male)	Age (y) Mean ± SD or Median (Range)	Inclusion Criteria	mRS Score ≤2 at 90 d	Recanalization (TICI)	Key Conclusion
PROACT II, 1999	I = IA r-proUK + IV heparin C = IV heparin	121 (58%) 59 (61%)	64 ± 14 64 ± 14	New focal neurologic signs in the MCA distribution allowing initiation of treatment within 6 h of the onset of symptoms, NIHSS ≥4	40%, P = .04 25%	Grade 2a–3 66%, P<.001 Grade 2a–3 18%	Improved good neurologic outcome (mRS score), recanalization with IA thrombolysis
SWIFT, 2012	I = Solitaire FR stent retriever C = MERCI clot retriever	58 (48%) 55 (51%)	67 ± 12 67 ± 11	NIHSS 8–29 and stroke onset ≤8 h with anterior/posterior large-vessel occlusion	58%, P = .017 33%	Grade 2a–3 61%, P<.0001 Grade 2a–3 24%	Improved good neurologic outcome (mRS score 0–2 or NIHSS improvement by ≥10 points), recanalization, and lower mortality with Solitaire
TREVO2, 2012	I = Trevo stent retriever C = MERCI clot retriever	88 (45%) 90 (40%)	70 (61–77) 71 (58–79)	NIHSS 8–29 and stroke onset ≤8 h with anterior/posterior large-vessel occlusion	40%, P = .013 22%	Grade 2a–3 86%, P<.0001 Grade 2a–3 60%	Improved good neurologic outcome (mRS score 0–2) and recanalization with Trevo; similar mortality rates

		N (%)	Age	Inclusion criteria	Good outcome	Recanalization	Outcome
IMS III, 2013	I = IV tPA + IV heparin ± MT	434 (50%)	69 (23–89)	NIHSS ≥10 without CTA/MRA or NIHSS ≥8 in patients with CTA/MRA showing large vessel occlusion	40.8%, P = .25	Grade 2b–3: ICA (38%), M1 (41%), single M2 (44%), multiple M2 (23%)	No difference in good neurologic outcome (mRS score 0–2), symptomatic ICH, or mortality
	C = IV tPA	222 (55%)	68 (23–84)		38.7%	NA	
MR RESCUE, 2013 (Penumbra)	I = IA/IV tPA ± MT	34 (50%)	66 ± 13	Stroke onset ≤8 h, NIHSS 6–29, anterior circulation large-vessel occlusion on MRA/CTA, infarct core on perfusion imaging ≤90 ml and pneumbral mismatch <70%	21%[a], P = .14	Grade 2a–3 at day 7 = 67%	No difference in good neurologic outcome (mRS score 0–2) among all 4 groups; smaller final infarct volume in good penumbral pattern groups
	C = IV tPA	34 (44%)	66 ± 17		26%[a]	Grade 2a–3 at day 7 = 93%	
SYNTHESIS-Expansion, 2013	I = IA tPA ± IV heparin ± MT	181 (59%)	66 ± 11	No defined NIHSS threshold; lack of confirmation of large-vessel occlusion before intervention	30.4%[b], P = .16	NA	No difference in good neurologic outcome (mRS score 0–2), symptomatic ICH, or mortality
	C = IV tPA	181 (57%)	67 ± 11		34.8%[b]	NA	

Abbreviations: CTA, computer tomography angiography; I, intervention; IA, irtraarterial; ICH, intracranial hemorrhage; IV, intravenous; MRA, magnetic resonance angiography; mRS, modified Rankin Score; MT, mechanical thrombectomy; NA, not applicable; NIHSS, NIH stroke scale; r-proUK, recombinant prourokinase; tPA, tissue plasminogen activator; TICI, thrombolysis in cerebral infarction.

[a] Improved in mRS score level in 90 days.

[b] mRS score 0 or 1.

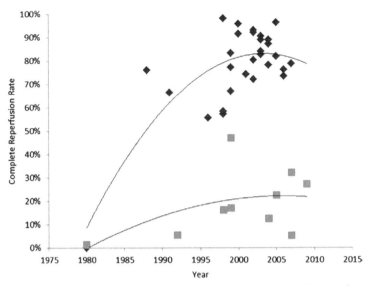

Fig. 3. Trends over time in complete reperfusion rates in active arms of coronary (*diamond*) and cerebral (*square*) reperfusion trials. (*From* Patel RD, Saver JL. Evolution of reperfusion therapies for acute brain and acute myocardial ischemia: a systematic, comparative analysis. Stroke 2013;44:94–8; with permission.)

had no mortality or morbidity benefits.[30] The optimal time or BP target to start antihypertensive treatment after acute stroke is also uncertain.

Aspirin

There is a small but statistically significant decline in mortality and unfavorable outcomes with the administration of aspirin (initial dose is 325 mg) within 24 to 48 hours after stroke. Early aspirin treatment leads to a 1% absolute reduction of stroke over the next 2 weeks.[31,32] If IV-tPA or acute endovascular therapy is administered, aspirin is initiated at approximately 24 hours and only after confirmation of no hemorrhagic transformation on 24-h CT head. Data regarding the utility of other antiplatelet agents, including clopidogrel alone or in combination with aspirin, for the treatment of acute ischemic stroke are limited. The Clopidogrel in High-Risk Patients with Acute Non-disabling Cerebrovascular Events trial compared clopidogrel plus aspirin versus aspirin alone started within 24 hours and continued for 21 days in Chinese patients with minor ischemic stroke or transient ischemic attack.[33] Over 90 days, 8.2% of patients in the clopidogrel + aspirin group, compared with 11.7% in the aspirin-only group, had a stroke (hazard ratio [HR] 0.68; 95% CI, 0.57–0.81; P<.001). The rate of ICH was 0.3% in each group.[33]

Statins

Statin therapy with intensive lipid-lowering effects is established for primary and secondary stroke

prevention.[34,35] There is emerging evidence favoring the neuroprotective effect of statins on ischemic stroke outcomes.[36,37] The only randomized trial on the topic was a small study involving 89 patients already taking chronic statins at the time of ischemic stroke. Patients were randomized within 24 hours of onset to statin withdrawal for 3 days or to continued statin therapy. Patients with statin withdrawal showed a higher frequency of mRS score greater than 2 at the end of follow-up (60.0% vs 39.0%; P = .043), which is associated with a 4.66-fold (1.46–14.91) increase in the risk of death or dependency and a 8.67-fold (3.05–24.63) increase in the risk of early neurologic deterioration compared with the nonstatin withdrawal group.[36] Similarly, in a large observation study, statin use before ischemic stroke hospitalization was associated with improved survival (HR 0.85; 95% CI, 0.79–0.93; P<.001), and use before and during hospitalization was associated with better rates of survival (HR 0.59; 95% CI, 0.53–0.65; P<.001).[37] Therefore, patients already taking statins at the time of ischemic stroke should continue this regimen. Those who are not on statin therapy should be; however, the impact on functional outcome is less certain.

Anticoagulation

Venous thromboembolism is a common but preventable complication of acute ischemic stroke. Without venous thromboembolism prophylaxis, up to 75% of patients with hemiplegia after stroke develop deep vein thrombosis and 20% develop pulmonary embolism,[38] which is fatal in 1% to 2% of patients with acute ischemic stroke and causes up to 25% of early deaths after strokes.[39] The Prevention of Venous Thromboembolism After Acute Ischemic Stroke (PREVAIL) study gives strong evidence of the superiority of low-molecular-weight heparin (LMWH) in prevention of venous thromboembolism over unfractionated heparin after ischemic stroke.[40] PREVAIL is an open-label, randomized comparison between enoxaparin (40 mg) subcutaneous daily versus unfractionated heparin (5000 U) subcutaneous every12 hours in patients with acute ischemic stroke. Enoxaparin reduced the risk of venous thromboembolism by 43% compared with unfractionated heparin (68 [10%] vs 121 [18%]; relative risk 0.57; 95% CI, 0.44–0.76; P = .0001; difference −7.9%, −11.6 to −4.2).[40] Hence, patients with acute ischemic stroke should be on LMWH for deep vein thrombosis prophylaxis on the day of admission or 24 hours after tPA administration.

On the other hand, urgent full anticoagulation for the management of noncerebrovascular conditions (ie, atrial fibrillation) is not recommended for patients with moderate-to-severe stroke because of an increased risk of symptomatic ICH. A meta-analysis of anticoagulants in patients with presumed cardioembolic stroke found that the agents were associated with a nonsignificant reduction in the rate of early recurrent stroke within 7 to 14 days (3.0% vs 4.9%; OR 0.68; 95% CI, 0.44–1.06; P = .09), a significant increase in symptomatic intracranial bleeding (2.5% vs 0.7%; OR 2.89; 95% CI, 1.19–7.01; P = .02), and a similar rate of death or disability at final follow-up (73.5% vs 73.8%; OR 1.01; 95% CI, 0.82–1.24; P = .9).[41]

STROKE SYSTEMS OF CARE

Rapid evaluation of stroke begins with community education to recognize signs and symptoms of stroke. The call to a 9-1-1 dispatcher is the first link in the stroke chain of survival (see **Fig. 1**).[42] Specific time frames have been established for the Emergency Medical Service System to follow on dispatch, response, and on-scene activities.[43] It then takes an organized system of care that involves EMS personnel, public safety agencies, emergency facilities, and hospital health care personnel, including acute and subacute stroke units, to enable delivery of acute stroke care.[4] Primary Stroke Centers, with certification by the Joint Commission based on demonstration of compliance with recommendations from the Brain Attack Coalition and American Heart Association guidelines,[4,44] are generally associated with lower mortality rates compared with noncertified hospitals.[45,46] Nationwide quality improvement initiatives include the American Heart Association's Get With The Guidelines program and the National Stroke Registry.

Hospitals that have implemented organized stroke care by following the Get With The Guidelines program have demonstrated sustained improvement in multiple measures of stroke care quality, including tPA administration.[47] To evaluate the impact of the Get With The Guidelines and Target: Stroke[48,49] programs on acute stroke care and outcomes, Fonarow and colleagues[50] compared door-to-needle (DTN) times of tPA administration in patients with acute ischemic stroke before (2003–2009; n = 27,319) and after (2010–2013; n = 43,850) the implementation of the initiative in 1030 participating hospitals (52.8% of total). The investigators found improvements in process measures, such as timeliness of tPA administration (DTN times improved from 77 minutes preintervention to 67 minutes postintervention), and the proportion of individuals with DTN times of less than or equal to 60 minutes increased from 26.5% to 41.3% (all P<.001). Clinical outcomes also improved: in-hospital mortality decreased from 9.9% to 8.2%, symptomatic ICH within 36 hours decreased fr006Fm 5.7% versus 4.7%, and percentage of patients discharged home increased from 37.6% to 42.7% (all P<.001).

SUMMARY

Rapid evaluation of stroke begins with community education to recognize signs and symptoms of acute ischemic stroke. It then takes an organized system of care that involves EMS personnel, emergency facilities, and hospital health care personnel all striving to achieve a DTN time of IV-tPA administration within less than or equal to 60 minutes. The FDA has approved the use of IV-tPA within 3 hours of symptom onset, and multiple randomized controlled trials have shown benefits up to 3 to 4.5 hours after symptom onset. For patients not eligible for IV-tPA or for those with persistent large-vessel occlusion, endovascular therapy should be considered within up to 6 hours of symptom onset. There are currently 4 devices cleared by the FDA for recanalization of arterial occlusion in patients with ischemic stroke. The IMS III, MR RESCUE, and SYNTHESIS-Expansion studies failed to show clinical outcome differences between endovascular retrieval devices and IV-tPA; therefore, no evidence has currently been presented showing superiority of endovascular clot retrieval over IV-tPA. Endovascular device technology and advanced imaging technology for patient selection, however, continue to evolve; newer devices have suggested greater recanalization success. Finally, postperfusion therapy care, including BP modulation and antiplatelet and neuroprotective agents (statins), is paramount for successful stroke outcome.

REFERENCES

1. Medical expenditure panel survey: household component summary data table: table 4: total expenses and percent distribution for selected conditions by source of payment: United States, 2008. Agency for Healthcare Research and Quality. Available at: http://meps.ahrq.gov/data_stats/. Accessed September 1, 2014.
2. Behavioral risk factor surveillance system: prevalence and trends data. Centers for Disease Control and Prevention. Available at: http://apps.nccd.cdc.gov/brfss/index.asp. Accessed September 1, 2014.
3. Murphy SL, Xu JQ, Kochanek KD. No 4. Deaths: final data for 2010. National Vital Statistics Report, vol. 61. Hyattsville (MD): National Center for Health Statistics; 2013.
4. Jauch EC, Saver JL, Adams HP, et al. Guidelines for the early management of patients with acute ischemic stroke: a guideline for healthcare professionals from the American Heart Association/American Stroke Association. Stroke 2013;44:870–947.
5. Tissue plasminogen activator for acute ischemic stroke. The National Institute of Neurological Disorders and Stroke rt-PA Stroke Study Group. N Engl J Med 1995;333:1581–7.
6. Rha JH, Saver JL. The impact of recanalization on ischemic stroke outcome: a meta-analysis. Stroke 2007;38:967–73.
7. Jerath NU, Reddy C, Freeman WD, et al. Gender differences in presenting signs and symptoms of acute ischemic stroke: a population-based study. Gend Med 2011;8:312–9.
8. Lisabeth LD, Brown DL, Hughes R, et al. Acute stroke symptoms: comparing women and men. Stroke 2009;40:2031–6.
9. Hand PJ, Kwan J, Lindley RI, et al. Distinguishing between stroke and mimic at the bedside: the brain attack study. Stroke 2006;37:769–75.
10. Hacke W, Donnan G, Fieschi C, et al, ATLANTIS Trials Investigators, ECASS Trials Investigators, NINDS rt-PA Study Group Investigators. Association of outcome with early stroke treatment: pooled analysis of ATLANTIS, ECASS, and NINDS rt-PA stroke trials. Lancet 2004;363:768–74.
11. Lees KR, Bluhmki E, von Kummer R, et al. Time to treatment with intravenous alteplase and outcome in stroke: an updated pooled analysis of ECASS, ATLANTIS, NINDS, and EPITHET trials. Lancet 2010;375:1695–703.
12. Zangerle A, Kiechl S, Spiegel M, et al. Recanalization after thrombolysis in stroke patients: predictors and prognostic implications. Neurology 2007;68:39–44.
13. Sillanpää N, Saarinen JT, Rusanen H, et al. Location of the clot and outcome of perfusion defects in acute anterior circulation stroke treated with intravenous thrombolysis. AJNR Am J Neuroradiol 2013;34:100–6.
14. Georgiadis AL, Memon MZ, Shah QA, et al. Comparison of partial (.6 mg/kg) versus full-dose (.9 mg/kg) intravenous recombinant tissue plasminogen activator followed by endovascular treatment for acute ischemic stroke: a meta-analysis. J Neuroimaging 2011;21:113–20.
15. Zaidat OO, Lazzaro MA, Liebeskind DS, et al. Revascularization grading in endovascular acute ischemic stroke therapy. Neurology 2012;79:S110–6.
16. The thrombolysis in myocardial infarction (TIMI) trial - phase I findings. TIMI Study Group. N Engl J Med 1985;312:932–6.
17. Zaidat OO, Yoo AJ, Khatri P, et al. Recommendations on angiographic reevascularization grading standards for acute ischemic stroke: a consensus statement. Stroke 2013;44:2650–63.
18. Furlan A, Higashida R, Wechsler L, et al. Intra-arterial prourokinase for acute ischemic stroke. The PROACT II study: a randomized controlled trial. JAMA 1999;282:2003–11.
19. Saver JL, Jahan R, Levy EI, et al. Solitaire flow restoration device versus the Merci Retriever in patients with acute ischaemic stroke (SWIFT): a randomised, parallel-group, non-inferiority trial. Lancet 2012;380:1241–9.
20. Nogueira RG, Lutsep HL, Gupta R, et al. Trevo versus Merci retrievers for thrombectomy revascularisation of large vessel occlusions in acute ischaemic stroke (TREVO 2): a randomised trial. Lancet 2012;380:1231–40.
21. Broderick JP, Palesch YY, Demchuk AM, et al. Endovascular therapy after intravenous t-PA versus t-PA alone for stroke. N Engl J Med 2013;368:893–903.
22. Kidwell CS, Jahan R, Gornbein J, et al. A trial of imaging selection and endovascular treatment for ischemic stroke. N Engl J Med 2013;368:914–23.
23. Ciccone A, Valvassori L, Nichelatti M, et al. Endovascular treatment for acute ischemic stroke. N Engl J Med 2013;368:904–13.
24. Mokin M, Khalessi A, Mocco J, et al. Endovascular treatment of acute ischemic stroke: the end or just the beginning? Neurosurg Focus 2014;36:E5.
25. Qureshi A, Abd-Allah F, Aleu A, et al. Endovascular treatment for acute ischemic stroke patients: implications and interpretation of IMS III, MR RESCUE, and SYNTHESIS EXPANSION trials: a report from the working group of international congress of

interventional Neurology. J Vasc Interv Neurol 2014; 7:56–75.

26. Patel RD, Saver JL. Evolution of reperfusion therapies for acute brain and acute myocardial ischemia: a systematic, comparative analysis. Stroke 2013;44: 94–8.

27. Khatri P. Evaluation and management of acute ischemic stroke. Continuum (Minneap Minn) 2014; 20:283–95.

28. Leonardi-Bee J, Bath PM, Phillips SJ, et al. Blood pressure and clinical outcomes in the international stroke trial. Stroke 2002;33:1315–20.

29. Sandset EC, Bath PM, Boysen G, et al. The angiotensin-receptor blocker candesartan for treatment of acute stroke (SCAST): a randomised, placebo-controlled, double-blind trial. Lancet 2011; 377:741–50.

30. He J, Zhang Y, Xu T, et al. Effects of immediate blood pressure reduction on death and major disability in patients with acute ischemic stroke: the CATIS randomized clinical trial. JAMA 2014; 311:479–89.

31. CAST: randomized placebo-controlled trial of early aspirin use in 20,000 patients with acute ischaemic stroke. CAST (Chinese Acute Stroke Trial) Collaborative Group. Lancet 1997;349:1641–9.

32. The International Stroke Trial (IST): a randomised trial of aspirin, subcutaneous heparin, both, or neither among 19435 patients with acute ischaemic stroke. Lancet 1997;349:1569–81.

33. Wang Y, Wang Y, Zhao X, et al. Clopidogrel with aspirin in acute minor stroke or transient ischemic attack. N Engl J Med 2013;369:11–9.

34. The Stroke Prevention by Aggressive Reduction in Cholesterol Levels (SPARCL) Investigators. High-dose atorvastatin after stroke or transient ischemic attack. N Engl J Med 2006;355:549–59.

35. Goldstein LB, Amarenco P, Zivin J, et al. Statin treatment and stroke outcome in the stroke prevention by aggressive reduction in cholesterol levels (SPARCL) trial. Stroke 2009;40:3520–31.

36. Blanco M, Nombela F, Castellanos M, et al. Statin treatment withdrawal in ischemic stroke: a controlled randomized study. Neurology 2007;69:904–10.

37. Flint AC, Kamel H, Navi BB, et al. Statin use during ischemic stroke hospitalization is strongly associated with improved poststroke survival. Stroke 2012;43:147–54.

38. McCarthy ST, Turner JJ, Robertson D, et al. Low-dose heparin as a prophylaxis against deep-vein thrombosis after acute strokE. Lancet 1977;310: 800–1.

39. Kelly J, Rudd A, Lewis R, et al. Venous thromboembolism after acute stroke. Stroke 2001;32:262–7.

40. Sherman DG, Albers GW, Bladin C, et al. The efficacy and safety of enoxaparin versus unfractionated heparin for the prevention of venous thromboembolism after acute ischemic stroke (PREVAIL Study): an open-label randomized comparison. Lancet 2007; 369:1347–55.

41. Paciaroni M, Agnelli G, Micheli S, et al. Efficacy and safety of anticoagulant treatment in acute cardioembolic stroke: a meta-analysis of randomized controlled trials. Stroke 2007;38:423–30.

42. Jauch EC, Cucchiara B, Adeoye O, et al. Part 11: adult stroke: 2010 American Heart Association guidelines for cardiopulmonary resuscitation and emergency cardiovascular care. Circulation 2010; 122:S818–28.

43. Acker JE, Pancioli AM, Crocco TJ, et al. Implementation strategies for emergency medical services within stroke systems of care: a policy statement from the American Heart Association/American Stroke Association Expert Panel on Emergency Medical Services Systems and the Stroke Council. Stroke 2007;38:3097–115.

44. Alberts MJ, Hademenos G, Latchaw RE, et al. Recommendations for the establishment of primary stroke centers. Brain attack coalition. JAMA 2000; 283:3102–9.

45. Lichtman JH, Jones SB, Wang Y, et al. Outcomes after ischemic stroke for hospitals with and without Joint Commission-certified primary stroke centers. Neurology 2011;76:1976–82.

46. Xian Y, Holloway RG, Chan PS, et al. Association between stroke center hospitalization for acute ischemic stroke and mortality. JAMA 2011;305(4):373–80.

47. Schwamm LH, Fonarow GC, Reeves MJ, et al. Get with the guidelines-stroke is associated with sustained improvement in care for patients hospitalized with acute stroke or transient ischemic attack. Circulation 2009;119:107–15.

48. Fonarow GC, Smith EE, Saver JL, et al. Improving door-to-needle times in acute ischemic stroke: the design and rationale for the American Heart Association/American Stroke Association's Target: stroke initiative. Stroke 2011;42:2983–9.

49. Fonarow GC, Reeves MJ, Smith EE, et al. Characteristics, performance measures, and in-hospital outcomes of the first one million stroke and transient ischemic attack admissions in get with the Guidelines-Stroke. Circ Cardiovasc Qual Outcomes 2010;3:291–302.

50. Fonarow GC, Zhao X, Smith EE, et al. Door-to-needle times for tissue plasminogen activator administration and clinical outcomes in acute ischemic stroke before and after a quality improvement initiative. JAMA 2014;311:1632–40.

Contemporary Medical Management of Peripheral Arterial Disease
A Focus on Risk Reduction and Symptom Relief for Intermittent Claudication

Kush Agrawal, MD[a], Robert T. Eberhardt, MD[b],*

KEYWORDS

- Peripheral arterial disease • Intermittent claudication • Supervised exercise therapy • Cilostazol
- Pentoxifylline • Atherosclerotic risk factors • Ankle-brachial index

KEY POINTS

- Peripheral arterial disease (PAD) due to lower limb atherosclerosis is a common problem that is often asymptomatic but associated with a high risk of adverse cardiovascular events and mortality.
- The classic symptom due to PAD is exertional leg discomfort or intermittent claudication, but most patients are asymptomatic or experience atypical leg symptoms.
- Diagnostic testing should include measurement of the ankle-brachial index in all patients plus physiologic testing and/or advanced imaging as needed to determine disease severity and location, and revascularization options.
- Treatment of modifiable risk factors, including smoking cessation, lipid-lowering therapy, antihypertensive therapy, and antiplatelet therapies, is essential to delay disease progression and prevent ischemic events.
- Symptomatic relief for intermittent claudication should focus on supervised exercise training and pharmacologic therapy (most notably with cilostazol in North America).

INTRODUCTION

Peripheral arterial disease (PAD) most commonly refers to disease affecting the lower extremities that is primarily caused by progressive atherosclerosis. The spectrum of disease manifestations encompasses asymptomatic individuals with impaired resting flow, those with *intermittent claudication (IC)* or leg symptoms during exertion, those progressing to advanced manifestations of rest pain and tissue loss, or *critical limb ischemia* (CLI), and those with sudden inadequate limb perfusion to jeopardize viability in *acute limb ischemia*. IC results from an arterial oxygen supply and demand mismatch, usually as a result of arterial obstruction causing inadequate blood flow to the muscles during activity.

Approaching the patient with suspected PAD often presents a formidable challenge to the clinician. Given the myriad manifestations of disease that often present in an atypical fashion, a low index of suspicion and thorough yet focused history

The authors have nothing to disclose.
[a] Cardiovascular and Endovascular Intervention, Section of Cardiovascular Medicine, Boston Medical Center, Boston, MA 02118, USA; [b] Vascular Medicine Program, Section of Cardiovascular Medicine, Boston Medical Center, Boston University School of Medicine, 88 East Newton Street, Boston MA 02118, USA
* Corresponding author.
E-mail address: robert.eberhardt@bmc.org

0733-8651/15/$ – see front matter © 2015 Elsevier Inc. All rights reserved.

cardiology.theclinics.com

and physical examination are critical. Although the term PAD may include stenosis, occlusion, or aneurysmal changes of the upper or lower extremities or other noncoronary vascular territories,[1] this review focuses on lower extremity arterial obstructive disease. There are various nonatherosclerotic etiologies of PAD, including trauma, vasculitis, and emboli (**Table 1**); however, atherosclerosis comprises the vast majority of PAD presentations and has the greatest epidemiologic impact.

The epidemiology, clinical presentation, workup, and medical management of PAD are reviewed here with a focus on IC. Key advances in the recognition of cardiovascular risk in asymptomatic individuals with mildly abnormal ankle-brachial index (ABI), newer reflections on exercise therapy, including the incremental value of home-based, nonsupervised programs and results from direct randomized comparisons to invasive management techniques, and a review of established and investigational agents for the treatment of PAD, such as cilostazol, statins, and angiotensin-converting enzyme (ACE) inhibitors, are also highlighted. With a limited role for medical management, the use of adjunct, noninvasive therapies for CLI is outside the scope of this review but the promise of angiogenesis is briefly discussed.

EPIDEMIOLOGY

PAD is highly prevalent, with estimates of disease burden in the United States alone at 8 million adults.[2] There is an expected increase in prevalence with aging, with an estimated 10% of adults 65 years or older affected by the spectrum of disease, and approximately 30% affected at 80 years or older,[3] which mirrors data in the diabetic and smoking cohorts from the PAD Awareness, Risk, and Treatment: New Resources for Survival (PARTNERS) program more than a decade ago.[4] There is a startling prevalence of PAD in patients newly diagnosed with coronary artery disease (CAD) or cerebrovascular disease (CVD); the diagnosis of concomitant PAD is a significant negative prognosticator for cardiovascular events.[5] Although the overlap between these comorbid conditions (PAD and CVD, PAD and CAD, and CAD and CVD) is well-recognized, patients often remain undertreated (**Fig. 1**).[6] In addition, analysis of the National Health and Nutrition Examination Survey (NHANES) data from 1999 to 2004 revealed an ethnic disparity disfavoring those of African American and Mexican American heritage, showcasing the need for maintaining a low index of suspicion in these groups.[3] Furthermore, despite controlling for traditional risk factors, PAD affects African Americans twofold more than it does others, as seen in the Multi-Ethnic Study of Atherosclerosis (MESA) study,[7] which suggests a need for greater screening efforts on a population-wide basis, but also perhaps the need for enhanced risk factor analysis and optimization, beyond traditional factors applied to the general population.

Risk Factors

Traditionally recognized risk factors for atherosclerosis play an important role in the risk of PAD onset, accelerated development, and overall disease severity. Among the myriad causative factors, smoking, diabetes mellitus (DM),

Table 1
Differential diagnoses in the patient with suspected PAD

Nonvascular Causes of PAD-like Symptoms	Vascular Causes
Orthopedic causes (joint disease, Baker cyst, bursitis)	Peripheral atherosclerosis
Compartment syndrome (from fracture or crush injury)	Thromboembolism (cardiogenic, related to aortoiliac aneurysm, or in situ thrombosis)
Peripheral neuropathy	Connective tissue disorders (Marfan syndrome or Ehlers-Danlos [type IV] syndrome)
Venous claudication (after iliofemoral DVT, such as in May-Thurner syndrome)	Fibromuscular dysplasia
Spinal stenosis or cauda equina pseudoclaudication	Buerger disease
	Heritable thrombophilias (Factor V Leiden, prothrombin gene mutation, antithrombin III deficiency, and protein C and S deficiency)
	Vasculitides (giant cell arteritis, polyarteritis nodosa, systemic lupus erythematosus)
	Entrapment syndromes (popliteal)

Abbreviation: DVT, deep vein thrombosis; PAD, peripheral arterial disease.

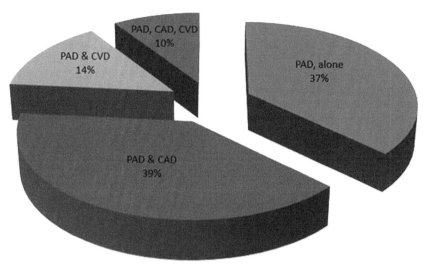

Fig. 1. Coexistent atherosclerotic disease in PAD. Data from the international Reduction of Atherothrombosis for Continued Health (REACH) registry of 7013 patients with PAD demonstrated a significant overlap in disease co-prevalence among PAD, CVD, and CAD. PAD alone, n = 2588; PAD and CAD, n = 2763; PAD and CVD, n = 666; and PAD, CAD, and CVD, n = 996. (*Data from* Boden WE, Cherr GS, Eagle KA, et al. Prior cardiovascular interventions are not associated with worsened clinical outcomes in patients with symptomatic atherothrombosis. Crit Pathw Cardiol 2010;9(3):116–25.)

hypertension, and hypercholesterolemia are by far the most impactful and well-recognized contributors to the development and progression of PAD (**Fig. 2**). In a prospective study of more than 20,500 high cardiovascular risk participants studied over 2 decades, the Heart Protection Study identified these aforementioned factors as contributing to more than 75% of the population-attributable risk for the development of PAD.[8] Stated differently, these factors were not responsible in only one-fourth of afflicted patients.

Tobacco smoking is by far the most potent and deleterious risk factor in the development of PAD. Observational studies attribute a greater potency of risk with tobacco use for the development of PAD than even for CAD, although the mechanism is poorly understood.[9] Up to a sixfold risk has been noted with a dose-dependent effect due to tobacco use over an individual's lifetime.[10] Smokers have a higher incidence of not only the onset of CLI and limb amputation, but also suffer from poorer outcomes of revascularization

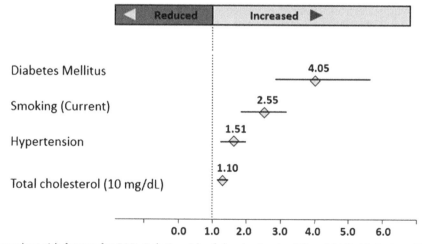

Fig. 2. Independent risk factors for PAD. Relative risk of developing traditional PAD risk factors. Defined by an ABI less than 0.9. (*Data from* Newman AB, Siscovick DS, Manolio TA, et al. Ankle-arm index as a marker of atherosclerosis in the Cardiovascular Health Study. Cardiovascular Heart Study (CHS) Collaborative Research Group. Circulation 1993;88:837–45.)

procedures and bypass graft patency.[11,12] Moreover, the inherent risk seems to extend to those suffering from secondhand smoke as well. In an observational study, among the approximately 40% of the 1200 nonsmoking Chinese women who reported secondhand smoke exposure either in the workplace or in the home, rates of incident CAD, CVD, or PAD (as defined by IC symptoms, an ABI less than 0.90, or both) were significantly higher and displayed a dose-dependent response (number of cigarettes per day and minutes of duration of exposure).[13] With the advent of popular electronic cigarettes being touted as a public health benefit by manufacturers, concerns have been raised regarding the actual benefit achieved with tobacco cessation by such means. Concerns also have been raised regarding the increased risk of secondhand smoke by introducing widespread battery vapor by-product and subverting the established successes of strict "no-smoking" policies, by softening the social stigma currently associated with smoking in public places.[14]

Diabetes Mellitus is at least twice as prevalent in those with incident PAD,[1,3] with a stepwise incremental risk seen in type 2 DM related to their glycemic controls. Higher glycosylated hemoglobin levels are associated with an increased risk of PAD, on the order of a 30% relative increase for incident PAD with a 1% increase in hemoglobin A1C level.[15] DM affects the macrovascular and microvascular circulation, with glycosylation end products accelerating atherosclerosis and oxidative stress, culminating in alterations in the rheologic properties of blood and impairing the local immune response.[16,17] PAD seen among diabetic individuals is often described as being diffuse and distal in distribution. It is not surprising that diabetic individuals suffer from a fivefold increased risk of limb loss through amputation when compared with their nondiabetic counterparts.[18] DM remains the leading cause of limb amputation, especially with concomitant PAD.

Hypertension is a well-recognized risk factor in the development of atherosclerosis and ischemic vascular events, especially stroke. In the presence of PAD, hypertension confers an increased risk of cardiovascular events. Hypertensive men were twice as likely, and women four times as likely, to develop PAD with IC in the Framingham Heart Study.[19] In the Cardiovascular Health Study, patients with a history of hypertension were 50% more likely to develop PAD.[20]

Dyslipidemia confers risk for the development of PAD and its complications by promotion of atherosclerotic mechanisms, and is a ready target for risk reduction. Dyslipidemia, including elevations in serum total cholesterol (TC) and triglycerides

(TG) and decreased high-density lipoprotein (HDL) levels, may all contribute to the development and acceleration of peripheral atherosclerosis.[21] The Framingham Heart Study found that higher cholesterol levels are associated with an increased risk of developing IC at a hazard ratio of 1.2 per 40 mg/dL of TC elevation.[22] Similarly, a population-level analysis demonstrated that in nonsmokers, elevated ratios of TC to HDL were independently associated with a low ABI of less than 0.9, suggesting a potentially greater role for lipid assessment as a screening tool for PAD, rather than simply as a risk marker.[23] In addition, in the more than 5000 participants free of baseline cardiovascular disease in the Cardiovascular Health Study, incident PAD (defined as an ABI of <0.9) was associated with increased TC levels, such that a 10 mg/dL increase in total cholesterol levels was associated with a 10% increase in the incidence of PAD.[20] There was a linear relationship between increased low-density lipoprotein (LDL) levels and decreased ABI levels in female participants.[20]

Emerging risk factors, such as sensitive serum biomarkers, can complement our traditional understanding of risk stratification in the preclinical stages of PAD. Among these, elevated homocysteine, lipoprotein(a), and C-reactive protein (CRP) levels have demonstrated a strong association with incident PAD and accelerated atherosclerosis.

- The benefit of inflammatory and pro-atherosclerotic biomarkers, such as CRP, interleukin-6, fibrinogen, and lipoprotein(a), is shown in the preclinical prediction of atherosclerotic events. The most useful seems to be CRP, as the addition of CRP to lipid profiles significantly improved risk prediction for incident PAD in a nested case-control analysis of the Physicians' Health Study.[24]
- Elevated homocysteine levels independently double the risk of incident PAD,[25] even demonstrating a stepwise and linear relationship with levels of elevation and both all-cause and cardiovascular mortality.[26] Unfortunately, lowering homocysteine levels with folic acid and B vitamins as an independent therapeutic target has not translated into improved cardiovascular or peripheral arterial outcomes.[27]
- Borderline abnormal and low-normal ABI values have not routinely been regarded as markers of atherosclerosis and functional decline, but they are now proving valuable in the recognition of patients with subclinical PAD. Subclinical disease with no symptoms

but an ABI of less than 0.9 was associated with a threefold increased risk of death from all causes at 4 years, compared with those without an abnormal ABI.[28] Accordingly, a borderline ABI should prompt enhanced follow-up and greater sensitivity to the sequelae of pan-atherosclerosis at an earlier stage.

In the pursuit of increasingly sensitive biochemical or serum markers of atherosclerosis and PAD, we have gained the ability to predict atherosclerotic events earlier; however, some markers have fallen short of the ideal of becoming an independent treatable risk factor, such as in the case of homocysteine levels. In contrast, a borderline abnormal ABI may be more useful.

Morbidity and Mortality

The presence of PAD is a well-recognized risk factor for both cardiovascular disease and ischemic events. In 2011, it was estimated that 14,000 deaths in the United States alone were due to PAD.[2] Even in asymptomatic individuals, an abnormal resting ABI ($\leq$0.9) is associated with a doubling of coronary events, cardiovascular mortality, and total mortality.[29–31] The insidious nature of slowly progressing atherosclerosis before the development of symptoms, explains the high co-morbid risks seen at diagnosis across other vascular beds, such as in the carotid, cerebral, and coronary distributions. If screened for broadly, such as in the primary care setting, early recognition of individuals with asymptomatic or symptomatic PAD could possibly confer a morbidity and mortality benefit, as this group is particularly vulnerable to severe vascular events, such as myocardial infarction, stroke, and limb loss.[32]

Aside from the recognized, deterministic cardiovascular risk over a lifetime, survival trends in patients with PAD are associated with the presence or absence of symptoms and the severity of symptoms when present (**Fig. 3**).[33] Fortunately, observations support a generally low risk of progression to limb-threatening disease. In patients followed over 5 years, those with PAD at the outset demonstrated the following natural history: 70% to 80% of PAD symptoms are stable at 5 years, 10% to 20% will suffer from progressive IC, and only 1% to 3% will progress to CLI.[1] The latter is a limb-threatening and life-threatening condition with dismal 1-year outcomes.[34]

CLINICAL PRESENTATION AND EVALUATION

The evaluation of the patient with suspected PAD requires a thorough history focused on exclusion of *pseudo-claudication* and other nonvascular causes (see **Table 1**), localization and timing of onset (duration of symptoms and estimation of both maximal and pain-free walking distance) of claudication symptoms, determination of relieving factors, and presence or absence of rest pain or ischemic tissue injury. Furthermore, types of leg pain, when the diagnosis of PAD is in doubt, should be clarified with regard to symptom quality, reproducibility, positional variability, and effects on quality of life.[35]

Most patients (ie, 90%) do not present with symptoms typical of IC (**Fig. 4**)[20] and, unfortunately, the use of a screening form to elicit a classic history, such as the Rose questionnaire (**Box 1**),[36] is often highly insensitive in diagnosing PAD.[4] Nuances extracted from the history can be helpful. In general, the level of obstruction is one

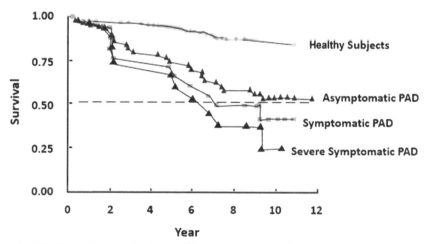

Fig. 3. Survival in PAD. Survival curves for those with asymptomatic and symptomatic PAD, as well as those with severe symptomatic PAD. (*From* Criqui MH, Langer RD, Fronek A, et al. Mortality over a period of 10 years in patients with peripheral arterial disease. N Engl J Med 1992;326:385; with permission.)

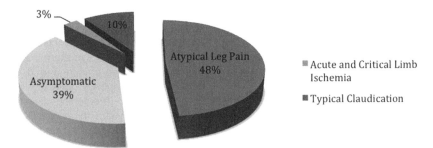

Fig. 4. Distribution of symptoms in patients diagnosed with PAD. The vast majority of patients do not present with typical symptoms. (*Data from* Newman AB, Siscovick DS, Manolio TA, et al. Ankle-arm index as a marker of atherosclerosis in the Cardiovascular Health Study. Cardiovascular Heart Study (CHS) Collaborative Research Group. Circulation 1993;88(3):837–45.)

joint above the affected muscle group and patients will often given a history of decreased walk time when climbing uphill or while carrying a load. As the walking pace slows, time and, distance to onset of pain can be delayed. Finally, asking about symptoms during infrequent periods of greater exertion, for example during vacation or a yearly activity, can yield helpful information as patients often have to step outside of their usual self-adjusted exercise regimen or usual physical capacity during these periods.[35]

Fortunately, fewer patients present with more advance forms of disease, such as CLI or acute limb ischemia. Patients with CLI present with ischemic symptoms at rest and frequently suffer from tissue loss in the form of ulceration or gangrene. Determining the character of the pain and alleviating factors, such as placing the limb in a dependent position, is useful in establishing a diagnosis. Patients presenting with acute limb ischemia have sudden compromise to limb perfusion that results in a threat to limb viability. This is characterized by the 6 "P's": pain, pulselessness, pallor, paresthesia, paralysis, and poikilothermia. Determining symptom onset and extent of any associated neurologic symptoms is essential for treatment. Once the diagnosis is made, disease severity for the chronic manifestations can be classified according to the Fontaine or Rutherford classification schemes, providing the clinician an effective method of staging for serial follow-up, as well as simplifying communication with a vascular specialist (**Table 2**).[37]

Physical Examination

Given the diffuse nature of disease in PAD, a thorough vascular examination is paramount in identifying both the extent and severity of disease. In the upper extremities, bilateral brachial artery blood pressures should be within 10 to 15 mm Hg, otherwise they are considered abnormal. Furthermore, palpation and quantification of the entire lower extremity arterial system is mandatory, including bilateral femoral, popliteal, dorsalis pedis (DP), and posterior tibial (PT) pulses, with a common grading system of 2+ being normal, 1+ diminished, and 0 as nonpalpable. The cardiac examination may be nonspecific. A focused abdominal examination should include palpation for a large aortic aneurysm and the presence of any bruits, which might help identify mesenteric and/or renal stenoses. The skin examination, particularly of the lower extremities, should include an assessment of color, temperature, hair growth, tissue loss or ulceration, and nail features. In the lower extremities, dependent rubor and elevation pallor are often noted in severe PAD, and the time to onset of pallor should be noted and recorded for purposes of surveillance. Distal embolization can result in *livedo reticularis*.

Box 1
Rose questionnaire

Symptoms of intermittent claudication

- Do you have pain involving 1 or both calves?
- Is your leg pain provoked by exertion?
- Do you have similar leg pain at rest? (Expected answer "no")
- Does your leg pain prompt you to stop exerting yourself?
- Does your pain improve within 10 minutes of rest? (Expected answer "yes")
- Does your pain continue to worsen with continued exertion? (Expected answer "yes")

Data from Rose GA. The diagnosis of ischaemic heart pain and intermittent claudication in field surveys. Bull World Health Organ 1962;27:645–58.

Table 2
Fontaine's and Rutherford's classification of peripheral arterial disease

	Fontaine		Rutherford		
Stage	Clinical	Grade	Category	Clinical	
I	Asymptomatic	0	0	Asymptomatic	
IIa	Mild claudication	I	1	Mild claudication	
IIb	Moderate to severe claudication	I	2	Moderate claudication	
		I	3	Severe claudication	
III	Rest pain	II	4	Rest pain	
IV	Ulcers or gangrene	III	5	Minor tissue loss	
		IV	6	Ulcers or gangrene	

Norgren L, Hiatt WR, Dormandy JA, et al. Inter-Society Consensus for the Management of Peripheral Arterial Disease (TASC II). Journal of Vascular Surgery 2007;45 (1S):S29A.

Serial comprehensive examinations can provide important insight into disease severity and progression, and can inform treatment decisions before the need for noninvasive testing.

Diagnostic Testing

Because the vast majority of patients with suspected PAD do not present with typical symptoms of IC, making the diagnosis requires a low threshold for testing in appropriately selected patients. It may be important to screen those with an intermediate to high pretest probability of disease to ensure appropriate yield and resource use. The joint American College of Cardiology/American Heart Association (ACC/AHA) taskforce updated guidelines from 2011 to identify the appropriate population to screen for PAD with a resting ABI examination (**Box 2**).[38] The resting ABI examination has excellent test characteristics, with over 90% sensitivity and a similar specificity for diagnosing PAD.[39] Notably, the use of ABI for screening was not endorsed by the US Preventive Service Task Force.[40]

An ABI assessment is a simple and inexpensive examination that is useful when diagnosing and assessing its severity. The higher of the two ankle systolic blood pressure measurements for a given limb is divided by the higher of the two brachial systolic blood pressure measurements to give the ABI, with normal defined as a ratio of 1.0–1.4 (**Fig. 5A**).[41] Blood pressure is usually 8% to 10% higher in the periphery due to wave reflection of systolic blood volume and peripheral augmentation.[42] Values greater than 1.4 are consistent with impaired vessel compressibility, a common occurrence in those with diabetes mellitus or chronic kidney disease and in the elderly. An abnormal ABI of 0.90 or lower is indicative of the presence of PAD, with severe disease correlating to an ABI of 0.50 or lower. An important adjunct test in this scenario is use of the toe brachial index (TBI), which is calculated from the highest toe systolic pressure divided by the higher brachial pressure; a ratio of 0.70 or higher is generally regarded as normal, and an absolute systolic toe pressure of 30 to 40 mm Hg or higher is a high yield predictor of viability of the ischemic foot.[43]

A borderline ABI, whether at low-normal values of 1.0 to 1.09 or borderline abnormal values of 0.91 to 0.99, is likely an independent marker of functional decline and accelerated pan-atherosclerosis, but not universally adopted on a population-screening basis. In the Walking and Leg Circulation Study (WALCS), participants with ABI values of 0.91 to 1.09 were prospectively

Box 2
Who should be screened for the diagnosis of peripheral arterial disease with a resting ankle-brachial index examination?

Patients with 1 or more of the following characteristics:

- Exertional leg symptoms
- Nonhealing wounds
- ≥65 years of age
- ≥50 years of age with history of diabetes mellitus or smoking

Class I, level of evidence B recommendations.
Adapted from Rooke TW, Hirsch AT, Misra S, et al. 2011 ACCF/AHA focused update of the guideline for the management of patients with peripheral artery disease (updating the 2005 guideline): a report of the American College of Cardiology Foundation/American Heart Association Task Force on Practice Guidelines: developed in collaboration with the Society for Cardiovascular Angiography and Interventions, Society of Interventional Radiology, Society for Vascular Medicine, and Society for Vascular Surgery. J Vasc Surg 2011;54(5):e32–58.

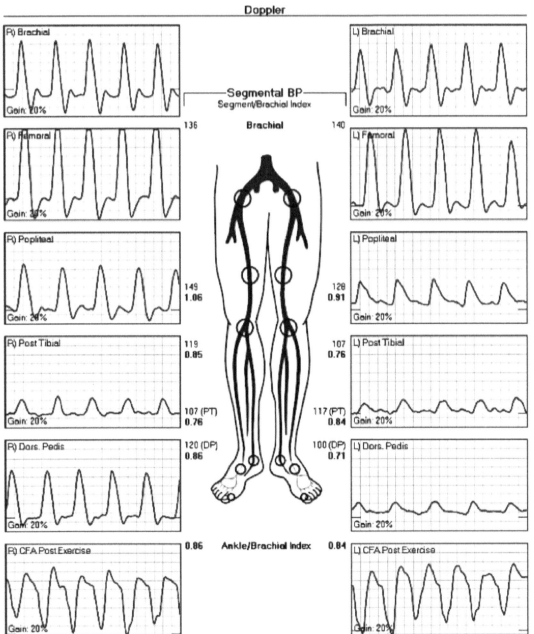

Fig. 5. Case example of testing and intervention for claudication. A 67-year-old man was treated for debilitating left leg claudication for 6 months. (*A, B*) ABI and pulse-volume recordings demonstrated loss of normal triphasic Doppler signal and diminished pulse amplitude at the femoral-popliteal level on the left, respectively. (*C*) Exercise ankle pressures were performed and confirmed more severe disease. (*D*) Duplex demonstrated a high-grade (>75%) stenosis near the mid-left superficial femoral artery based on peak flow velocities of 70-80 cm/s in the non-stenosed segment, increasing five-fold to 5 m/s within the mid-vessel (*middle panel*). (*E*) Peripheral contrast angiography revealed a severe left superficial femoral artery stenosis. Treatment of the culprit lesion (E1) with orbital atherectomy and balloon angioplasty (E2, E3). The final result (E4) demonstrated patency with a small non–flow-limiting intimal dissection that did not require further treatment.

B

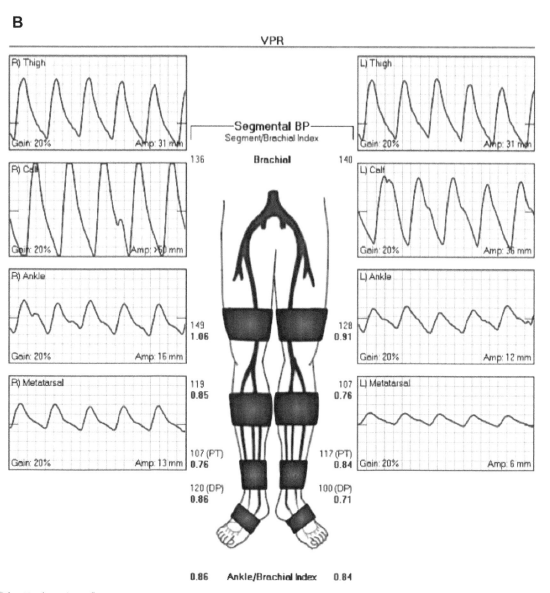

Fig. 5. (continued)

studied for 5 years to determine the incidence of functional decline, as defined by self-reported loss of walking distance.[44] Subjects with a border-line ABI (0.91–0.99) had a threefold increased risk of functional decline at 5 years and 50% of this group went on to have a "truly" abnormal ABI of less than 0.90 at study conclusion. This reclassification of previously "normal" individuals highlights the need for readjustment of the ABI assessment in those at highest risk, especially with the goals of delaying functional impairment and preserving quality-of-life measures.

A postexercise ankle pressure (see **Fig. 5C**) can be used for patients with a high index of suspicion of PAD but who have a normal resting ABI. Not only does this test serve to distinguish exertional from nonexertional causes of leg pain, it also provides important prognostic data on pain-free walking time and walking distance, and maximal walking time and walking distance. It also may assess for the presence of any associated symptoms, such as electrocardiogram changes (if assessed), to suggest concomitant coronary atherosclerosis manifested at a lower total workload. The postexercise ankle pressure is particularly useful in the longitudinal assessment of the PAD patient following limb revascularization.

C

Exercise Pressures

	Rest	1	2	3	4	5	6	7	8	9	10
R Ankle (DP):	120	90				98					109
L Ankle (PT):	117	52				63					81
L Brachial:	140	181				140					117
R ABI:	0.86	0.50				0.70					0.93
L ABI:	0.84	0.29				0.45					0.69

12 5% Grade
2 M.P.H.
3 Min

Bilateral calf pain noted 1 minute into exercise L>R.

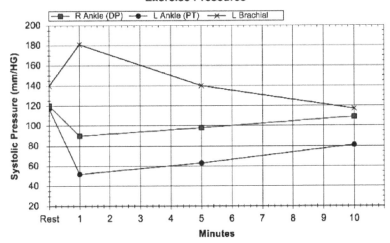

D

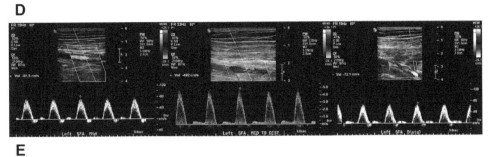

E

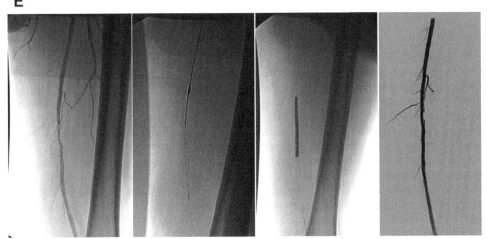

Fig. 5. (*continued*)

Additional noninvasive physiologic and imaging modalities, including segmental limb pressures, pulse volume recording (see **Fig. 5**B), Doppler waveform analysis, arterial duplex ultrasound (DUS) (see **Fig. 5**D), computerized tomography (CT), and MRI, play important adjunct roles in patient care once the diagnosis of PAD has been made. However, care must be taken to apply these modalities where they offer the highest yield from their judicious use (**Fig. 6**).

- Physiologic testing, including segmental limb pressures, pulse volume recording, and Doppler waveforms, complements the ABI in the localization of the level of disease and quantification of disease severity.
- Imaging with DUS may be used before consideration of limb revascularization (see **Fig. 5**D). It also may help characterize vessels and flow dynamics following revascularization, and is especially useful for longitudinal surveillance. After graft placement, it is often recommended that DUS be performed at least at 3, 6, and 12 months, then yearly afterward for surveillance.[45]
- The use of advanced imaging techniques, including MR angiography (MRA), and CT angiography (CTA), is typically reserved for planning revascularization. MRA allows excellent visualization of the arterial tree, tissue characterization, and vessel calcium. There is no radiation related to the procedure, but

caution must be taken in light of the risk of nephrogenic systemic fibrosis, however infrequent. Limitations include associated claustrophobia, preclusion of patients with implanted metallic devices (eg, pacemakers, defibrillators, and loop recorders), and limited space precluding the severely obese. The 2011 American College of Cardiology Foundation/AHA guidelines give a strong recommendation (Class I, level of evidence [LOE] A) to MRI/MRA for initial angiographic localization, and a reasonably confident (Class I, LOE B) recommendation for the concomitant use of gadolinium contrast enhancement.[45] The use of CTA as a means of imaging allows for a "real-feel" view of the arterial tree and multiplane reconstruction for more accurate depth perception, but at the cost of ionizing radiation, the need for iodinated contrast, and potentially lengthy acquisition times.

PATIENT MANAGEMENT

The fundamental goals of patient management stem first from prevention of myocardial infarction, cerebrovascular accident (CVA), and death, then extend to optimal and goal-directed medical therapy of PAD to achieve deferred symptoms; improved quality-of-life measures, such as pain-free activities, walking ability, and delaying the need for limb amputation (or amputation-free survival); and, when limb salvage becomes

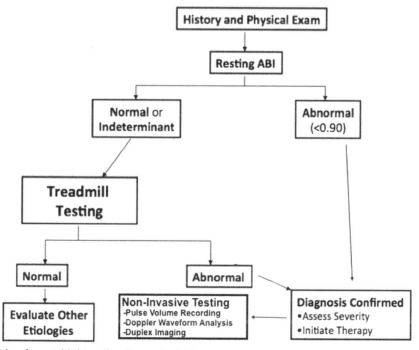

Fig. 6. Algorithm for establishing the diagnosis of IC.

necessary, the use of salvage for CLI selectively and with combined wound care. The surplus benefit of risk factor modification is seen in the inherent benefit to multiple levels of atherosclerosis and likely prophylaxis against strokes and heart attacks. Subsumed benefits from lifestyle modification should become an explicit component of the recurring patient visit to encourage patients to incorporate lifestyle changes to achieve a body mass index of less than 25 kg/m^2 and to adopt a heart healthy diet.

An initial strategy of patient management involves participation in an exercise program (preferably supervised) along with risk factor optimization and the use of carefully selected pharmacologic therapy to supplement care as needed. The consideration of invasive management options is appropriate in patients who have failed optimal medical management, and in those with continued disabling or lifestyle-limiting symptoms. An in-depth discussion of revascularization, however, is out of the scope of this review. Treatment objectives for the optimized contemporary management plan[1,38,46] are summarized in **Table 3**.

Prevention of Cardiovascular Events and Delayed Disease Progression

Tobacco cessation

Smoking cessation is key in reducing the progression of PAD and its symptoms, but also in preventing ischemic cerebrovascular and cardiovascular events. One can readily appreciate the great obstacle patients encounter in achieving cessation; not only is quitting extremely difficult to achieve, but relapse rates are very high. In accordance with the importance of repeated encouragement, the 2011 ACC/AHA guidelines (see **Table 3**) make the following strong recommendations (Class I, LOE A):

- Any current or former smoker should be asked about tobacco status at every visit.
- Counseling and developing a cessation plan, including referral to a program for help and/or pharmacologic therapy, should be addressed.
- One or more of the following pharmacologic therapies should be offered, if no medical contraindications exist:
  ○ Nicotine replacement
  ○ Bupropion
  ○ Varenicline

Repeat counseling, however brief the advice, aimed at complete cessation is the ultimate goal, and is encouraged during multiple patient visits. A plan combining intensive counseling and structured behavioral intervention can achieve cessation rates as high as 20% at 1 year.[47] This recommendation is derived partly from success seen in a high-risk PAD population. In a randomized controlled trial, participants were treated to either an intensive counseling arm, including 6 therapy sessions over 5 months, education, cognitive behavioral therapy, setting a quit date, and social support, or point-of-care unstructured counseling by the clinician.[48] Those in the intensive counseling session were 3 times more likely to be abstinent from smoking at 6 months by self-survey compared with those in the minimal counseling group, a promising conclusion that merits further long-term study. **Table 4** incorporates various therapies and their relative merits toward tobacco cessation.[48,49] An offer of use of one or more of the recommended agents should be included in the efforts to help a patient quit smoking.

The use of electronic cigarettes (ECs) has rapidly expanded over the past 3 years due to robust marketing and unfounded health claims, such as lower nicotine consumption per cigarette, use as a cessation aid, and lack of secondhand smoke from the emitted vapor.[14] Major contributions to the rapid expansion can be explained by the fact that ECs have penetrated beyond the accepted limitations placed on traditional cigarettes: full-color ads on billboards, television and print media showing customers actively engaged in the act of smoking an EC, permitted use in public places, such as bars, restaurants, and airports, and widespread endorsement by public figures and celebrities. Significant concerns that have not yet been scientifically disproven exist regarding (1) the inconsistency of inhaled nicotine per puff; (2) active secondhand exposure to toxic chemicals, such as formaldehyde, acetone, and propylene (by-products of the chemical used to generate the vapor); and (3) initiation of the habit of smoking in never-smokers (in particular, at-risk and impressionable adolescent youth) because of the belief that ECs are a safe and healthy alternative to traditional cigarettes. Furthermore, data regarding the facilitation of tobacco cessation using ECs are inconsistent and meta-analyses are plagued by heterogeneity, from which clear signals of benefit cannot be derived.[14,50,51] Finally, the individual and societal dangers from "dual use" of concomitant EC consumption and traditional cigarettes have not been fully analyzed.

Diabetes mellitus

The impact of DM management on microvascular and macrovascular end points has been extensively investigated, and a few important lessons have been learned. The Diabetes Control and Complications Trial (DCCT) demonstrated microvascular benefits (delay to onset and slowed progression of retinopathy, nephropathy, and neuropathy) with diabetes control, but a lack of overall macrovascular benefits with intensive control of hyperglycemia.[52] As a result, an important goal for glucose control set forth in the guidelines is a target hemoglobin A1C (HgbA1C) of less than 7.0%. However, results from the Action to Control Cardiovascular Risk in Diabetes (ACCORD) study of intensive (with a goal HgbA1C of <6.0%) versus regular glucose control (with a target HgbA1C of 7.0%–7.9%)[53] unveiled a previously unrecognized harm. A significantly higher number of patients in the intensive control group died or suffered from hypoglycemia requiring assistance or had greater than 10 kg of weight gain at 3.5 years of follow-up, prompting early termination of the trial. The benefits of modest glycemic control may extend beyond microvascular events; the United Kingdom Prospective Diabetes Study's (UKPDS) survivor cohort followed for 10 years[54] showed emerging reduction in myocardial infarction, but no benefit in reduction of PAD development or progression, with a target glucose of less than 108 mg/dL. Overall, macrovascular end points with intensive hyperglycemic control have not been convincingly achieved, and societal recommendations exist only for microvascular benefits. Because of the increased risk of PAD and peripheral neuropathy, proper foot care and hygiene are major focuses of the 2005 and 2011 ACCF/AHA guidelines in the diabetic population. This includes meticulous attention to overall nail length and character (frequently requiring management by podiatric specialists), skin or tissue loss to suggest ulceration or gangrene, and serial (every 6 months) surveillance for small fiber sensory neuropathy (with use of diabetic monofilament tool). Patients are reminded to remain vigilant for fissures and cracks (especially near the heels and pads of the feet) that could become secondarily infected. The goal is to reduce the risk of toe and limb amputation.

Hypertension

Hypertension is a well-recognized atherosclerotic risk factor. In the survivor cohort of the UKPDS, a 12% reduction in all-cause mortality was observed for each 10-mm Hg reduction in systolic blood pressure. Remarkably, the risk of PAD complications, such as limb amputation or PAD-related death, was reduced by 16% for the same blood pressure reduction.[55] In the Heart Outcomes Prevention Evaluation (HOPE) study, those with atherosclerosis or DM and one additional cardiovascular risk factor benefited from the use of ramipril versus placebo

with a 20% relative risk reduction in a composite end point of myocardial infarction, stroke, or vascular death.[56] The 2011 ACCF/AHA PAD guidelines update provides a strong recommendation (Class I, LOE A) that the goal blood pressure on treatment should be less than 140/90 mm Hg in nondiabetic patients and less than 130/80 in those with DM or chronic kidney disease.[38] The use of ACE inhibitors is given a moderate, reasonable recommendation (Class IIa, LOE B). Importantly, despite historic concern regarding the use of beta-adrenergic blockade in those with symptomatic PAD, two meta-analyses of randomized, controlled studies suggested there was no need to avoid this class of drugs.[57,58] Given the high co-prevalence of CAD and proven reduction in myocardial infarction with derived mortality benefit,[59] the use of beta-adrenergic blockade therapy in PAD accordingly carries a high-grade recommendation (Class I, LOE A) as being effective and not contraindicated in PAD.

Hyperlipidemia

The mechanisms by which hyperlipidemia contributes to coronary atherosclerosis are well understood and its treatment well established for primary and secondary prevention. In PAD, the role of lipid-reduction therapy is less appreciated and significantly underused. In the Heart Protection Study (HPS), simvastatin 40 mg daily was compared with placebo, with mean LDL levels of 89 mg/dL on treatment versus 127 mg/dL in the placebo group, and an overall significant reduction in cardiovascular events.[8] Patients with PAD within the study demonstrated a 24% relative risk reduction to the onset of the first major vascular event, an outcome independent of baseline LDL level.[60] Despite these profound gains, HMG-CoA-reductase (statin) therapy is often underused in those with PAD. The Bypass versus Angioplasty in Severe Ischaemia of the Leg (BASIL) trial demonstrated that nearly two-thirds of patients with severe PAD were not on statin therapy at the time of study enrollment.[61] In a large, single-center, retrospective review of patients with diagnoses of CAD and/or PAD, statin use and mean lipid levels were compared.[62] Of the 10,000 patients studied, 5% had a PAD diagnosis alone, and 10% had both diagnoses. The mean LDL level in the PAD cohort was significantly higher than in the CAD cohort (LDL mean 92 mg/dL vs 83 mg/dL); fewer PAD patients were treated to targets of LDL less than 100 mg/dL (62% vs 78%) and less than 70 mg/dL (30% vs 39%). However, patients with both diagnoses (approximately 10%) were found to have a normalization of this discrepancy, suggesting greater statin administration and on-target attainment in those with the

Table 3
Treatment goals in the contemporary medical management of the patient with peripheral arterial disease

Category[a,b]	Recommendation	Strength of Recommendation	Level of Evidence
Smoking cessation	1. Advise to stop at each visit.	Class I	A
	2. Offer comprehensive options, including behavior modification, nicotine replacement, or other (bupropion or varenicline)		
Treat hyperlipidemia[c]	1. Statin therapy for goal LDL <100 mg/dL, or	Class I	B (LDL <100 mg/dL)
	2. <70 mg/dL with pan-atherosclerosis	Class IIa	B (LDL <70 mg/dL)
	3. In 2013, ACCF/AHA guidelines, secondary prevention with moderate to high-intensity statin recommended	Class I	A (secondary prevention)
Diabetes treatment	1. Proper foot care	Class I	B
	2. HgbA1c <7.0%	Class IIa	C (to reduce microvascular complications only)
Treat hypertension	1. <140/90 mm Hg (nondiabetic)	Class I	A
	2. <130/80 mm Hg (diabetic and/or CKD)	Class I	A
	3. Beta-blockers are effective and not contraindicated in PAD	Class I	A
Antiplatelet and antithrombotic therapy	1. Antiplatelet agent indicated in symptomatic pt	Class I	A
	2. Use ASA 75–325 mg daily monotherapy	Class I	B
	3. Use Plavix 75 mg daily as ASA alternative	Class I	B
	4. Use antiplatelet in asymptomatic patient with ABI <0.90	Class IIa	C
	5. Use antiplatelet in asymptomatic patient with ABI 0.91–0.99	Class IIb	A
	6. Use ASA + Plavix in high-risk symptomatic patient at low bleed risk and high CV risk	Class IIb	B
	7. *Anticoagulation (warfarin) + antiplatelet in absence of any other indication is ineffective and harmful*	*Class III*	*B*

Improve claudication symptoms and quality of life	1. Supervised exercise program as initial treatment, 30–45 min per session, 3–4 sessions per week, minimum 12 wk	Class I	A
	2. Unsupervised exercise program of questionable benefit	Class IIb	B
	3. Cilostazol 100 mg BID trial in all patients (in absence of heart failure)	Class I	A
	4. Pentoxifylline 400 mg TID as alternative, but effectiveness marginal	Class IIb	A (alternative to cilostazol) C (effectiveness)

Abbreviations: ABI, Ankle-Brachial Index; ACCF/AHA, American College of Cardiology/American Heart Association; ASA, aspirin; BID, twice a day; CKD, chronic kidney disease; CV, cardiovascular; LDL, low-density lipoprotein; TID, 3 times a day; PAD, peripheral arterial disease.

[a] Hirsch AT, Haskal ZJ, Hertzer NR, et al. ACC/AHA 2005 guidelines for the management of patients with peripheral arterial disease (lower extremity, renal, mesenteric, and abdominal aortic): executive summary a collaborative report from the American Association for Vascular Surgery/Society for Vascular Surgery, Society for Cardiovascular Angiography and Interventions, Society for Vascular Medicine and Biology, Society of Interventional Radiology, and the ACC/AHA Task Force on Practice Guidelines (Writing Committee to develop guidelines for the management of patients with peripheral arterial disease) endorsed by the American Association of Cardiovascular and Pulmonary Rehabilitation; National Heart, Lung, and Blood Institute; Society for Vascular Nursing; TransAtlantic Inter-Society Consensus; and Vascular Disease Foundation. J Am Coll Cardiol 2006;47(6):1239–312.

[b] Rooke TW, Hirsch AT, Misra S, et al. 2011 ACCF/AHA focused update of the guideline for the management of patients with peripheral artery disease (updating the 2005 guideline): a report of the American College of Cardiology Foundation/American Heart Association Task Force on Practice Guidelines: developed in collaboration with the Society for Cardiovascular Angiography and Interventions, Society of Interventional Radiology, Society for Vascular Medicine, and Society for Vascular Surgery. J Vasc Surg 2011;54(5):e32–58.

[c] Stone NJ, Robinson JG, Lichtenstein AH, et al. 2013 ACC/AHA guideline on the treatment of blood cholesterol to reduce atherosclerotic cardiovascular risk in adults: a report of the American College of Cardiology/American Heart Association Task Force on Practice Guidelines. J Am Coll Cardiol 2014;63(25 Pt B):2889–934.

Table 4
Comparison of nonpharmacologic and pharmacologic agents for smoking cessation

Intervention	Details	Considerations
Structured counseling[a]	Intense multifactorial counseling.	Six-month survey based results with 3× benefit in those in intense counseling group. Long-term studies needed.
Nicotine replacement[b]	Systematic review 150 trials; 50%–70% reduction at 6 mo compared with placebo. Method (gum, patch, spray) did not affect efficacy.	Caution selection bias: only studies with cessation success were analyzed.
Bupropion (Wellbutrin)	Aminoketone antidepressant inhibits norepinephrine and dopamine reuptake. Twelve-month quit rates 35% with nicotine, 30% alone, vs 15% for placebo in randomized trial.[115]	Exact mechanism of action uncertain. No significant difference in quit rates at 1 y when nicotine added to bupropion.
Varenicline (Chantix)	Partial nicotinic acetylcholine receptor agonist, stimulates dopamine release, reduces reinforcement and reward cycle.	Superior results in 2 randomized trials at 7 wk[116] and at 1 y[117] compared with placebo or bupropion. FDA black box warning regarding risk of worsening depression and suicidality from nicotine withdrawal.
E-cigarettes[c]	Battery-powered chemical-based atomization of nicotine in a handheld plastic device.	Concerns exist regarding safety of generated vapor, inconsistent nicotine absorption, and recruitment of nonsmokers to habitual smoking. Value of ECs in tobacco cessation not established, with inconsistent data.

Abbreviations: EC, electronic cigarette; FDA, Food and Drug Administration.
 [a] Hennrikus D, Joseph A, Lando H, et al. Effectiveness of a smoking cessation program for peripheral artery disease patients: a randomized controlled trial. J Am Coll Cardiol 2010;56(25):2105–12.
 [b] Silagy C, Lancaster T, Stead L, et al. Nicotine replacement therapy for smoking cessation. Cochrane Database Syst Rev 2004;(3):CD000146.
 [c] Grana R, Benowitz N, Glantz S. Contemporary reviews in cardiovascular medicine. Circulation 2014;129(19):1972–86.

concomitant diagnosis of CAD. This study, although limited by a retrospective review and single-center bias, highlights the importance of greater attention being given to aggressive lipid control for secondary prevention of coronary disease and the current discrepant rates of hyperlipidemia treatment disfavoring patients with PAD. Society guidelines have consistently highlighted the need for attainment of low LDL levels (<100 mg/dL) in patients with PAD and more aggressive targets (goal LDL <70 mg/dL) in those considered high risk (see **Table 3**).[46,63] In addition, the most current cholesterol guidelines of 2013 include PAD as a clinical atherosclerotic cardiovascular disease condition and favor either moderate or high-potency statin based on age and other clinical metrics.[46]

Antiplatelet therapy

The role of antiplatelet therapy in atherosclerosis is well established for the prevention of cardiovascular events, especially in secondary prevention. There is also a benefit of antiplatelet therapies,

including aspirin and clopidogrel, in symptomatic PAD. This benefit was demonstrated in the Antithrombotic Trialists' Collaboration, which showed a 23% reduction in major vascular events defined as nonfatal myocardial infarction, nonfatal stroke, or vascular death, in a pooled PAD population of 9214 patients.[64] In this high-risk population, the risk of revascularization was significantly reduced for those on antiplatelet therapy (primarily aspirin but including other classes of agents, such as the thienopyridines).

The specific role of aspirin in PAD is less robust than it once was. In a recent meta-analysis of 5269 patients with PAD, the use of aspirin resulted in a 12% reduction in combined ischemic cardiovascular events and death, but this failed to reach statistical significance.[65] In addition, aspirin failed to show a benefit in reducing events in those with asymptomatic, borderline to low ABI.[66] However, the use of antiplatelet therapy, including aspirin, is still highly recommended in the prevention of ischemic events in those with symptomatic PAD (Class 1, LOE B).

In addition to aspirin, the thienopyridine class of antiplatelet agents may be used in PAD. Clopidogrel has the most abundant safety and efficacy data among this class and is generically available. In the Clopidogrel versus Aspirin in Patients at Risk of Ischaemic Events (CAPRIE) trial, clopidogrel was compared with 325 mg of aspirin therapy in more than 19,000 high-risk patients. Clopidogrel was associated with a significant 8.7% overall relative risk reduction in the combined end point (ischemic stroke, myocardial infarction, and/or vascular death) compared with aspirin (5.32% vs 5.83%, an absolute risk reduction of 0.51%, P<.04) Importantly, in the PAD subgroup (6452 patients), a 24% relative risk reduction was seen with clopidogrel over aspirin.[1] As a result, clopidogrel is strongly recommended as an alternative to aspirin in those with PAD (Class 1, LOE B).

Given the positive results of the CAPRIE study, the impact of dual antiplatelet therapy with both aspirin and clopidogrel was evaluated in high-risk patients in the Clopidogrel and Aspirin versus Aspirin Alone for the Prevention of Atherothrombotic Events (CHARISMA) trial. Dual antiplatelet therapy versus low-dose aspirin alone was evaluated in 15,603 patients with established atherosclerotic disease or numerous high-risk features. Overall, the dual antiplatelet treatment group had the same number of events within the primary composite end point of myocardial infarction, stroke, and cardiovascular death, with no significant between-group differences in the prespecified analyses, including those with PAD.[67] The use of dual antiplatelet therapy is given a weak recommendation (Class IIb, LOE B), with the warning to use only in those at low risk of gastrointestinal and central nervous system bleeding disorders and high cardiovascular risk (see **Table 3**). The use of dual antiplatelet therapy should be limited to those with absolute indications, such as in the use of intracoronary stents.

A systematic review from the Cochrane Peripheral Vascular Diseases Group conducted in 2011 pooled the effects of aspirin, clopidogrel, and picotamide versus placebo from 12 randomized, double-blinded and controlled trials that enrolled more than 12,000 claudicants but excluded patients on either extremes of the Fontaine classification scheme (see **Table 2**). In those with IC, when compared with placebo, the use of antiplatelet agents significantly reduced all-cause mortality, cardiovascular mortality, and the risk of limb deterioration requiring revascularization, but also significantly increased drug-related adverse effects, such as dyspepsia, which lead to treatment discontinuation.[68]

The use of warfarin with antiplatelet therapy in the absence of other primary indications for systemic anticoagulation is not indicated (Class III, LOE B) and is considered a definite harm, in light of the observed major bleeding events when antiplatelet and anticoagulant therapies are combined (see **Table 3**). The substitution of the novel oral anticoagulants, such as dabigatran, rivaroxaban, edoxaban, or apixaban, for warfarin in the absence of a primary indication for anticoagulation has not yet been evaluated in a rigorous clinical trial. Absent these data, recommendations for their use cannot be made at the present time.

Reducing Symptoms and Improving Quality of Life

Improving functional status and quality of life is a formidable challenge in the management of patients with symptomatic PAD, especially when aimed at improving symptoms of IC. Established therapies for the symptomatic treatment of IC include exercise training and two approved pharmacologic agents in North America: cilostazol and pentoxifylline. We discuss the relative merits of each of these established options (**Fig. 7**), followed by emerging and investigational therapies.

Pharmacologic therapy

Cilostazol (Pletal; Otsuka Pharmaceutical Company, Tokyo, Japan) is an inhibitor of phosphodiesterase-3, whose action causes an increase in intracellular cyclic adenosine mono phosphate (cAMP), leading to arterial smooth muscle dilatation, increased nitric oxide signaling, and, to a lesser extent, decreased platelet aggregation.[69] Additional pleiotropic effects include increased HDL levels and lower triglyceride levels.[70] In a pooled analysis of 9 randomized clinical trials, cilostazol (100 mg taken twice daily) was associated with a twofold improvement in maximal walking distance from baseline at 20 weeks compared with placebo, with an absolute improvement of 42 meters.[71] Notably, these effects were found to be independent of age, gender, smoking status, DM, PAD duration, prior myocardial infarction, and beta-blocker use. Importantly, the investigators concluded that there was no observed difference in all-cause mortality with the addition of cilostazol. Although patients with congestive heart failure were included in all but one of the randomized clinical trials evaluated in this meta-analysis, they comprised only 3% of the pooled participants. Because of a similar mechanism of action to the inotropic agents amrinone and milrinone, which demonstrated an adverse effect on mortality in advanced heart failure, the US Food and Drug Administration has established a boxed

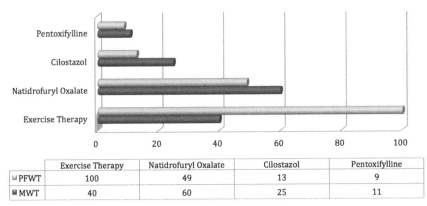

	Exercise Therapy	Natidrofuryl Oxalate	Cilostazol	Pentoxifylline
▦ PFWT	100	49	13	9
▦ MWT	40	60	25	11

Fig. 7. Placebo-controlled comparison of percentage improvement in walking performance at 6 months. MWT, maximum walking time in minutes; PFWT, pain-free walking time. (*Data for pharmacologic therapies from* Stevens JW, Simpson E, Harnan S, et al. Systematic review of the efficiency of cilostazol, naftidrofuryl oxalate and pentoxifylline for the treatment of intermittent claudication. Br J Surg 2012;99(12):1630–8; and *Data for exercise therapy from* Lane R, Ellis B, Watson L, et al. Exercise for intermittent claudication. Cochrane Database Syst Rev 2014;(7):CD000990.)

warning for cilostazol, prohibiting its use in patients with congestive heart failure. Treatment discontinuation is unfortunately quite common; it has been estimated that up to 60% of patients stop taking cilostazol by 36 months because of treatment side effects,[72] such as headache, palpitations, and diarrhea.[73,74] Cilostazol is highly recommended in the symptomatic treatment of IC (Class I, LOE A) in the absence of heart failure (see **Table 3**). The usual dosage is 100 mg twice daily, but because of its inhibitory effects on the cytochrome P450 enzymes 3A4 (co-inhibited by diltiazem) and 2C19 (co-inhibited by omeprazole), a dosage adjustment to 50 mg twice daily is advised.[75,76]

Pentoxifylline (Trental; Sanofi, Paris, France), in contrast, has marginal efficacy in the relief of PAD symptoms. Pentoxifylline, a rheologic modifier, is a methylxanthine metabolized at the red blood cell membrane level. It increases erythrocyte flexibility, increases fibrinogen levels, and reduces blood viscosity.[77] Placebo-controlled trials have historically demonstrated significant benefit of pentoxifylline for symptomatic PAD, both in terms of improved walking distance and hospital cost savings.[78] However, a recent systematic review of 23 randomized controlled trials with data on more than 2800 patients highlighted the overall poor quality of these historical data. Significant heterogeneity was noted in the interventions and in the results, which lead to the inability to clearly demonstrate a signal of benefit in those with claudication (Fontaine class II),[79] thereby softening the stance on its independent use. Accordingly, its use carries a weak recommendation (Class IIb, LOE C) for overall effectiveness, but is a reasonable alternative to cilostazol (Class IIb, LOE A; see **Table 3**).

Naftidrofuryl oxalate (Praxilene; Merck Serono, Middlesex, UK) is a serotonin receptor antagonist with vasoactive properties in vascular smooth muscle; it inhibits vasoconstriction, reduces platelet aggregation, and decreases cell proliferation. It also improves glucose aerobic metabolism and thus reduces ischemic arterial wall injury.[80] It has been used for claudication primarily in the UK and throughout Europe since its approval in 1972, but is not available in the United States. This likely stems from legal difficulties and the lengthy drug-approval processes, high marketing costs in a competitive environment, and limited market exclusivity (protection of only 5 years from generic competition).[81] The dosage is 100 to 200 mg 3 times daily with a treatment duration of 5 to 6 months.[82] Comparing the relative efficacies of cilostazol, pentoxifylline, and naftidrofuryl oxalate, a 2012 systematic review pooled data from 11 trials and networked trials of cilostazol and pentoxifylline to allow a direct head-to-head comparison of the two drugs.[83] Naftidrofuryl oxalate had the maximum therapeutic effect, although only one trial using this drug was included in the pooled analysis. At 24 weeks, naftidrofuryl oxalate increased maximal walking time and pain-free walking time by 60% and 49% over placebo, respectively. When using cilostazol, maximal walking time and pain-free walking time were improved by 25% and 13%, respectively. In contrast, the benefit of pentoxifylline remained questionable, with paltry 11% and 9% improvements seen in these walking parameters compared with placebo. Adverse effect profiles were similar across these agents. Concerns about heterogeneity and lack of confounding were noted, in particular the inability to separate from the meta-analysis (1) those who may have received exercise therapy before the trial, (2) patient follow-up lasting more than 24 weeks in the trials of cilostazol versus placebo, (3) censoring of health-related quality-of-life data for those who prematurely discontinued drug therapies in the final analysis,[81] and (4) among others, a lack of standardized exercise protocols for assessing maximal walking distance. Ultimately, naftidrofuryl oxalate, with its enhanced safety profile, may be the most efficacious drug in this setting. It is the only drug recommended for PAD symptom reduction in the United Kingdom, as cilostazol is not approved for use in part because of the enhanced safety profile of naftidrofuryl oxalate. A cost-sensitivity analysis revealed that naftidrofuryl oxalate, when compared with cilostazol, is also at least sevenfold more cost-effective when comparing incremental cost-effectiveness ratios (ICER) per quality-adjusted life year (QALY).[84] Despite these findings, however, naftidrofuryl is likely not to be approved in the United States any time soon.

Exercise therapy

Exercise training is arguably the most important intervention for the patient with IC, in terms of overall benefit (see **Fig. 7**). This benefit is noted in the increased maximal and pain-free walk distances, as well as improvements in quality of life and overall cardiovascular health.[85] Participation in a supervised exercise-training program (SET) is the preferred method to achieve these benefits.

Exercise therapy is postulated to benefit limb perfusion through promotion of angiogenesis[86] and improved endothelial function,[87] as well as increased muscle strength through enhanced nutrient delivery to skeletal muscle.[88] Regular exercise also has been shown to reduce cardiovascular risk through improvements in glucose metabolism, blood pressure, lipid metabolism, and systemic inflammation.[89]

There are several components of the SET that have been shown to provide the greatest benefit: the frequency (at least 3 times per week), duration (at least 30 minutes per session), method (using interval training with moderate claudication at rest point), and mode of exercise (most commonly walking). Key components of the exercise program are outlined in **Box 3**. The ACCF/AHA 2011 guidelines update highly recommends SET for all patients with IC (Class I, LOE A) (see **Table 3**).

Supervised exercise programs

Remarkable gains are made with exercise training for IC, most notably supervised exercise. In a recent Cochrane Database Systematic Review, Lane and colleagues[90] evaluated combined data from 30 trials of exercise versus placebo or usual care, encompassing a total of 1816 patients with stable IC symptoms. Exercise was performed in

---

> **Box 3**
> **Components of a supervised exercise training program for intermittent claudication**
>
> - At least three 30–45-minute sessions per week, for a total of at least 12 weeks.
> - Warm up and cool down for 5 minutes.
> - Walking on a track or treadmill (preferred) with intensity designed to elicit moderate claudication pain in 3–5 minutes, then initiate a period of sitting or standing rest until pain subsides, then exercise again until claudication symptoms ("exercise-rest-exercise" or interval training method).
> - Determine walk performance at entrance and exit from program using 6-min walk (best approximation of walking in daily living).
> - Monitor for angina, arrhythmias, and significant changes in blood pressure with increasing workloads of exercise.

---

a supervised fashion at least twice per week in most trials with variable follow-up. Follow-up ranged from 2 weeks to 2 years, and exercise type, including treadmill, strength training, and pole-striding, as well as upper limb exercises, were performed. Although exercise, partly due to insufficient data, did not demonstrate an improvement in the ABI, mortality, amputation, peak exercise calf blood flow, and improvements in walking ability were astounding (in the range of 50%–200%). Compared with placebo, SET resulted in a greater improvement in the following areas: mean change in maximal walking time of 4.5 minutes (95% CI 3.11–9.52), a pain-free walking distance of 82 m (95% CI 71.86–92.72), and a maximum walking distance of 109 m (95% CI 38.20–179.78) at up to 2 years. Even when compared with overall pharmacologic therapies, exercise based interventions achieve the greatest improvements in walking performance (see **Fig. 7**).

Exercise therapy for asymptomatic individuals with peripheral arterial disease

Considering the overall cardiovascular benefits, exercise training is, not surprisingly, beneficial to those without symptoms of IC, but at elevated risk of future events, as defined by an abnormal resting ABI. In a randomized, controlled trial comparing placebo, lower extremity resistance training, and treadmill training, asymptomatic patients at risk (ABI <0.95) were enrolled in respective treatment arms and followed to 6 months. A significant improvement in the 6-minute walk test (21 m) compared with the placebo group (–15 m) for a net gain of 36 m (95% CI 15–56, P<.001) was noted in the treadmill arm, with no statistically significant improvement in the resistance-training arm for the 6-minute walk test.[91] Importantly, a sizable number of screened participants were excluded from the randomization, because they could not participate 3 times weekly in the study protocol or failed to keep the study appointment before randomization, which cautioned a selection bias in interpreting the results. Approximately 50 patients were enrolled in each study arm, with excellent follow-up. Exploratory analyses suggested a signal of benefit in global cardiovascular health as judged by improvements ($P<.02$) in flow-mediated dilatation in the brachial artery, although sample sizes were too small to make definitive conclusions.

Unsupervised (home-based) exercise programs

Home-based or community-based, unsupervised exercise programs could play an important supplementary role in the medical management of the treatment of IC. However, controversy has arisen regarding the use of this alternative versus supervised training, and only limited conclusions can be drawn from the heterogeneous data. Currently the ACCF/AHA guidelines give a weaker recommendation (Class IIb, LOE B) for the use of unsupervised exercise training.

A Cochrane systematic review from 2013 evaluated 14 studies (with a total of 1002 participants) that compared supervised and unsupervised exercise training programs. Programs using SET maintained an effect size of 0.48 (95% CI 0.32–0.64) over unsupervised programs, which translates to an approximately 180-m gain in maximal walking distance, again providing evidence for the benefit of exercise for symptomatic PAD, and confirming that the delivery of exercise therapy through a structured intervention is superior to an unstructured one.[92]

Inability to participate, however, in a thrice-weekly exercise setting is a common drawback of traditional SET programs, which is ultimately reflected in the lack of benefit derived by the symptomatic patient. Lack of insurance coverage significantly limits the patient enrollment into these programs, it constricts the programs' growth and success in the long-term, and ultimately discourages physicians from using all of their potential resources. Despite the impressive gains seen with SET, this is not a feasible reality for most patients. In an online survey of vascular surgeons (most respondents were from Europe), accessibility to SET programs was judged to be as low as 30%.[93]

How do unsupervised programs fare? An observational study of a community-based exercise program provided mixed reviews; it showed significant improvements in absolute claudication distance, but disappointingly high dropout rates. The dropout rate was approximately 50%, for a variety of reasons, including satisfaction with the achieved improvements, lack of motivation, dissatisfaction with the results, and concurrent nonvascular illness.[94] In a rigorous, randomized controlled trial setting, the results were significantly better. In the Group Oriented Arterial Leg Study (GOALS), investigators randomized patients to a rigorous and multifaceted home-based exercise regimen (group-based cognitive behavioral support and self-regulatory behavioral support) versus a traditional "educate only" control group.[95] At 6 months of follow-up, a mean improvement of 54 m (95% CI 33–74, $P<.001$) was demonstrated on the 6-minute walk test in the treatment group compared with the control group. Important precautions to interpreting the data include a significant referral bias, as study participants were enrolled from responses to print and online advertisements, physicians within the health system conducting the study, and previous participants in vascular outcomes research at that institution; a performance bias for those trained to use the treadmill and cognitively modify their performance; and finally the ever-present Hawthorne effect of those who are under greater scrutiny performing more closely to the expected outcomes. Home-based programs in which participants were even outfitted with motion detectors, biofeedback devices, or pedometers provided mixed results both for and against home-based regimens in comparison with SET programs,[96,97] thereby further polluting a clear signal of benefit.

Given the lack of proven benefit with unsupervised programs and the lack of access to SET in large part because of lack of insurance coverage, could government payers be influenced to cover appropriate individuals if SET were proven cost-effective? In a cost-effectiveness assessment of trials comparing supervised versus unsupervised training programs for symptomatic PAD, an average ICER of approximately $2000 per QALY was gained,[98] a value that is well below the accepted $50,000 per QALY threshold in the United States.[99] Adoption of centralized reimbursements, through the Centers for Medicaid and Medicare Services, ought to be considered for the payment of supervised exercise programs in patients with the appropriate indications, as the public health burden widens and treatment options remain limited.

Exercise compared with revascularization

Although the aim of this review is to summarize current knowledge and relevant opinions in the noninvasive, medical management of the patient with PAD, recent results challenge the traditional paradigm that invasive therapy should bypass or replace medical therapy in certain lesion subsets. On the contrary, SET may trump the value of invasive management (ie, revascularization) and also has shown benefit when used concomitantly with revascularization.

In the Claudication: Exercise versus Endoluminal Revascularization (CLEVER) study, Murphy and colleagues[100] randomized 119 participants with moderate to severe claudication symptoms and hemodynamically significant aortoiliac disease in a 2:2:1 fashion to stent-based revascularization, supervised exercise training, and optimal medical management. The primary end point of the study was an improvement in the peak, or maximum, walking time 6 months after the allotted treatment. Supervised exercise was a 26-week standardized regimen, with hour-long sessions thrice weekly. All stent procedures were technically successful, with a mean aortoiliac stenosis of 83% before revascularization and 5% after revascularization, and ABI readings 0.66 at baseline and improving by 0.29 at 6 months after revascularization. The results defied the investigators' initial hypothesis that stenting would be superior, as improvements in peak walking time were 5.8, 3.7, and 1.2 minutes for exercise, stenting, and optimal medical management, respectively. When comparing them directly, there was a 2.1-minute greater improvement in mean maximal walking time with exercise over stenting (95% CI 0.0–4.2 minutes, $P = .04$). Secondary end points demonstrated that both exercise and stenting groups had improvement in pain-free walking time and quality-of-life measurements.

In a meta-analysis incorporating 8 randomized controlled trials comparing exercise versus stenting, including 1 aortoiliac, 3 femoropopliteal, and 5 trials with both lesions addressed, despite significant heterogeneity preventing pooling of data, the conclusion could still be made that percutaneous angioplasty approximated the benefits of exercise therapy. However, used synergistically, revascularization and exercise enhanced maximal walking distance and quality-of-life outcomes.[101] An assessment of QALYs when comparing SET, percutaneous transluminal angioplasty (PTA), or both in a randomized, controlled fashion showed that the use of PTA first or alone was nearly twice as costly per QALY in comparison with the use of SET first or in combination with PTA,[102] yet again endorsing the need for widespread support for SET for the management of claudication.

Investigational therapies for symptom improvement

Statins There are data to suggest that statin therapy may favorably influence walking abilities in PAD. In a randomized trial of 354 patients treated with placebo, atorvastatin 10 mg daily, or atorvastatin 80 mg daily, statin therapy showed improvement in pain-free walk times of 25% above baseline. This improvement in pain-free walking time was seen with 80 mg of atorvastatin compared with placebo at 1 year (providing an approximately 40-second longer time), but no improvement in maximal walking time.[103] Although no statistical interaction existed in this trial between the primary finding and LDL levels, or the ABI in either treatment group, a purported mechanism for the finding that pain-free walk time improved with high-potency statin dose may be due to improvements in endothelin-derived nitric oxide signaling leading to improved local smooth muscle vasodilation.[104] Conclusions made from this trial were echoed in a systematic analysis of 18 trials with more than 10,000 participants. In an analysis of the pooled data (on a variety of lipid-lowering agents), total walking distance (weighted mean difference +152 m) and pain-free walking distance improved (weighted mean difference +90 m) with statin therapy compared with placebo, but without a significant impact on the ABI.[105] In those already at goal on less than or equal to moderate intensity statin therapy, the use of post hoc moderate to high-dose statin therapy to improve symptomatic PAD may have an emerging role.

Angiotensin-converting enzyme inhibition
ACE inhibitor therapy, particularly with ramipril, has shown promise in symptom reduction for PAD. In a randomized trial evaluating ramipril, 212 patients were randomized to either 10 mg per day of ramipril or placebo for 24 weeks, to primarily study the effects on maximal and pain-free walk time, as well as quality-of-life assessments, such as the Short-Form 36 (SF-36) Health Survey.[106] At 6 months, ramipril-treated patients had a significantly improved pain-free walking time (75 seconds longer than placebo, 95% CI 60–89 seconds, $P<.001$), maximum walking time (255 seconds longer than placebo, 95% CI 215–295, $P<.001$), and overall physical component summary score on the SF-36 ($P = .02$). Notably, significant improvements in systolic (-3.1 mm Hg, $P<.001$) and diastolic blood pressure (-4.3 mm Hg, $P<.001$) were seen in the treatment group. In addition, there were improvements in resting and postexercise ABI measurements

(0.10, $P<.001$ and 0.11, $P<.001$, respectively), with the resting improvement attributed to reductions in brachial systolic pressures. Positive effects of ACE inhibition have been attributed to improved vaso-dilatation and blood flow through reduction in angiotensin II, improved endothelial dysfunction through preservation of bradykinin, and sympathetic inhibition.

Based on this potential improvement in function and the previously noted robust cardio-protective effect seen in the HOPE trial independent of blood pressure reduction, a recommendation was made by the TransAtlantic Inter-Society Consensus (TASC) II group for the use of ACE inhibitors in patients with PAD.[107]

Propionyl-L-carnitine

Carnitine is a critical amino acid component of free fatty acid oxidation as well as pyruvate dehydrogenase-mediated glucose oxidation,[108] whose metabolism is altered and dysfunctional in advanced PAD.[109] Supplementation with propionyl-L-carnitine (PLC) reduces oxidative stress brought on by tissue hypoxia, and delays muscle fatigue in an animal model.[110] When analyzed in a placebo-controlled clinical trial of 239 patients with moderate to severe PAD, the administration of 2 g per day orally of PLC led to significant improvements in maximum walking time (1.6 minutes more than placebo, $P<.05$) and pain-free walking time, with no significant difference in the ABI and no independent serious adverse effects from the treatment.[111] A meta-analysis of 2013 subjects from 18 experimental studies using varying doses and routes of PLC administration showed mixed results, with the overall trend toward a modest benefit from PLC, with some signal toward improved results with intravenous therapy over oral therapy and in those with severe claudication versus moderate claudication.[112] Before routine supplementation, the investigators recommend a randomized analysis to determine optimal dose, route, and cost-effectiveness of this supplement.

Therapeutic angiogenesis

Stem cell and gene therapies are promising, newer options aimed at inducing therapeutic angiogenesis for PAD, but primarily in advanced PAD. In a meta-analysis, autologous stem cell therapy and gene transfer therapy in 543 patients in 6 randomized controlled trials showed minimal improvement in those with claudication, but a significant benefit in those with CLI with ulceration, rest pain, or tissue loss. In addition, this potential benefit was seen with only a slightly higher rate of nonserious adverse effects like edema, hypotension, and proteinuria, thus making this a tolerable and potentially efficacious therapy in advanced PAD.[113] However, caution is advised by the investigators of a more inclusive systematic review published in 2013, whereby 12 randomized trials with 1494 patients (64% with CLI) were assessed.[114] In this analysis, no single end point (all-cause mortality, amputations, ulcer healing) was met in most studies, despite positive findings in individual randomized controlled trials. No differences were noted in those with IC or CLI. Thus, the role of therapeutic angiogenesis remains uncertain in PAD but is unlikely to have a role in IC symptom management.

SUMMARY

PAD due to lower limb atherosclerosis is a common problem that is often overlooked by the medical community. PAD is associated with a high risk of adverse cardiovascular events and mortality, even in the asymptomatic state. Classic symptoms due to PAD are exertional leg discomfort or IC, but most patients are asymptomatic or experience atypical leg symptoms. The use of diagnostic testing should include measurement of the ABI in all patients plus physiologic testing and/or advanced imaging as needed to determine disease severity and location and determine revascularization options. The treatment of PAD should focus on treatment of modifiable risk factors, including smoking cessation, lipid-lowering therapy, and antihypertensive therapy, and antiplatelet therapies to delay disease progression and prevent ischemic events. Treatment to provide symptomatic relief for IC should focus on supervised exercise training and pharmacologic therapy, most notably with cilostazol (in North America).

REFERENCES

1. Hirsch AT, Haskal ZJ, Hertzer NR, et al. ACC/AHA 2005 guidelines for the management of patients with peripheral arterial disease (lower extremity, renal, mesenteric, and abdominal aortic): executive summary a collaborative report from the American Association for Vascular Surgery/Society for Vascular Surgery, Society for Cardiovascular Angiography and Interventions, Society for Vascular Medicine and Biology, Society of Interventional Radiology, and the ACC/AHA Task Force on Practice Guidelines (Writing Committee to develop guidelines for the management of patients with peripheral arterial disease) endorsed by the American Association of Cardiovascular and Pulmonary Rehabilitation; National Heart, Lung, and Blood Institute; Society for Vascular Nursing;

1. TransAtlantic Inter-Society Consensus; and Vascular Disease Foundation. J Am Coll Cardiol 2006;47(6):1239–312.

2. Roger VL, Go AS, Lloyd-Jones DM, et al. Heart disease and stroke statistics–2012 update: a report from the American Heart Association. Circulation 2012;125(1):e2–220. Available at: http://www.ncbi.nlm.nih.gov/pubmed/22179539.

3. Ostchega Y, Paulose-Ram R, Dillon CF, et al. Prevalence of peripheral arterial disease and risk factors in persons aged 60 and older: data from the National Health and Nutrition Examination Survey 1999-2004. J Am Geriatr Soc 2007;55(4):583–9.

4. Hirsch AT, Criqui MH, Treat-Jacobson D, et al. Peripheral arterial disease detection, awareness, and treatment in primary care. JAMA 2001;286(11):1317–24.

5. Agnelli G, Cimminiello C, Meneghetti G, et al. Low ankle-brachial index predicts an adverse 1-year outcome after acute coronary and cerebrovascular events. J Thromb Haemost 2006;4(12):2599–606.

6. Boden WE, Cherr GS, Eagle KA, et al. Prior cardiovascular interventions are not associated with worsened clinical outcomes in patients with symptomatic atherothrombosis. Crit Pathw Cardiol 2010;9(3):116–25.

7. Allison MA, Criqui MH, McClelland RL, et al. The effect of novel cardiovascular risk factors on the ethnic-specific odds for peripheral arterial disease in the Multi-Ethnic Study of Atherosclerosis (MESA). J Am Coll Cardiol 2006;48(6):1190–7.

8. Heart Protection Study Collaborative Group. MRC/BHF Heart Protection Study of cholesterol lowering with simvastatin in 20,536 high-risk individuals: a randomised placebo-controlled trial. Lancet 2002;360(9326):7–22.

9. Fowkes FG, Housley E, Riemersma RA, et al. Smoking, lipids, glucose intolerance, and blood pressure as risk factors for peripheral atherosclerosis compared with ischemic heart disease in the Edinburgh Artery Study. Am J Epidemiol 1992;135(4):331–40.

10. Krupski WC. The peripheral vascular consequences of smoking. Ann Vasc Surg 1991;5(3):291–304.

11. Shammas NW. Epidemiology, classification, and modifiable risk factors of peripheral arterial disease. Vasc Health Risk Manag 2007;3(2):229–34.

12. Bartholomew JR, Olin JW. Pathophysiology of peripheral arterial disease and risk factors for its development. Cleve Clin J Med 2006;73(Suppl 4):S8–14.

13. He Y, Lam TH, Jiang B, et al. Passive smoking and risk of peripheral arterial disease and ischemic stroke in Chinese women who never smoked. Circulation 2008;118(15):1535–40.

14. Grana R, Benowitz N, Glantz SA. E-cigarettes: a scientific review. Circulation 2014;129(19):1972–86.

15. Selvin E, Marinopoulos S, Berkenblit G, et al. Meta-analysis: glycosylated hemoglobin and cardiovascular disease in diabetes mellitus. Ann Intern Med 2004;141(6):421–31.

16. American Diabetes Association. Peripheral arterial disease in people with diabetes. Diabetes Care 2003;26(12):3333–41.

17. Pedicino D, Giglio AF, Galiffa VA, et al. Type 2 diabetes, immunity and cardiovascular risk: A Complex Relationship, Pathophysiology and Complications of Diabetes Mellitus. In: Oguntibeju O, editor. InTech; 2012.

18. Jude EB, Oyibo SO, Chalmers N, et al. Peripheral arterial disease in diabetic and nondiabetic patients: a comparison of severity and outcome. Diabetes Care 2001;24(8):1433–7.

19. Kannel WB, McGee DL. Update on some epidemiologic features of intermittent claudication: the Framingham Study. J Am Geriatr Soc 1985;33(1):13–8.

20. Newman AB, Siscovick DS, Manolio TA, et al. Ankle-arm index as a marker of atherosclerosis in the Cardiovascular Health Study. Cardiovascular Heart Study (CHS) Collaborative Research Group. Circulation 1993;88(3):837–45.

21. Cardia G, Grisorio D, Impedovo G, et al. Plasma lipids as a risk factor in peripheral vascular disease. Angiology 1990;41(1):19–22.

22. Murabito JM, D'Agostino RB, Silbershatz H, et al. Intermittent claudication. A risk profile from The Framingham Heart Study. Circulation 1997;96(1):44–9.

23. Zhan Y, Yu J, Ding R, et al. Triglyceride to high density lipoprotein cholesterol ratio, total cholesterol to high density lipoprotein cholesterol ratio and low ankle brachial index in an elderly population. Vasa 2014;43(3):189–97.

24. Ridker PM, Stampfer MJ, Rifai N. Novel risk factors for systemic atherosclerosis: a comparison of C-reactive protein, fibrinogen, homocysteine, lipoprotein(a), and standard cholesterol screening as predictors of peripheral arterial disease. JAMA 2001;285(19):2481–5.

25. Boushey CJ, Beresford SA, Omenn GS, et al. A quantitative assessment of plasma homocysteine as a risk factor for vascular disease. Probable benefits of increasing folic acid intakes. JAMA 1995;274(13):1049–57.

26. Taylor LM, Moneta GL, Sexton GJ, et al. Prospective blinded study of the relationship between plasma homocysteine and progression of symptomatic peripheral arterial disease. J Vasc Surg 1999;29(1):8–19 [discussion: 19–21].

27. Lonn E, Yusuf S, Arnold MJ, et al. Homocysteine lowering with folic acid and B vitamins in vascular disease. N Engl J Med 2006;354(15):1567–77.

28. Newman AB, Tyrrell KS, Kuller LH. Mortality over four years in SHEP participants with a low ankle-arm index. J Am Geriatr Soc 1997;45(12):1472–8.

29. Resnick HE, Lindsay RS, McDermott MM, et al. Relationship of high and low ankle brachial index to all-cause and cardiovascular disease mortality: the Strong Heart Study. Circulation 2004;109(6):733–9.

30. Heald CL, Fowkes FG, Murray GD, et al. Risk of mortality and cardiovascular disease associated with the ankle-brachial index: systematic review. Atherosclerosis 2006;189(1):61–9.

31. Fowkes FG, Murray GD, Butcher I, et al. Ankle brachial index combined with Framingham Risk Score to predict cardiovascular events and mortality: a meta-analysis. JAMA 2008;300(2):197–208.

32. Diehm C, Allenberg JR, Pittrow D, et al. Mortality and vascular morbidity in older adults with asymptomatic versus symptomatic peripheral artery disease. Circulation 2009;120(21):2053–61.

33. Criqui MH, Langer RD, Fronek A, et al. Mortality over a period of 10 years in patients with peripheral arterial disease. N Engl J Med 1992;326(6):381–6.

34. Weitz JI, Byrne J, Clagett GP, et al. Diagnosis and treatment of chronic arterial insufficiency of the lower extremities: a critical review. Circulation 1996;94(11):3026–49.

35. Wennberg PW. Approach to the patient with peripheral arterial disease. Circulation 2013;128(20):2241–50.

36. Rose GA. The diagnosis of ischaemic heart pain and intermittent claudication in field surveys. Bull World Health Organ 1962;27:645–58.

37. Dormandy JA, Rutherford RB. Management of peripheral arterial disease (PAD). TASC Working Group. TransAtlantic Inter-Society Consensus (TASC). J Vasc Surg 2000;31(1 Pt 2):S1–296.

38. Rooke TW, Hirsch AT, Misra S, et al. 2011 ACCF/AHA focused update of the guideline for the management of patients with peripheral artery disease (updating the 2005 guideline): a report of the American College of Cardiology Foundation/American Heart Association Task Force on Practice Guidelines: developed in collaboration with the Society for Cardiovascular Angiography and Interventions, Society of Interventional Radiology, Society for Vascular Medicine, and Society for Vascular Surgery. J Vasc Surg 2011;54(5):e32–58.

39. Feigelson HS, Criqui MH, Fronek A, et al. Screening for peripheral arterial disease: the sensitivity, specificity, and predictive value of noninvasive tests in a defined population. Am J Epidemiol 1994;140(6):526–34.

40. Beckman JA, Jaff MR, Creager MA. The United States Preventive Services Task Force recommendation statement on screening for peripheral arterial disease: more harm than benefit? Circulation 2006;114(8):861–6.

41. Aboyans V, Criqui MH, Abraham P, et al. Measurement and interpretation of the ankle-brachial index: a scientific statement from the American Heart Association. Circulation 2012;126(24):2890–909.

42. McDermott MM. The magnitude of the problem of peripheral arterial disease: epidemiology and clinical significance. Cleve Clin J Med 2006;73(Suppl 4):S2–7.

43. Ramsey DE, Manke DA, Sumner DS. Toe blood pressure. A valuable adjunct to ankle pressure measurement for assessing peripheral arterial disease. J Cardiovasc Surg (Torino) 1983;24(1):43–8.

44. McDermott MM, Guralnik JM, Tian L, et al. Associations of borderline and low normal ankle-brachial index values with functional decline at 5-year follow-up: the WALCS (Walking and Leg Circulation Study). J Am Coll Cardiol 2009;53(12):1056–62.

45. Rooke TW, Hirsch AT, Misra S, et al. Management of patients with peripheral artery disease (compilation of 2005 and 2011 ACCF/AHA Guideline Recommendations): a report of the American College of Cardiology Foundation/American Heart Association Task Force on Practice Guidelines. J Am Coll Cardiol 2013;61(14):1555–70.

46. Stone NJ, Robinson JG, Lichtenstein AH, et al. 2013 ACC/AHA guideline on the treatment of blood cholesterol to reduce atherosclerotic cardiovascular risk in adults: a report of the American College of Cardiology/American Heart Association Task Force on Practice Guidelines. J Am Coll Cardiol 2014;63(25 Pt B):2889–934.

47. Clinical Practice Guideline Treating Tobacco Use and Dependence 2008 Update Panel, Liaisons, and Staff. A clinical practice guideline for treating tobacco use and dependence: 2008 update. A U.S. Public Health Service report. Am J Prev Med 2008;35(2):158–76.

48. Hennrikus D, Joseph AM, Lando HA, et al. Effectiveness of a smoking cessation program for peripheral artery disease patients: a randomized controlled trial. J Am Coll Cardiol 2010;56(25):2105–12.

49. Silagy C, Lancaster T, Stead L, et al. Nicotine replacement therapy for smoking cessation. Cochrane Database Syst Rev 2004;(3):CD000146.

50. Odum LE, O'Dell KA, Schepers JS. Electronic cigarettes: do they have a role in smoking cessation? J Pharm Pract 2012;25(6):611–4.

51. Goniewicz ML, Kuma T, Gawron M, et al. Nicotine levels in electronic cigarettes. Nicotine Tob Res 2013;15(1):158–66.

52. The effect of intensive treatment of diabetes on the development and progression of long-term complications in insulin-dependent diabetes mellitus. The Diabetes Control and Complications Trial Research Group. N Engl J Med 1993;329(14):977–86.

53. Gerstein HC, Miller ME, Byington RP, et al. Effects of intensive glucose lowering in type 2 diabetes. N Engl J Med 2008;358(24):2545–59.

54. Holman RR, Paul SK, Bethel MA, et al. 10-year follow-up of intensive glucose control in type 2 diabetes. N Engl J Med 2008;359(15):1577–89.

55. Adler AI, Stratton IM, Neil HA, et al. Association of systolic blood pressure with macrovascular and microvascular complications of type 2 diabetes (UKPDS 36): prospective observational study. BMJ 2000;321(7258):412–9.

56. Hoogwerf BJ, Young JB. The HOPE study. Ramipril lowered cardiovascular risk, but vitamin E did not. Cleve Clin J Med 2000;67(4):287–93.

57. Radack K, Deck C. Beta-adrenergic blocker therapy does not worsen intermittent claudication in subjects with peripheral arterial disease. A meta-analysis of randomized controlled trials. Arch Intern Med 1991;151(9):1769–76.

58. Paravastu SC, Mendonca DA, da Silva A. Beta blockers for peripheral arterial disease. Eur J Vasc Endovasc Surg 2009;38(1):66–70.

59. Hennekens CH, Albert CM, Godfried SL, et al. Adjunctive drug therapy of acute myocardial infarction–evidence from clinical trials. N Engl J Med 1996;335(22):1660–7.

60. Heart Protection Study Collaborative Group. Randomized trial of the effects of cholesterol-lowering with simvastatin on peripheral vascular and other major vascular outcomes in 20,536 people with peripheral arterial disease and other high-risk conditions. J Vasc Surg 2007;45(4):645–54 [discussion: 653–4].

61. Adam DJ, Beard JD, Cleveland T, et al. Bypass versus Angioplasty in Severe Ischaemia of the Leg (BASIL): multicentre, randomised controlled trial. Lancet 2005;366(9501):1925–34.

62. Sharma S, Thapa R, Jeevanantham V, et al. Comparison of lipid management in patients with coronary versus peripheral arterial disease. Am J Cardiol 2014;113(8):1320–5.

63. Expert Panel on Detection, Evaluation, and Treatment of High Blood Cholesterol in Adults. Executive summary of the third report of the National Cholesterol Education Program (NCEP) expert panel on detection, evaluation, and treatment of high blood cholesterol in adults (adult treatment panel III). JAMA 2001;285(19):2486–97.

64. Antithrombotic Trialists' Collaboration. Collaborative meta-analysis of randomised trials of antiplatelet therapy for prevention of death, myocardial infarction, and stroke in high risk patients. BMJ 2002;324(7329):71–86.

65. Berger JS, Krantz MJ, Kittelson JM, et al. Aspirin for the prevention of cardiovascular events in patients with peripheral artery disease: a meta-analysis of randomized trials. JAMA 2009; 301(18):1909–19.

66. Fowkes FG, Price JF, Stewart MC, et al. Aspirin for prevention of cardiovascular events in a general population screened for a low ankle brachial index: a randomized controlled trial. JAMA 2010;303(9): 841–8.

67. Bhatt DL, Fox KA, Hacke W, et al. Clopidogrel and aspirin versus aspirin alone for the prevention of atherothrombotic events. N Engl J Med 2006; 354(16):1706–17.

68. Wong PF, Chong LY, Mikhailidis DP, et al. Antiplatelet agents for intermittent claudication. Cochrane Database Syst Rev 2011;(11):CD001272.

69. Ota H, Eto M, Kano MR, et al. Cilostazol inhibits oxidative stress-induced premature senescence via upregulation of Sirt1 in human endothelial cells. Arterioscler Thromb Vasc Biol 2008;28(9):1634–9.

70. Elam MB, Heckman J, Crouse JR, et al. Effect of the novel antiplatelet agent cilostazol on plasma lipoproteins in patients with intermittent claudication. Arterioscler Thromb Vasc Biol 1998;18(12):1942–7.

71. Pande RL, Hiatt WR, Zhang P, et al. A pooled analysis of the durability and predictors of treatment response of cilostazol in patients with intermittent claudication. Vasc Med 2010;15(3):181–8.

72. Hiatt WR, Money SR, Brass EP. Long-term safety of cilostazol in patients with peripheral artery disease: the CASTLE study (Cilostazol: a study in long-term effects). J Vasc Surg 2008;47(2):330–6.

73. Beebe HG, Dawson DL, Cutler BS, et al. A new pharmacological treatment for intermittent claudication: results of a randomized, multicenter trial. Arch Intern Med 1999;159(17):2041–50.

74. Chapman TM, Goa KL. Cilostazol: a review of its use in intermittent claudication. Am J Cardiovasc Drugs 2003;3(2):117–38.

75. Schrör K. The pharmacology of cilostazol. Diabetes Obes Metab 2002;4(Suppl 2):S14–9.

76. Drugs for intermittent claudication. Med Lett Drugs Ther 2004;46(1176):13–5.

77. Aviado DM, Porter JM. Pentoxifylline: a new drug for the treatment of intermittent claudication. Mechanism of action, pharmacokinetics, clinical efficacy and adverse effects. Pharmacotherapy 1984;4(6): 297–307.

78. Gillings DB. Pentoxifylline and intermittent claudication: review of clinical trials and cost-effectiveness analyses. J Cardiovasc Pharmacol 1995;25(Suppl 2):S44–50.

79. Salhiyyah K, Senanayake E, Abdel-Hadi M, et al. Pentoxifylline for intermittent claudication. Cochrane Database Syst Rev 2012;(1):CD005262.

80. Wiernsperger NF. Serotonin, 5-HT2 receptors, and their blockade by naftidrofuryl: a targeted therapy of vascular diseases. J Cardiovasc Pharmacol 1994;23(Suppl 3):S37–43.

81. Hong H, Mackey WC. The limits of evidence in drug approval and availability: a case study of

cilostazol and naftidrofuryl for the treatment of intermittent claudication. Clin Ther 2014;36(8):1290–301.

82. Barradell LB, Brogden RN. Oral naftidrofuryl. A review of its pharmacology and therapeutic use in the management of peripheral occlusive arterial disease. Drugs Aging 1996;8(4):299–322.

83. Stevens JW, Simpson E, Harnan S, et al. Systematic review of the efficacy of cilostazol, naftidrofuryl oxalate and pentoxifylline for the treatment of intermittent claudication. Br J Surg 2012;99(12):1630–8.

84. Shalhoub J, Davies AH. Adjunctive pharmacotherapies for intermittent claudication–NICE guidance. Heart 2012;98(3):244–5.

85. Bendermacher BL, Willigendael EM, Nicolaï SP, et al. Supervised exercise therapy for intermittent claudication in a community-based setting is as effective as clinic-based. J Vasc Surg 2007;45(6):1192–6.

86. Gustafsson T, Kraus WE. Exercise-induced angiogenesis-related growth and transcription factors in skeletal muscle, and their modification in muscle pathology. Front Biosci 2001;6:D75–89.

87. Brendle DC, Joseph LJ, Corretti MC, et al. Effects of exercise rehabilitation on endothelial reactivity in older patients with peripheral arterial disease. Am J Cardiol 2001;87(3):324–9.

88. Hiatt WR, Regensteiner JG, Wolfel EE, et al. Effect of exercise training on skeletal muscle histology and metabolism in peripheral arterial disease. J Appl Physiol (1985) 1996;81(2):780–8.

89. Tisi PV, Shearman CP. The evidence for exercise-induced inflammation in intermittent claudication: should we encourage patients to stop walking? Eur J Vasc Endovasc Surg 1998;15(1):7–17.

90. Lane R, Ellis B, Watson L, et al. Exercise for intermittent claudication. Cochrane Database Syst Rev 2014;(7):CD000990.

91. McDermott MM, Ades P, Guralnik JM, et al. Treadmill exercise and resistance training in patients with peripheral arterial disease with and without intermittent claudication: a randomized controlled trial. JAMA 2009;301(2):165–74.

92. Fokkenrood HJ, Bendermacher BL, Lauret GJ, et al. Supervised exercise therapy versus non-supervised exercise therapy for intermittent claudication. Cochrane Database Syst Rev 2013;(8):CD005263.

93. Makris GC, Lattimer CR, Lavida A, et al. Availability of supervised exercise programs and the role of structured home-based exercise in peripheral arterial disease. Eur J Vasc Endovasc Surg 2012;44(6):569–75 [discussion: 576].

94. Kruidenier LM, Nicolaï SP, Hendriks EJ, et al. Supervised exercise therapy for intermittent claudication in daily practice. J Vasc Surg 2009;49(2):363–70.

95. McDermott MM, Liu K, Guralnik JM, et al. Home-based walking exercise intervention in peripheral artery disease: a randomized clinical trial. JAMA 2013;310(1):57–65.

96. Gardner AW, Parker DE, Montgomery PS, et al. Efficacy of quantified home-based exercise and supervised exercise in patients with intermittent claudication: a randomized controlled trial. Circulation 2011;123(5):491–8.

97. Collins TC, Lunos S, Carlson T, et al. Effects of a home-based walking intervention on mobility and quality of life in people with diabetes and peripheral arterial disease: a randomized controlled trial. Diabetes Care 2011;34(10):2174–9.

98. Bermingham SL, Sparrow K, Mullis R, et al. The cost-effectiveness of supervised exercise for the treatment of intermittent claudication. Eur J Vasc Endovasc Surg 2013;46(6):707–14.

99. Simoens S. Health economic assessment: a methodological primer. Int J Environ Res Public Health 2009;6(12):2950–66.

100. Murphy TP, Cutlip DE, Regensteiner JG, et al. Supervised exercise versus primary stenting for claudication resulting from aortoiliac peripheral artery disease: six-month outcomes from the Claudication: Exercise versus Endoluminal Revascularization (CLEVER) study. Circulation 2012;125(1):130–9.

101. Frans FA, Bipat S, Reekers JA, et al. Systematic review of exercise training or percutaneous transluminal angioplasty for intermittent claudication. Br J Surg 2012;99(1):16–28.

102. Mazari FA, Khan JA, Carradice D, et al. Economic analysis of a randomized trial of percutaneous angioplasty, supervised exercise or combined treatment for intermittent claudication due to femoropopliteal arterial disease. Br J Surg 2013;100(9):1172–9.

103. Mohler ER, Hiatt WR, Creager MA. Cholesterol reduction with atorvastatin improves walking distance in patients with peripheral arterial disease. Circulation 2003;108(12):1481–6.

104. Kinlay S, Plutzky J. Effect of lipid-lowering therapy on vasomotion and endothelial function. Curr Cardiol Rep 1999;1(3):238–43.

105. Aung PP, Maxwell HG, Jepson RG, et al. Lipid-lowering for peripheral arterial disease of the lower limb. Cochrane Database Syst Rev 2007;(4):CD000123.

106. Ahimastos AA, Walker PJ, Askew C, et al. Effect of ramipril on walking times and quality of life among patients with peripheral artery disease and intermittent claudication: a randomized controlled trial. JAMA 2013;309(5):453–60.

107. Norgren L, Hiatt WR, Dormandy JA, et al. Inter-society consensus for the management of peripheral arterial disease (TASC II). J Vasc Surg 2007;45(Suppl S):S5–67.

108. Stephens FB, Constantin-Teodosiu D, Greenhaff PL. New insights concerning the role of carnitine in the regulation of fuel metabolism in skeletal muscle. J Physiol 2007;581(Pt 2):431–44.

109. Hiatt WR, Wolfel EE, Regensteiner JG, et al. Skeletal muscle carnitine metabolism in patients with unilateral peripheral arterial disease. J Appl Physiol (1985) 1992;73(1):346–53.

110. Dutta A, Ray K, Singh VK, et al. L-carnitine supplementation attenuates intermittent hypoxia-induced oxidative stress and delays muscle fatigue in rats. Exp Physiol 2008;93(10):1139–46.

111. Luo T, Li J, Li L, et al. A study on the efficacy and safety assessment of propionyl-L-carnitine tablets in treatment of intermittent claudication. Thromb Res 2013;132(4):427–32.

112. Delaney CL, Spark JI, Thomas J, et al. A systematic review to evaluate the effectiveness of carnitine supplementation in improving walking performance among individuals with intermittent claudication. Atherosclerosis 2013;229(1):1–9.

113. De Haro J, Acin F, Lopez-Quintana A, et al. Meta-analysis of randomized, controlled clinical trials in angiogenesis: gene and cell therapy in peripheral arterial disease. Heart Vessels 2009; 24(5):321–8.

114. Hammer A, Steiner S. Gene therapy for therapeutic angiogenesis in peripheral arterial disease—a systematic review and meta-analysis of randomized, controlled trials. Vasa 2013;42(5):331–9.

115. Jorenby DE, Leischow SJ, Nides MA, et al. A controlled trial of sustained-release bupropion, a nicotine patch, or both for smoking cessation. N Engl J Med 1999;340(9):685–91.

116. Nides M, Oncken C, Gonzales D, et al. Smoking cessation with varenicline, a selective alpha4beta2 nicotinic receptor partial agonist: results from a 7-week, randomized, placebo- and bupropion-controlled trial with 1-year follow-up. Arch Intern Med 2006;166(15):1561–8.

117. Jorenby DE, Hays JT, Rigotti NA, et al. Efficacy of varenicline, an alpha4beta2 nicotinic acetylcholine receptor partial agonist, vs placebo or sustained-release bupropion for smoking cessation: a randomized controlled trial. JAMA 2006;296(1): 56–63.

Preoperative Cardiovascular Evaluation in Patients Undergoing Vascular Surgery

Parveen K. Garg, MD, MPH*

KEYWORDS

- Peripheral vascular disease • Revised cardiac risk index • Perioperative cardiovascular guidelines
- Noninvasive stress testing • Coronary revascularization • β-blockers • Statins • Antiplatelet therapy

KEY POINTS

- Vascular surgery is associated with a higher incidence of perioperative cardiovascular morbidity and mortality. The overwhelming perioperative cardiac event is myocardial infarction.
- Patients undergoing vascular surgery represent a higher-risk population. Careful preoperative cardiovascular evaluation involves an assessment of the urgency of surgery, active cardiac conditions, functional capacity, and clinical risk predictors.
- Various cardiac risk indices are available to estimate perioperative cardiovascular risk in the setting of vascular surgery. Awareness of these indices and a careful understanding of their limitations are crucial.
- Noninvasive stress testing in patients undergoing major vascular surgery is often required but not necessary, and knowledge of the appropriate indications is important.
- Although the benefit of coronary revascularization or initiation of β-blockade before vascular surgery on reducing perioperative cardiovascular morbidity is still unproved, there is a reported benefit for the perioperative use of statin therapy.

INTRODUCTION

Major vascular surgery is associated with an increased risk of postoperative major adverse cardiac events (MACE), with the most common being myocardial infarction (MI). Postoperative cardiovascular morbidity and mortality rates for aortic and lower extremity arterial surgeries are reported to be greater than 20%.[1–4] Vascular surgery is associated with the highest 30-day postsurgical Medicare rehospitalization rate at almost 25%.[5] In an analysis of nationwide, surgery-specific, postoperative mortality rates in the Netherlands, vascular surgery was associated with the highest mortality incidence at nearly 6%.[6] The demand for vascular surgery will only increase in parallel with the aging United States population. It is expected that 1 to 2 million such procedures will be performed annually in the United States by the year 2030, resulting in an estimated 18,000 deaths.[7]

There are several key features inherent to vascular surgery, particularly procedures that are open, which account for the increased cardiovascular risk. These include prolonged duration of surgery, large shifts in intravascular and extravascular fluid volumes, cross-clamping of the

The author has nothing to disclose.
Division of Cardiology, Keck School of Medicine, University of Southern California, 1520 San Pablo Street, Suite 322, Los Angeles, CA 90033, USA
* 1510 San Pablo Street, Suite 322, Los Angeles, CA 90033.
E-mail address: parveeng@usc.edu

aorta, and hypothermia induction. These factors can lead to a state of high stress and low flow across major vascular beds. The result is increased inflammation, hypercoagulability, catecholamines, and hypoxia, all of which can precipitate the occurrence of acute coronary thrombosis and myocardial ischemia.[8]

In addition to the risks posed by the procedure itself, typical patients undergoing vascular surgery also have certain factors in common that further contribute to the high risk of postoperative cardiovascular complications.[9] Patients with vascular disease already have many of the major risk factors associated with development of coronary artery disease (CAD). The prevalence of significant CAD in patients undergoing elective peripheral vascular surgery is reported to be 25%.[10] In addition, symptoms of CAD are often difficult to assess in this population because of exercise limitations from advanced age, associated comorbidities, and severe lower extremity arterial disease. Patients with flow-limiting lesions or vulnerable lesions in the coronary vasculature are also more susceptible to the significant hemodynamic shifts commonly associated with vascular surgery.

Characteristic features of the patient and the surgical procedure itself contribute to the increased risk of perioperative cardiovascular complications associated with major vascular surgery. A careful preoperative cardiovascular evaluation is crucial in reducing the risk of perioperative events. Such an evaluation includes assessing surgical and patient risk, determining the need for noninvasive stress testing or preoperative coronary revascularization, and implementing appropriate medical therapy.[11] This article offers an approach to preoperative management of patients undergoing vascular surgery in the context of the most recent literature and the most current guidelines and recommendations.

PREOPERATIVE ALGORITHM FOR PATIENTS UNDERGOING VASCULAR SURGERY

The evaluation and management of cardiovascular risk associated with vascular surgery is primarily based on the 2014 American College of Cardiology/American Heart Association (ACC/AHA) guidelines on perioperative cardiovascular evaluation and care for noncardiac surgery.[12] **Fig. 1** is a specific algorithm depicting preoperative cardiovascular management for patients undergoing vascular surgery, whereas recommendations refer to the ACC/AHA guidelines.

Emergency Surgery

A complete preoperative cardiovascular assessment is often impossible in the setting of emergent (<6 hours) or urgent (6–24) vascular surgery, such as aortic dissection, aneurysmal rupture of the aorta, or acute limb ischemia. In such circumstances, the patient requires vascular surgery without delay. A bedside evaluation, including electrocardiogram (EKG) by the cardiology consultant, should be performed if time permits and the focus should be on providing recommendations for postoperative monitoring and medical management.

Active Cardiac Conditions

If a patient is found to have an active cardiac condition (**Box 1**), elective vascular surgery may be postponed. The postoperative cardiovascular event risk is substantially increased in the presence of an active cardiac condition. Treatment of the cardiac condition and maintenance of hemodynamic stability must precede surgery.[13]

Unstable coronary syndromes
In addition to acute coronary syndrome, this category includes patients with severe angina. Severe angina refers to those individuals with Canadian Cardiovascular Society class III or class IV angina. The risk of a recurrent MI is very high if the time between the initial MI and surgery is less than 30 days (32.8%) or between 31 and 60 days (18.7%) and declines to less than 10% after this time frame.[14]

Congestive heart failure
The presence of decompensated or worsening congestive heart failure also elevates perioperative cardiovascular event risk. Among individuals undergoing surgery within 4 weeks of a diagnosed heart failure episode, perioperative mortality exceeds 13%.[15] Preoperative B-type natriuretic peptide levels have also been shown to independently predict the occurrence of cardiovascular events within the first 30 days after vascular surgery; however, further randomized studies are needed to validate the clinical utility of such testing.[16] Treatment should focus on achieving euvolemic status and improving heart failure signs and symptoms before surgery. In cases of new-onset heart failure, a search for underlying cause is also warranted because it may guide perioperative management.

Significant cardiac arrhythmias
Arrhythmias that cause or place the patient at risk for hemodynamic instability should be managed immediately. Examples include high-grade or third-degree atrioventricular block, symptomatic

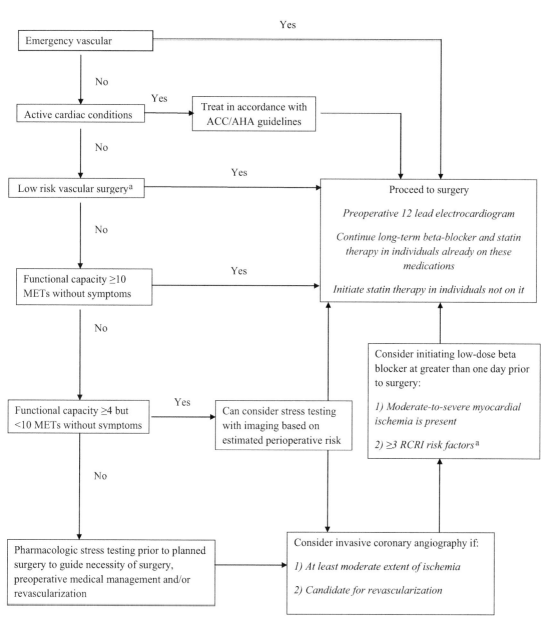

Fig. 1. Suggested approach to the preoperative evaluation of patients undergoing vascular surgery. Risk factors include insulin-dependent diabetes mellitus, heart failure, coronary artery disease, cerebrovascular disease, and creatinine greater than or equal to 2 mg/dL. [a] Assessment based on estimated perioperative combined clinical/surgical risk of major adverse cardiac events. MET, metabolic equivalents; RCRI, Revised Cardiac Risk Index. (*Adapted from* Fleisher LA, Fleischmann KE, Auerbach AD, et al. 2014 ACC/AHA guidelines on perioperative cardiovascular evaluation and management for patients undergoing noncardiac surgery: a report of the ACC/AHA task force on practice guidelines. Circulation 2014;[Epub ahead of print].)

bradycardias, and ventricular and supraventricular tachyarrhythmias.

Advanced valvular disease

Mitral and aortic valve disease should be corrected before elective vascular surgery for patients who meet indications for intervention based on the severity and/or presence of symptoms as per the 2014 ACC/AHA guidelines on valvular disease. A preoperative echocardiogram should be performed in patients with known valvular disease that is at least moderate in severity if no prior echocardiography has been performed in the past year or there has been a change in clinical status. In the

---

Box 1
Active cardiac conditions requiring urgent management

Unstable coronary syndromes

Unstable or severe angina

Acute myocardial infarction

Congestive heart failure

Decompensated heart failure (New York Heart Association class IV)

Worsening heart failure

New-onset heart failure

Significant cardiac arrhythmias

High-grade or third-degree atrioventricular block

Symptomatic bradycardia

Supraventricular tachyarrhythmia

Ventricular tachyarrhythmia

Advanced valvular disease

Severe aortic valve disease

Severe mitral valve disease

Adapted from Fleisher LA, Beckman JA, Brown KA, et al. 2009 ACCF/AHA focused update on perioperative beta blockade incorporated into the ACC/AHA 2007 guidelines on perioperative cardiovascular evaluation and care for noncardiac surgery: a report of the ACCF/AHA task force on practice guidelines. Circulation 2009;120:e169–276.

---

setting of severe aortic or mitral valvular disease that does not meet standard criteria for intervention, it is recommended to proceed with elective vascular surgery.

Perhaps most important in terms of increased cardiovascular risk for surgery is aortic stenosis.[17] In circumstances where the stenosis is at least moderate but the patient does not meet standard indications for intervention, the best approach to preoperative cardiovascular management is still unclear. Even when valvular correction is indicated, patients often either refuse the surgery or are not candidates for aortic valve replacement. In these situations, the increased-risk surgery can be performed but perioperative cardiovascular event rates are 10% to 20%.[18] For patients who are either not candidates or are deemed high risk for surgical aortic valve replacement, transcatheter aortic valve replacement has recently been shown to be an effective alternative to traditional surgery.[19–22] In the future, this may become a recommended option to help reduce perioperative cardiovascular event rates in this patient subset.

ASSESSMENT OF CARDIOVASCULAR RISK

After the need for emergent or urgent vascular surgery and the presence of active cardiac conditions have been excluded, careful preoperative assessment initially focuses on accurately identifying the cardiovascular risk associated with the surgery. This is done most effectively by integrating the procedure-associated risk and the patient-associated risk to determine the perioperative MACE risk.

Procedure-Specific Risk

There have been numerous advances in surgery and improvements made in surgical technique. Vascular surgery, in particular, has experienced significant advances with endovascular interventions and substantial improvements in open surgical techniques. Risk-adjusted mortality after high-risk surgery has declined significantly as a result.[23] **Box 2** stratifies perioperative cardiovascular risk for common vascular surgical procedures into low, intermediate, and high categories. In general, with the exception of carotid endarterectomy, open repair or reconstruction of the aorta or major branch vessels are regarded as high risk, whereas endovascular interventions are

---

Box 2
Cardiac risk stratification for common vascular surgical procedures

High risk (≥5%)

Open repair or reconstruction involving the thoracic or abdominal aorta

Open reconstruction of the mesenteric or renal arteries

Lower extremity bypass surgery

Intermediate risk (1%–5%)

Carotid endarterectomy

Major amputation (above hand or foot)

Endovascular intervention of aorta or major branch arteries (carotid, mesenteric, renal, iliac)

Low risk (<1%)

Arteriovenous fistula formation

Minor amputation (restricted to hand or foot)

Cardiac risk is defined as 30-day incidence of cardiovascular death or nonfatal myocardial infarction.

---

considered intermediate risk. Major amputations are intermediate risk and minor amputations are low risk. Arteriovenous fistula formations and venous surgeries are low risk.

Patient-Specific Risk

The history and physical examination is essential in determining whether patient risk is low or has increased. Important features of the patient's evaluation include assessment of functional capacity, identification of the presence of clinical risk predictors, and performance of a complete cardiovascular physical examination. An EKG is also indicated in individuals with peripheral arterial disease.

ACC/AHA guidelines recommend a preoperative echocardiogram only when structural heart disease is suspected based on abnormal clinical or electrocardiographic findings. In a prospective study of more than 1000 patients undergoing preoperative echocardiography before elective vascular surgery, 40% of patients were found to have asymptomatic left ventricular (LV) systolic dysfunction. The perioperative cardiovascular event rate was 23% in those with asymptomatic systolic LV dysfunction compared with 10% in those with normal LV function.[24] These findings suggest a potential role for routine preoperative echocardiography before vascular surgery;

however, further study is needed to validate the clinical utility of such a strategy translating into reduced perioperative cardiovascular events.

If the combined clinical and surgical risk of vascular surgery is low (<1%) or if the patient has a good baseline functional capacity ($\geq$4 metabolic equivalents [METs]), then the patient can usually proceed to vascular surgery without considering further preoperative cardiovascular evaluation (ACC/AHA class I). Patients able to achieve greater than or equal to four METs before vascular surgery have a significantly lower risk of perioperative cardiovascular events.[25] Most often, however, vascular surgeries are not low risk and patients do not have good functional capacity because of their severe vascular disease and multiple comorbidities. Clinical risk prediction indices can be helpful to quantify perioperative MACE likelihood, differentiate between low risk (<1%) and increased risk (>1%), and determine need for additional testing (ACC/AHA class IIA).

CLINICAL RISK PREDICTION MODELS
Revised Cardiac Risk Index

Many efforts have been made to predict cardiac risk before noncardiac surgery. The Revised Cardiac Risk Index (RCRI) (**Table 1**) is the most well-established and most commonly used cardiac

Table 1
Comparison of the Revised Cardiac Risk Index, NSQIP myocardial infarction cardiac arrest calculator, and Vascular Study Group Cardiac Risk Index

Revised Cardiac Risk Index		NSQIP Myocardial Infarction Cardiac Arrest Calculator	Vascular Study Group Cardiac Risk Index	
Risk Factor	Points	Risk Factor[a]	Risk Factor	Points
Coronary heart disease	1	Increasing age	Age	
Congestive heart failure	1	Creatinine >1.5 mg/dL	$\geq$80	4
Insulin-dependent diabetes	1	Dependent functional status	70–79	3
Creatinine >2.0 mg/dL	1	ASA physical status class	60–69	2
Cerebrovascular disease	1	Surgery type	Coronary heart disease	1
High-risk surgery	1		Congestive heart failure	1
			Chronic obstructive pulmonary disease	1
			Creatinine >1.8 mg/dL	1
			Smoking	1
			Insulin-dependent diabetes	1
			Long-term β-blockade	1
			History of coronary revascularization	−1

Abbreviation: NSQIP, National Surgical Quality Improvement Program.
[a] The NSQIP myocardial infarction cardiac arrest calculator is a risk calculator and does not use points to estimate perioperative cardiovascular event risk.

risk stratification tool.[26] The RCRI stratifies patients into low and elevated risk based on the presence of six clinical risk predictors: (1) coronary heart disease, (2) congestive heart failure, (3) cerebrovascular disease, (4) insulin-dependent diabetes mellitus, (5) renal insufficiency with a serum creatinine greater than 2 mg/dL, and (6) high-risk surgery (suprainguinal vascular, intraperitoneal, or intrathoracic). A patient with two or more clinical risk predictors has elevated risk. Although the RCRI has been the most validated risk index, its applicability to specific surgical categories or patient subsets is limited. The RCRI was derived from a very diverse patient population undergoing a wide range of surgical procedures. Vascular procedures comprised only one-fifth of the entire RCRI derivation cohort.

The RCRI consistently underestimates perioperative cardiac events in vascular surgery patients. A large meta-analysis reported that the RCRI did significantly worse at discriminating risk for cardiac events, as measured by the receiver operating characteristic area under the curve (AUC), between patients at low versus high risk for cardiac events after vascular noncardiac surgery (AUC = 0.64), than mixed noncardiac surgery (AUC = 0.75).[27] In a separate analysis the discriminatory value of the RCRI in vascular surgery patients reduced with age (age >75, AUC = 0.62; age 56–75, AUC = 0.64; age ≤55, AUC = 0.75).[28]

Vascular Surgery Group Cardiac Risk Index

Because of the limitations of the RCRI, the Vascular Study Group of New England derived the Vascular Surgery Group Cardiac Risk Index (VSG-CRI) (see **Table 1**), a risk prediction index specific to vascular surgery.[29] Their cohort included more than 10,000 patients undergoing carotid endarterctomy, lower extremity bypass, endovascular abdominal aortic aneurysm repair, and open infrarenal abdominal aortic aneurysm repair. Although the Vascular Study Group of New England used a slightly different composite outcome for perioperative cardiac events for this cohort, the RCRI again was found to underestimate cardiac complications based on actual event rates across all categories of risk. Factoring in additional clinical variables, such as age, pulmonary disease, smoking, β-blocker use, and history of revascularization, the VSG-CRI more accurately predicted perioperative cardiac event risk for all four procedures.

Myocardial Infarction and Cardiac Arrest Risk Calculator

An MI and cardiac arrest risk calculator (see **Table 1**) using data from the National Surgical Quality Improvement Program database is also available as an alternative to the RCRI.[30] Incorporating patient data regarding type of surgery, functional status, serum creatinine, American Society of Anesthesiologist class, and age, this model reported a discriminatory ability for perioperative MI and cardiac arrest risk superior to the RCRI in patients undergoing noncardiac vascular surgery (AUC = 0.75 vs 0.59). This discriminatory ability was comparable with that reported by the VSG-CRI (AUC = 0.75 vs 0.71). Surgery-specific risk models for infrainguinal bypass surgery, carotid endarterectomy, and open aortic aneurysm repair are also available using National Surgical Quality Improvement Program data.[31–33]

Although the VSG-CRI and MI and cardiac arrest risk calculator are not as well established, the RCRI has clearly been shown to underestimate cardiovascular risk in vascular surgery patients. These alternative models may be particularly helpful in patients undergoing vascular surgery who are low risk according to the RCRI to more appropriately guide preoperative cardiovascular management.

ASSESSMENT AND TREATMENT OF CARDIOVASCULAR ISCHEMIA
Noninvasive Stress Testing

Moderate to large areas of inducible ischemia on noninvasive stress tests have been consistently shown to be an independent predictor of perioperative cardiac events in patients undergoing major vascular surgery.[34–36] More importantly, these tests have shown a very high negative predictive value in the absence of any inducible ischemia. The positive predictive value of an abnormal stress test result, however, is limited and it is difficult to determine which patients with inducible ischemia will experience a cardiac event. Based on the available evidence, current guidelines advocate the consideration of noninvasive stress testing in patients undergoing elevated-risk surgery with poor or unknown functional capacity on the assumption that it will potentially change management (ACC/AHA class IIA).

Although exercise EKG is a recommended diagnostic test for assessment of coronary ischemia in individuals with interpretable resting EKGs, vascular patients are often unable to exercise to an adequate level and pharmacologic measures are needed. Dobutamine stress echocardiography and myocardial perfusion scintigraphy should be considered for these patients. In a meta-analysis of patients undergoing noncardiac surgery, dobutamine stress echocardiography was slightly superior to myocardial perfusion scintigraphy in predicting postoperative cardiac events; however, randomized control trial data are lacking.[36] Dobutamine stress echocardiography has the additional benefit of detecting baseline valvular or LV dysfunction.

Coronary Angiography and Revascularization

Preoperative angiography is indicated in the presence of active cardiac conditions or other standard indications as per the ACC/AHA guidelines in patients who otherwise required it. Monaco and colleagues[37] randomized more than 200 patients undergoing elevated-risk vascular surgery to a selective strategy of coronary angiography based on the results of noninvasive testing or a routine strategy of coronary angiography. Myocardial revascularization occurred more frequently in the routine strategy; however, there was no difference in postoperative cardiovascular events. Patients in the routine strategy did have significantly better long-term cardiac outcomes.

Current ACC/AHA class I indications for coronary revascularization before surgery are similar to those for the nonoperative setting and include significant left main stenosis, ischemia-driven life-threatening arrhythmias, and acute coronary syndrome. The complete list of indications for coronary revascularization is found in the 2011 American College of Cardiology Foundation/AHA Guideline for Coronary Artery Bypass Graft Surgery and in the 2011 American College of Cardiology Foundation/AHA/Society for Cardiovascular Angiography and Interventions Guideline for Percutaneous Coronary Intervention. Routine coronary revascularization before noncardiac surgery is not recommended (ACC/AHA class III).

Published literature has not demonstrated an improvement in cardiovascular outcomes with coronary artery revascularization before vascular surgery. The Coronary Artery Revascularization Prophylaxis trial randomized more than 500 patients with obstructive CAD on angiography to revascularization or no revascularization before elective major vascular surgery.[38] After a mean follow-up of more than 30 months there was no difference in long-term survival between the two groups. In this study most patients were found to have one- or two-vessel disease (approximately two-thirds of the population). Patients with left main disease, an LV ejection fraction less than 20%, and severe aortic stenosis were excluded.

MEDICAL THERAPY
β-Blocker Therapy

The Perioperative Ischemic Evaluation (POISE) trial randomized more than 8000 patients to receive β-blockers or placebo before noncardiac surgery and found preoperative β-blocker initiation to be associated with a reduction in nonfatal MIs but with an increase in the risk of nonfatal stroke, significant bradycardia, and perioperative hypotension.[39] Perhaps most importantly, there was a significant increase in all-cause mortality. More than 40% of these patients underwent vascular surgery. A recent systematic review of the available literature corroborated these results.[40]

Randomized trials of preoperative β-blocker therapy in patients only undergoing major vascular surgery have reported similar results to those from the POISE trial.[41,42] The Perioperative Beta-Blocker trial included more than 100 patients undergoing infrarenal vascular surgery, whereas the Metoprolol after Vascular Surgery trial included nearly 500 patients undergoing abdominal aortic surgery and infrainguinal or axillofemoral revascularizations. Both of these trials randomized patients to receive either preoperative β-blocker therapy or placebo. Both of these studies found no difference in perioperative cardiovascular event rates between the two groups.

Current guidelines recommend that β-blockers be continued in patients undergoing surgery who are already on them chronically (ACC/AHA class I) but offer no compelling indications for initiating β-blocker therapy in patients undergoing increased-risk vascular surgery. Because β-blocker therapy has been consistently associated with a reduction in perioperative MI incidence, it may be reasonable to start if benefits are thought to outweigh risks in patients with significant inducible ischemia on noninvasive testing, three or more RCRI risk factors, or a compelling long-term indication for β-blocker use (ACC/AHA class IIB). The initiation of low-dose β-blocker therapy should occur at least 1 day before the scheduled surgery. There is no evidence of benefit with dose titration.

Statin Therapy

In patients undergoing vascular surgery, statins should either be initiated (ACC/AHA class IIA) or continued in those already taking them (ACC/AHA class I). Multiple randomized and observational studies have demonstrated a consistent reduction in cardiovascular events with perioperative statin use before vascular surgery.[43-47] Durazzo and colleagues[43] randomized 100 patients to 20 mg of atorvastatin or placebo within 30 days of vascular surgery and reported a threefold decrease in cardiovascular events at 6-month follow-up in the atorvastatin-treated group. Similarly, observational studies have reported improved cardiovascular outcomes with statin therapy after carotid endarterectomy, critical limb ischemia revascularization, and aortic aneurysm repair.[44–47]

Antiplatelet Therapy

Although aspirin therapy is routinely indicated in patients with noncoronary atherosclerotic disease, the benefit of either continuing or initiating perioperative aspirin therapy in patients undergoing vascular surgery who have not been recently stented is not clear. The largest and most influential trial to date, POISE-2, randomized more than 10,000 patients undergoing noncardiac surgery to perioperative aspirin therapy or placebo.[48] Patients already on aspirin therapy comprised the continuation stratum. Patients not already on aspirin therapy but who met the standard indications for it comprised the initiation stratum. There was no difference in the primary outcome (30-day postoperative mortality and nonfatal MI) or the secondary outcome, which additionally included nonfatal stroke, between the two groups. Results were consistent when each stratum was assessed separately. There was, however, a significant increase in major bleeding postoperatively among individuals on aspirin therapy.

In this trial only 6% of patients underwent vascular surgery, whereas those undergoing carotid endarterectomy were excluded. Therefore, generalizations of these findings to patients undergoing vascular surgery may be limited and a potential benefit to perioperative aspirin therapy may still exist. A randomized trial of patients undergoing carotid endarterectomy found that low-dose aspirin reduced the risk of perioperative strokes without complete recovery compared with placebo.[49] In a study of 191 patients on chronic aspirin undergoing vascular surgery, lower platelet responsiveness was associated with a decreased risk of cardiovascular events.[50] A retrospective analysis of patients undergoing vascular surgery found that the combination of aspirin, β-blockers, and statin therapy was associated with better 30-day cardiovascular outcomes than any of the three medications taken separately.[51] In patients undergoing major vascular surgery, including lower extremity bypass, carotid endarterectomy, and abdominal aortic aneurysm repair, perioperative bleeding risk was similar among patients on aspirin plus clopidogrel, aspirin or clopidogrel alone, or no antiplatelet therapy.[52] There are no randomized studies, however, that have been able to demonstrate a reduction in MACE with perioperative aspirin therapy in patients undergoing vascular surgery.

Based on the available evidence, current clinical practice guidelines state that no benefit has been found with initiation or continuation of aspirin in patients undergoing elective noncardiac noncarotid surgery unless the risk of cardiac events outweighs the risk of surgical bleeding (ACC/AHA class III).[12] Therefore, a careful assessment of risks versus benefits of perioperative aspirin use before vascular surgery needs to be performed on a patient-by-patient basis.

Antiplatelet therapy following percutaneous coronary revascularization

Fig. 2 is a suggested algorithm for duration of antiplatelet therapy in patients who have undergone coronary stenting before vascular surgery. Perioperative in-stent thrombosis risk is highest for bare metal stents (BMS) and drug-eluting stents (DES) in the first 4 to 6 weeks following percutaneous coronary intervention.[53–55] Premature discontinuation of dual antiplatelet therapy (DAPT) is also strongly associated with stent thrombosis.[56,57] Clinical practice guidelines recommend that elective vascular surgery be delayed to 14 days after balloon angioplasty, 30 days after BMS implantation, and 365 days after DES implantation to reduce cardiovascular risk and allow for adequate DAPT (ACC/AHA class I). In situations where the risks of delaying the surgery outweigh the risks of ischemia and stent thrombosis, vascular surgery can be considered in patients after 180 days of DES implantation (ACC/AHA class IIB). The decision to continue DAPT or aspirin alone, irrespective of the timing of surgery, needs to be individualized based on the relative risk of ischemia and stent thrombosis versus bleeding (ACC/AHA class IIA).

If vascular surgery is emergent or urgent then the risk of ischemia versus bleeding and absolute benefit of coronary revascularization needs to be considered. Coronary artery bypass graft combined with noncardiac surgery is a possibility if revascularization must be performed. If the procedure is time-sensitive (delay >1 week but <6 weeks) then balloon angioplasty is a safe option. In situations where the surgery is elective, then BMS or DES is recommended depending on the acceptable length of surgical delay.

Recent studies with newer-generation DESs in particular demonstrate that elective noncardiac surgery performed as early as 6 months after stent implantation does not significantly increase perioperative cardiovascular risk.[58,59] Similarly, other studies with primarily newer-generation DESs have found that DAPT duration less than 12 months does not significantly increase cardiovascular risk.[60,61] The Optimize Duration of Clopidogrel Therapy Following Treatment With the Zotarolimus-Eluting Stent in Real-World Clinical

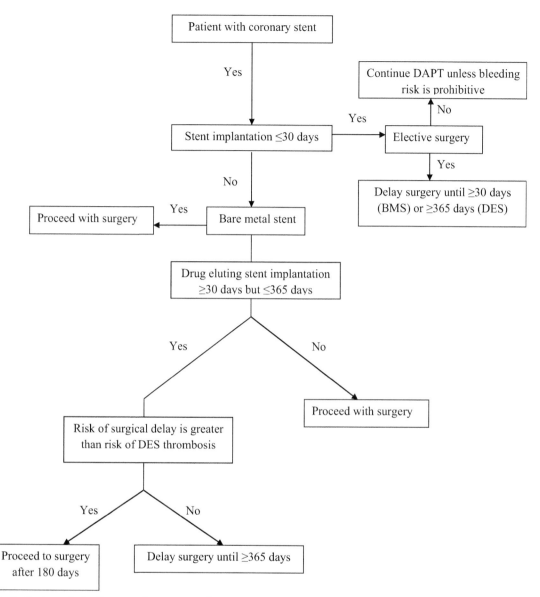

Fig. 2. Timing of elective vascular surgery after percutaneous coronary intervention. BMS, bare metal stents; DAPT, dual antiplatelet therapy; DES, drug-eluting stent. (*Adapted from* Fleisher LA, Fleischmann KE, Auerbach AD, et al. 2014 ACC/AHA guidelines on perioperative cardiovascular evaluation and management for patients undergoing noncardiac surgery: a report of the ACC/AHA task force on practice guidelines. Circulation 2014;[Epub ahead of print].)

Practice trial randomized individuals to 3 versus 12 months of DAPT after zotarolimus DES implantation.[60] There was no difference in the composite outcome of all-cause mortality, MI, stroke, or major bleeding between the groups at 1-year follow-up. The Prolonging Dual-Antiplatelet Treatment after Grading Stent-induced Intimal Hyperplasia Study investigators randomized more than 2000 patients to receive BMS, paclitaxel DES, everolimus DES, and zotoralimus DES.[61] Individuals in each stent group were then randomized to either 6 months or 24 months of DAPT. No difference was found in the composite outcome of total mortality, MI, or stroke between the two groups.

NOVEL THERAPIES

Although adherence to guideline-approved preoperative measures helps reduce the risk of perioperative cardiovascular complications associated with vascular surgery, the risk remains high. Novel preoperative therapies have been proposed to further reduce perioperative cardiovascular risk of vascular surgery. These therapies are still considered experimental and require further study in humans. Remote ischemic preconditioning involves a brief exposure to nonlethal ischemia in one tissue before surgery to protect against a prolonged ischemic insult to a distant tissue.[62] In a study of 82 individuals undergoing elective abdominal aortic aneurysm repair, those randomized to remote ischemic preconditioning had a significantly reduced incidence of postoperative myocardial injury and critical care length of stay compared with those who did not. Remote ischemic preconditioning in this study involved cross-clamping each iliac artery for 10 minutes followed by 10 minutes of reperfusion.[63] Dietary preconditioning or dietary restriction involves a reduction in caloric intake before surgery to help decrease the oxidative stress, neurohormonal release, and inflammation associated with surgery.[64] Experimental models in rats have demonstrated that reduction in caloric intake, particularly in protein or amino acid intake, substantially reduces surgical stress associated with renal and hepatic reperfusion injury.[65]

REFERENCES

1. Prinssen M, Verhoeven HL, Buth J, et al. A randomized trial comparing conventional and endovascular repair of abdominal aortic aneurysms. N Engl J Med 2004;351:1607–18.
2. Adam DJ, Beard JD, Cleveland T, et al. Bypass versus angioplasty in severe ischaemia of the leg (BASIL): multicentre, randomised controlled trial. Lancet 2005;366:1925–34.
3. Birkmeyer JD, Siewers AE, Finlayson EV, et al. Hospital volume and surgical mortality in the United States. N Engl J Med 2002;346:1128–37.
4. Krupski WC, Layug EL, Reilly LM, et al. Comparison of cardiac morbidity rates between aortic and infrainguinal operations: two-year follow-up. Study of Perioperative Ischemia Research Group. J Vasc Surg 1993;18:609–15.
5. Jencks SF, Willams MV, Coleman EA. Rehospitalizations among patients in the Medicare fee-for-service program. N Engl J Med 2009;360:1418–28.
6. Noordzij PG, Poldermans D, Schouten O, et al. Postoperative mortality in the Netherlands. Anesthesiology 2010;112:1105–15.
7. Anderson PL, Gelijns A, Moskowitz A, et al. Understanding trends in inpatient surgical volume: vascular interventions, 1980-2000. J Vasc Surg 2004;39:1200–8.
8. Devereaux PJ, Goldman L, Cook DJ, et al. Perioperative cardiac events in patients undergoing noncardiac surgery: a review of the magnitude of the problem, the pathophysiology of the events and methods to estimate and communicate risk. CMAJ 2005;173:627–34.
9. Ashton CM, Petersen NJ, Wray NP, et al. The incidence of perioperative myocardial infarction in men undergoing noncardiac surgery. Ann Intern Med 1993;118:504–10.
10. Hertzer NR, Beven EG, Young JR, et al. Coronary artery disease in peripheral vascular patients. A classification of 1,000 coronary angiograms and results of surgical management. Ann Surg 1984 199:223–33.
11. Faggiano P, Bonardelli S, De Feo S, et al. Preoperative cardiac evaluation and perioperative cardiac therapy in patients undergoing open surgery for abdominal aortic aneurysms: effects on cardiovascular outcome. Ann Vasc Surg 2012;26:156–65.
12. Fleisher LA, Fleischmann KE, Auerbach AD, et al. 2014 ACC/AHA guidelines on perioperative cardiovascular evaluation and management for patients undergoing noncardiac surgery: a report of the ACC/AHA task force on practice guidelines. Circulation 2014. [Epub ahead of print].
13. Fleisher LA, Beckman JA, Brown KA, et al. 2009 ACCF/AHA focused update on perioperative beta blockade incorporated into the ACC/AHA 2007 guidelines on perioperative cardiovascular evaluation and care for noncardiac surgery: a report of the ACCF/AHA task force on practice guidelines. Circulation 2009;120:e169–276.
14. Livhits M, Ko CY, Leonardi MJ, et al. Risk of surgery following recent myocardial infarction. Ann Surg 2011;253:857–64.
15. Van Diepen S, Bakal JA, McAlister FA, et al. Mortality and readmission of patients with heart failure, atrial fibrillation, or coronary artery disease undergoing noncardiac surgery: an analysis of 38047 patients. Circulation 2011;124:289–96.
16. Rodseth RN, Lurati Buse GA, Bolliger D, et al. The predictive ability of pre-operative B-type natriuretic peptide in vascular patients for major adverse cardiac events. J Am Coll Cardiol 2011;58:522–9.
17. Otto CM. Valvular aortic stenosis: disease severity and timing of intervention. J Am Coll Cardiol 2006; 47:2141–51.
18. Agarwal S, Rajamanickam A, Bajaj NS, et al. Impact of aortic stenosis on postoperative outcomes after noncardiac surgeries. Circ Cardiovasc Qual Outcomes 2013;6:193–200.
19. Leon MB, Smith CR, Mack M, et al. Transcatheter aortic-valve implantation for aortic stenosis in patients who cannot undergo surgery. N Engl J Med 2010;363:1597–607.

20. Smith CR, Leon MB, Mack MJ, et al. Transcatheter versus surgical aortic-valve replacement in high-risk patients. N Engl J Med 2011;346:2187–98.

21. Popma JJ, Adams DH, Reardon MJ, et al. Transcatheter aortic valve replacement using a self-expanding bioprosthesis in patients with severe aortic stenosis at extreme high risk for surgery. J Am Coll Cardiol 2014;63:1972–81.

22. Adams DH, Popma JJ, Reardon MJ, et al. Transcatheter aortic-valve replacement with a self-expanding prosthesis. N Engl J Med 2014;370:1790–8.

23. Finks JF, Osborne NH, Birkmeyer JD. Trends in hospital volume and operative mortality for high-risk surgery. N Engl J Med 2011;364:2128–37.

24. Flu WJ, van Kuijk JP, Hoeks SE, et al. Prognostic implications of asymptomatic left ventricular dysfunction in patients undergoing vascular surgery. Anesthesiology 2010;112:1316–24.

25. Sgura FA, Kopecky SL, Grill JP, et al. Supine exercise-capacity identifies patients at low risk for perioperative cardiovascular events and predicts long-term survival. Am J Med 2000;108:334–6.

26. Lee TH, Marcantonio ER, Mangione CM, et al. Derivation and prospective validation of a simple index for prediction of cardiac risk of major noncardiac surgery. Circulation 1999;100:1043–9.

27. Ford MK, Beattie WS, Wijeysundera DN. Systematic review: prediction of perioperative cardiac complications and mortality by the Revised Cardiac Risk Index. Ann Intern Med 2010;152:26–35.

28. Welten GM, Schouten O, van Domburg RT, et al. The influence of aging on the prognostic value of the revised cardiac risk index for postoperative cardiac complications in vascular surgery patients. Eur J Vasc Endovasc Surg 2007;34:632–8.

29. Bertges DJ, Goodney PP, Zhao Y, et al. The Vascular Study Group of New England Cardiac Risk Index (VSG-CRI) predicts cardiac complications more accurately than the Revised Cardiac Risk Index in vascular surgery patients. J Vasc Surg 2010;52:674–83.

30. Gupta PK, Gupta H, Sundaram A, et al. Development and validation of a risk calculator for prediction of cardiac risk after surgery. Circulation 2011;124:381–7.

31. Gupta PK, Ramanan B, Lynch TG, et al. Development and validation of a risk calculator for prediction of mortality after infrainguinal bypass surgery. J Vasc Surg 2012;56:372–9.

32. Gupta PK, Ramanan B, Mctaggart JN, et al. Risk index for predicting perioperative stroke, myocardial infarction, or death risk in asymptomatic patients undergoing carotid endarterectomy. J Vasc Surg 2013;57:318–26.

33. Ramanan B, Gupta PK, Sundaram A, et al. Development of a risk index for prediction of mortality after open aortic aneurysm repair. J Vasc Surg 2013;58:871–8.

34. Eichelberger JP, Schwarz KQ, Black ER, et al. Predictive value of dobutamine echocardiography just before noncardiac vascular surgery. Am J Cardiol 1993;72:602–7.

35. Cohen MC, Siewers AE, Dickens JD, et al. Perioperative and long-term prognostic value of dipyridamole Tc-99m sestamibi myocardial tomography in patients evaluated for elective vascular surgery. J Nucl Cardiol 2003;10:464–72.

36. Beattie WS, Abdelnaem E, Wijeysundera DN, et al. A meta-analytic comparison of preoperative stress echocardiography and nuclear scintigraphy imaging. Anesth Analg 2006;69:558–63.

37. Monaco M, Stassano P, Di Tommaso L, et al. Systemic strategy of prophylactic coronary angiography improves long-term outcome after major vascular surgery in medium- to high-risk patients: a prospective, randomized study. J Am Coll Cardiol 2009;54:989–96.

38. McFalls EO, Ward HB, Moritz TE, et al. Coronary artery revascularization before elective major vascular surgery. N Engl J Med 2004;351:2795–804.

39. Devereaux PJ, Yang H, Yusuf S, et al, POISE Study Group. Effects of extended-release metoprolol succinate in patients undergoing non-cardiac surgery (POISE trial): a randomized controlled trial. Lancet 2008;371:1839–47.

40. Wijeysundera DN, Duncan D, Nkonde-Price C, et al. Perioperative beta-blockade in noncardiac surgery: a systematic review for the 2014 ACC/AHA guideline on perioperative cardiovascular evaluation and management of patients undergoing noncardiac surgery: a report of the ACC/AHA task force on practice guidelines. Circulation 2014. [Epub ahead of print].

41. POBBLE Trial Investigators. Perioperative b-blockade (POBBLE) for patients undergoing infrarenal vascular surgery: results of a randomized double-blind controlled trial. J Vasc Surg 2005;41:602–9.

42. Yang H, Raymer K, Butler R, et al. The effects of perioperative beta-blockade: results of the Metoprolol after Vascular Surgery (MaVS) study, a randomized controlled trial. Am Heart J 2006;4:139–43.

43. Durazzo AE, Machado FS, Ikeoka DT, et al. Reduction in cardiovascular events after vascular surgery with atorvastatin: a randomized trial. J Vasc Surg 2004;39:967–75.

44. Kennedy J, Quan H, Buchan AM, et al. Statins are associated with better outcomes after carotid endarterectomy in symptomatic patients. Stroke 2005;36:2072–6.

45. Aiello FA, Khan AA, Meltzer AJ, et al. Statin therapy is associated with superior clinical outcomes after endovascular treatment of critical limb ischemia. J Vasc Surg 2012;55:371–80.

46. Raux M, Cochennec F, Becquemin JP, et al. Statin therapy is associated with aneurysm sac regression after endovascular aortic repair. J Vasc Surg 2012; 55:1587–92.

47. De Bruin JL, Baas AF, Heymans MW, et al. Statin therapy is associated with improved survival after endovascular and open aneurysm repair. J Vasc Surg 2014;59:39–44.

48. Devereaux PJ, Mrkobrada M, Sessler DI, et al. Aspirin in patients undergoing noncardiac surgery. N Engl J Med 2014;370:1494–503.

49. Lindblad B, Persson NH, Takolander R, et al. Does low-dose acetylsalicyclic acid prevent stroke after carotid surgery? A double-blind, placebo-controlled randomized trial. Stroke 1993;24:1125–8.

50. Calderaro D, Pastana AF, Flores da Rocha TR, et al. Aspirin responsiveness safely lowers perioperative cardiovascular risk. J Vasc Surg 2013;58:1593–9.

51. Lau WC, Froehlich JB, Jewell ES, et al. Impact of adding aspirin to beta-blocker and statin in high-risk patients undergoing major vascular surgery. Ann Vasc Surg 2013;27:537–45.

52. Stone DH, Goodney PP, Schanzer A, et al. Clopidogrel is not associated with major bleeding complications during peripheral arterial surgery. J Vasc Surg 2011;54:779–84.

53. Tokushige A, Shiomi H, Morimoto T, et al. Incidence and outcome of surgical procedures after coronary bare-metal and drug-eluting stent implantation: a report from CREDO-Kyoto PCI/CABG registry cohort-2. Circ Cardiovasc Interv 2012;63:141–5.

54. Berger PB, Kleiman NS, Pencina MJ, et al. Frequency of major noncardiac surgery and subsequent adverse events in the year after drug-eluting stent placement results from the EVENT Registry. JACC Cardiovasc Interv 2010;3:920–7.

55. Cruden NL, Harding SA, Flapan AD, et al. Previous coronary stent implantation and cardiac events in patients undergoing noncardiac surgery. Circ Cardiovasc Interv 2010;3:236–42.

56. Van Werkum JW, Heestermans AA, Zomer AC, et al. Predictors of coronary stent thrombosis: the Dutch Stent Thrombosis Registry. J Am Coll Cardiol 2009; 53:1399–409.

57. Iakovou I, Schmidt T, Bonizzoni E, et al. Incidence, predictors, and outcome of thrombosis after successful implantation of drug-eluting stents. JAMA 2005;293:2126–30.

58. Wijeysundera DN, Wijeysundera HC, Yun L, et al. Risk of elective major noncardiac surgery after coronary stent insertion: a population-based study. Circulation 2012;126:1355–62.

59. Hawn MT, Graham LA, Richman JS, et al. Risk of major adverse cardiac events following noncardiac surgery in patients with coronary stents. JAMA 2013;210:1462–72.

60. Feres F, Costa RA, Abizaid A, et al. Three vs twelve months of dual antiplatelet therapy after zotarolimus-eluting stents: the OPTIMIZE randomized trial. JAMA 2013;310:2510–22.

61. Valgimigli M, Campo G, Monti M, et al. Short- versus long-term duration of dual antiplatelet therapy after coronary stenting: a randomized multicenter trial. Circulation 2012;125:2015–26.

62. Walsh SR, Tang TY, Sadat U, et al. Remote ischemic preconditioning in major vascular surgery. J Vasc Surg 2009;49:240–3.

63. Ali ZA, Callaghan CJ, Lim E, et al. Remote ischaemic preconditioning reduces myocardial and renal injury after elective abdominal aortic aneurysm repair: a randomized controlled trial. Circulation 2007;116: 95–106.

64. Mitchell JR, Beckman JA, Nguyen LL. Reducing elective vascular surgery perioperative risk with brief preoperative dietary restriction. Surgery 2013;153: 594–8.

65. Peng W, Robertson L, Gallinetti J, et al. Surgical stress resistance induced by single amino acid deprivation requires Gcn2 in mice. Sci Transl Med 2012;4:118ra11.

Peripheral Drug-Eluting Technology

Anna Franzone, MD, Eugenio Stabile, MD, PhD*, Bruno Trimarco, MD, Giovanni Esposito, MD, PhD

KEYWORDS

- Peripheral artery disease • Drug-eluting balloon • Restenosis • Femoropopliteal • Below-the-knee
- Drug-coated balloons • Drug-eluting stents • In-stent restenosis

KEY POINTS

- Drug-eluting devices have been developed to overcome restenosis, the major limitation of conventional angioplasty, by achieving effective drug transfer into the arterial wall and by exerting antirestenotic effects.
- A large body of evidence supports the safety and efficacy of drug-eluting stents in below-the-knee arteries.
- Drug-eluting balloons are found to be superior to conventional angioplasty for the treatment of de novo femoropopliteal and below-the-knee diseases.
- Accurate lesion preparation before use of drug-eluting balloons is essential for effective drug transfer into the arterial wall.
- The use of drug-eluting technologies (drug-eluting stents and drug-eluting balloons) for the treatment of femoropopliteal in-stent restenosis seems to provide good long-term patency rates, as reported by registries and a randomized clinical trial.

INTRODUCTION

The endovascular approach has emerged as a valid therapeutic option for patients with peripheral artery disease (PAD), causing intermittent claudication or critical limb ischemia (CLI), with reduced morbidity and costs compared to surgical bypass grafting.[1] Despite marked improvements in materials and techniques, maintaining long-term patency after percutaneous transluminal angioplasty (PTA) of femoropopliteal (FP) or below-the-knee (BTK) lesions is still a real challenge because of the occurrence of restenosis. Indeed, mechanical stresses, heavy calcification, and extensive atherosclerotic lesions make the FP bed typically prone to PTA failure. Patency at 1 year after balloon angioplasty (plain old balloon angioplasty, POBA) is only near 40%.[2] Superior vessel scaffolding provided by nitinol stents has markedly improved the patency rates (65%–80%) over conventional angioplasty or atherectomy.[3,4] In-stent restenosis (ISR), however, has been reported to occur in up to 40% of FP lesions treated with bare metal stents (BMS) within 1 year of treatment, with an increasing number of patients requiring re-intervention.[5] Moreover, the diffuse nature of atherosclerotic disease and compromised general status make patients with BTK lesions more difficult to treat. In this scenario, drug-eluting technologies seem to offer promising tools to overcome the limitations of peripheral POBA or stenting and to manage ISR. Because drug-eluting balloons (DEB) and drug-eluting stents (DES) have major application in the treatment of FP or BTK tracts, this review

The authors have no conflict to disclose.
Division of Cardiology, Department of Advanced Biomedical Sciences, University of Napoli "Federico II", Via S. Pansini 5, Napoli 80131, Italy
* Corresponding author.
E-mail address: geko50@hotmail.com

Cardiol Clin 33 (2015) 151–162
http://dx.doi.org/10.1016/j.ccl.2014.09.005
0733-8651/15/$ – see front matter
© 2015 Elsevier Inc. All rights reserved.

focuses on the currently available evidence of their use in these arterial territories.

PERFORMANCE OF CONVENTIONAL PERCUTANEOUS TRANSLUMINAL ANGIOPLASTY DEVICES

Low complication rates (0.5%–4%) and high technical success (90%) are the major advantages of the percutaneous approach to PAD over surgery.[6]

Conventional Balloon Angioplasty

POBA has been the cornerstone of endovascular therapy for the FP region. However, despite good early angiographic results, balloon injury is associated with the occurrence of adverse events such as elastic recoil, negative remodeling, and vessel dissection accounting for disappointing long-term primary patency.[7] For these reasons, as a standalone therapy, POBA is indicated for short, focal lesions (<4 or 5 cm).

Low-profile, long balloons with long inflation times provide good acute angiographic results when used in BTK arteries of patients suffering from CLI. Despite a 90% rate of limb salvage, restenosis at 6 months is extremely high (up to 80%) with a 1-year re-intervention rate of 59%.[1]

Stents

Because of their peculiar features (radial strength and crush recoverability), self-expanding nitinol stents have been found to improve the patency rates compared with PTA only in the treatment of long lesions (≥8 cm) of the FP tract.[4,8,9] Growing evidence from randomized trials has changed the previous common paradigm that limited stenting of shorter FP lesions to bailout indications (flow-limiting dissections, acute or subacute recoil, or reocclusion) after POBA. Primary nitinol stenting now represents the first-line strategy for the treatment of intermediate-length superficial femoral artery (SFA) lesions with a restenosis rate at 1 and 2 years 20% to 30% lower than conventional angioplasty.[10] Technologic advances in stent design provide more flexibility and crush resistance to second-generation nitinol stents that is associated with improved clinical and angiographic outcomes.[11,12] Furthermore, covered stent grafts may be a valid option for longer and more complex SFA lesions, showing results comparable to those of prosthetic bypass surgery.[13]

The role of metal stents (mostly balloon-expandable coronary stents) for BTK lesions has been historically restricted to bailout indications after failure of PTA. In a small, randomized trial comparing the performance of different metal stents and balloon-only angioplasty in 38 limbs, no difference in survival, limb salvage, and primary and secondary patency was seen at 1 year.[14] In a pooled analysis of 640 patients treated with infragenicular stent implantation, sirolimus-eluting stents showed superiority in terms of binary restenosis and primary patency over BMS.[15]

RATIONALE FOR DRUG-ELUTING TECHNOLOGIES

Successful application of drug-eluting devices in coronary vasculature has encouraged their use in peripheral arteries. The addition of a drug layer to common endovascular devices (balloons or stents) aims mainly to hinder the occurrence of restenosis.

Balloon injury–induced arterial recoil, negative remodeling, and vessel dissection can limit the acute gain of conventional angioplasty. Improved mechanical scaffolding provided by nitinol stents, however, is associated with an increased risk of late vessel injury and neointimal hyperplasia.[16] Regardless of the underling mechanism, the occurrence of neointimal hyperplasia is caused by smooth muscle cell (SMC) proliferation as a result of sustained inflammatory response and therefore invalidates long-term patency of PTA. Against this background, the concept of drug delivery directly into the vessel wall is attractive for 2 main reasons: (1) it ensures effective and steady concentration of chemotherapeutic drugs able to prevent neointimal hyperplasia by inhibiting SMC migration and proliferation of pharmacologic agents and (2) there is minimal associated risk of systemic toxicity.[17]

DRUG-ELUTING STENTS

The introduction of DES has added substantial benefit to the clinical outcomes of patients undergoing percutaneous coronary revascularization, driven mainly by a significant reduction of target lesion revascularization (TLR) rates compared with those of BMS.[18] DES combine sustained local drug delivery with vessel scaffolding to prevent recoil and to solve vessel dissection.

An extensive, off-label use of balloon-expandable coronary stents has been made for the treatment of BTK lesions. Furthermore, dedicated self-expanding stents were developed for the FP arteries.

Two categories of antiproliferative (chemotherapeutic) drugs can be eluted on stent platform: macrolide antibiotics (rapamycin), such as sirolimus and its analogues (everolimus, zotarolimus, tacrolimus, biolimus A9) or paclitaxel. Rapamycin compounds bind to the mammalian target of rapamycin receptor thereby stopping mitosis at the G1 phase and inhibiting cellular growth.[19] Paclitaxel (Taxol) is a mitotic inhibitor (halts the cell cycle in the M phase of the mitotic cycle) that disrupts normal microtubule function and cytoskeleton arrangement and prevents neointimal hyperplasia by inhibiting SMC proliferation (this effect is not associated with the inhibition of endothelial cell proliferation and results in prevention of restenosis without stopping re-endothelization). Beyond the specific eluted drug, stent material and design, polymer coating, and strut thickness play important roles in defining the performance of different devices.

As reported in a later discussion, DES have shown excellent results in BTK arteries, whereas their effectiveness in the FP bed is still uncertain.

DRUG-ELUTING STENTS IN FEMOROPOPLITEAL LESIONS

Performance of BMS in FP arteries is hampered by the occurrence of restenosis as a consequence of neointimal hyperplasia and of the mechanical forces exerted by surrounding musculature that favors stent fracture and compression. Adding an antiproliferative drug to the abluminal surface of the devices has the potential to inhibit SMC proliferation. Devices that have been investigated for the use in FP arteries include the SMART stent (Cordis, Miami, FL), a sirolimus-eluting self-expanding nitinol stent; the Zilver PTX (Cook Medical, Bloomington, IN), a polymer-free, paclitaxel-coated stent; and the Dynalink E (Abbott Vascular, Santa Clara, CA), an everolimus-eluting stent.

SIROCCO Trial

SIROCCO (Sirolimus-eluting vs bare nitinol stent for obstructive superficial femoral artery disease) was a double-blind, randomized, trial that compared the efficacy of the SMART stent to that of a BMS for the treatment of SFA lesions. The high rates of stent fracture reported at 9 and 18 months (19% and 31%, respectively) led to an amendment to the protocol (SIROCCO II) to shorten the maximum lesion length from 20 cm to 14.5 cm. A total of 93 patients was included (47 assigned to DES, 46 to BMS); at 24 months follow-up, no differences in restenosis rates, TLR, and target vessel revascularization were reported. DES did not show superiority over BMS probably because of the low rate of restenosis in the BMS arm, as highlighted by the authors.[20,21]

Zilver PTX

In the Zilver PTX trial, patients were randomly assigned to standard PTA (n = 238) or DES treatment (n = 236). The primary patency was 83.1% and 74.8% in the DES arm and 64.5% and 57.8% in the PTA arm, at 12 and 24 months, respectively. At long-term follow-up (2 years), freedom from TLR was 83% in the DES group versus 70.2% in the BMS group. Moreover, in the subgroup of patients with long lesions (mean length, 226 mm), primary patency was 77.6%.[22–24]

Superficial Femoral Artery Treatment with Drug-Eluting Stents Trial

STRIDES (Superficial Femoral Artery Treatment with Drug-Eluting Stents) was a prospective, nonrandomized, multicenter, trial that enrolled 104 patients with FP lesions (mean length, 9 cm) treated with the Dynalink E stent (Abbott Vascular, Redwood City, CA). The primary patency rate at 12 months was 68.5% without the occurrence of stent fracture.[25]

The better performance shown in the Zilver trial compared with the other 2 randomized DES studies is probably attributable to specific characteristics of the Zilver PTX stent: beyond a peculiar strut design, it has no polymer or carriers within the drug coating that could trigger an inflammatory vessel reaction and further induce neointimal hyperplasia.

DRUG-ELUTING STENTS IN BELOW-THE-KNEE LESIONS

Although multilevel disease is frequently encountered in patients with CLI, BTK arteries are mostly involved. Atherosclerotic disease of tibioperoneal arteries is peculiar because of a large intimal lipid burden and medial calcification. As a consequence, vessels are often totally occluded and more prone to rupture or thrombosis.[26] Because of similar sizes, the pioneering use of drug-eluting devices in BTK arteries has been based on balloons and stents designed for coronary interventions. However, design modifications are needed to ensure more pushability and to comply with the typical anatomic features of these arteries.

Several nonrandomized studies first explored the use of first-generation DES (sirolimus- or paclitaxel-eluting, stainless steel) in BTK lesions showing a primary patency superior compared with the use of metal stents (**Table 1**). Randomized data have come from the trials discussed in the following sections.

Table 1
Summary of nonrandomized studies evaluating the performance of drug-eluting stents in below-the-knee lesions

Author, Year	Drug	Bailout or Primary Stenting	Limbs	Limb Salvage (mo)	Primary Patency (mo)
Commeau et al,[49] 2006	Sirolimus	Bailout	30	100% (7)	97% (7)
Scheinert et al,[50] 2006	Sirolimus	Primary	30	100% (6)	100% (6)
Bosiers et al,[51] 2006	Sirolimus	Primary	18	94% (6)	100% (6)
Feiring et al,[52] 2007	Sirolimus	Primary	11	100% (29)	100% (29)
Siablis et al,[53] 2007	Sirolimus	Bailout	29	96% (12)	86% (12)
Siablis et al,[54] 2007	Paclitaxel	Bailout	32	88.5% (12)	23 (12)
Grant et al,[55] 2008	60% Sirolimus 40% Paclitaxel	Primary	10	—	90 (12)
Rosales et al,[56] 2008	Sirolimus	Primary	24	83% (12)	95% (12)
Siablis et al,[57] 2009	Sirolimus	Bailout	75	80.3% (36)	32.9% (36)
Rastan et al,[58] 2010	Sirolimus	Primary	104	100% (12)	84% (12)
Balzer et al,[59] 2010	Sirolimus	Primary	128	96.9 (18)	83% (18)
Feiring et al,[30] 2010	83% Sirolimus 17% Paclitaxel	Primary	118	94% (36)	88% (36)
Karnabatidis et al,[60] 2011	Everolimus	Primary	51	77.1% (36)	29.7% (36)
Werner et al,[61] 2012	Sirolimus	Primary	158	96.3% (12)	87% (12)

YUKON-BTK

In the YUKON Drug-eluting Stent Below the Knee trial, 161 patients (mean lesion length, 31 mm) were randomly assigned to treatment with the polymer-free, 2% sirolimus-coated, YUKON stent (Translumina GmbH, Hechingen, Germany) or with the same uncoated stent. At 1-year of follow-up, primary patency was 80.6% for the DES group versus 55.6% for the BMS group ($P = .004$); a trend toward less TLR was also observed with the use of DES. At a longer follow-up (2.8 years), the primary endpoint of freedom from target vessel revascularization, myocardial infarction, and death favored the DES group.[27]

Destiny

The Destiny trial randomly assigned 140 patients with CLI to treatment with the everolimus polymer-coated Xience V stent (Abbott Vascular, Redwood City, CA) or with the Multilink Vision BMS (Abbott Vascular, Redwood City, CA) with findings at 1 year in favor of DES: higher primary patency (85.2% vs 54.4%; $P = .0001$); lower late lumen loss (0.78 vs 1.41; $P = .0001$) and TLR (8% vs 35%; $P = .005$).[28]

Achilles

The Achilles study involved 200 patients with CLI (mean lesion length, 27 mm) randomly assigned to receive the sirolimus- and polymer-coated CYPHER SELECT stent (Cordis, Johnson & Johnson, Bridgewater, NJ) or conventional, balloon-only PTA. The occurrence of angiographic binary restenosis at 1 year (primary endpoint) was observed in 22.4% of the DES group compared with 41.9% from the BMS group. The optimal performance of DES was confirmed in the diabetic subgroup. However, no significant differences were reported for TLR and limb salvage.[29]

Below

Sixty patients with CLI and ulcers were randomly assigned to receive abciximab plus the sirolimus-coated CYPHER stent (Cordis, Johnson & Johnson, Bridgewater, NJ) abciximab plus a BMS, abciximab plus PTA, or PTA alone. Angiographic control showed restenosis rates of 9%, 45.5%, 67%, and 46%, respectively, at 2 months and restenosis rates of 9%, 67%, 75%, and 58%, respectively, at 6 months; 14% of all patients had major amputations within 6 months. DES use was associated with the higher patency rate.

Despite several differences in study design, the findings from these studies are uniform and support the safety of DES in BTK arteries, their efficacy in significantly reducing TLR, and binary restenosis compared with either balloon angioplasty or BMS. No significant benefit resulted from the use of abciximab.

Long-term data support durable arterial repair by DES and come from the nonrandomized PReventing Amputations using Drug eluting StEnts (PaRADISE) trial: the 3-year cumulative incidence of amputation was about 6% (14% in patients in Rutherfod class 6) compared with the expected 40% to 50% rate with the standard therapy.[30]

Furthermore, in a recent meta-analysis including 5 randomized trials (611 patients; mean lesion length, 26.8 mm), the use of DES reduced the risk of re-intervention and amputation at 1 year follow-up compared with BMS or POBA, without any difference in mortality and Rutherford class improvement.[31]

DRUG-ELUTING BALLOONS

Nonstent local drug delivery offers the opportunity to avoid the implant of a foreign body and consequent chronic inflammatory reaction while providing adequate local release of antiproliferative agents. DEBs are the main tools of the "leave nothing behind" strategy that showed excellent results in the coronary bed, especially for the management of ISR. Most of them have Conformité Européene- (and not US Food and Drug Administration) mark approval. **Table 2** lists currently available DEBs for peripheral interventions.

Potential advantages of DEBs over DES include a more homogenous and broader drug delivery per square millimeter, the absence of a permanent implant constituting an inflammatory trigger, and an early restoration of normal vessel function. Moreover, DEBs may be used in anatomic locations that are not suitable for stents (bifurcations, distal arteries).

Drug-eluting Balloon Composition

The 3 major components of DEBs, whose synergistic action is crucial, are the following:

1. The platform that is the balloon itself can be either compliant or semicompliant.
2. Paclitaxel (Taxol) is the most frequently used antiproliferative agent because of its specific features: its lipophilic properties prevent adventitial washout and prolong antiproliferative effects, enhancing the interactions with lipids in the vessel wall; a single low-dose of paclitaxel ($3 \ \mu g/mm^2$) provides prolonged inhibition of SMCs proliferation. A balloon inflation of 30 to 45 seconds ensures high tissue concentration of drug without additional side effects

Table 2
Currently available peripheral drug-eluting balloons

Device (Company)	Drug (Dose-$\mu g/mm^2$)	Carrier	Diameter (mm)	Lengths (mm)
Elutax (Aachen Resonance, Aachen, Germany)	Paclitaxel (2)	None	2–6	10, 13, 16, 18, 21, 24, 27, 30, 33, 36, 39
Lutonix (BARD, New Hope, MN, USA)	Paclitaxel (2)	Polysorbate and Sorbitol	4–6	40, 60, 100
Passeo-18 LUX (Biotronik, Bülach, Switzerland)	Paclitaxel (3)	Butyryl-tri-hexyl citrate (BTHC)	3–7	40, 80, 120
Legflow (Cardionovum, Warsaw, Poland)	Paclitaxel (3)	Shelloic acid	2–4	20, 40, 60, 80, 100, 120, 150
Advance 18 PTX (Cook Medical, Bloomington, IN)	Paclitaxel (3)	None	3–7	40, 80, 100
Freeway 014 (Eurocor, Bonn, Germany)	Paclitaxel (3)	Shelloic acid	2–4	40, 80, 120, 150
Freeway 035 (Eurocor, Bonn, Germany)	Paclitaxel (3)	Shelloic acid	4–8	20, 40, 60, 80, 100, 120, 150
Moxy DCB (Lutonix-Bard, Murray Hill, NJ, USA)	Paclitaxel (2)	—	2–4	18, 30
IN.PACT Admiral (Medtronic Inc, Minneapolis, MN, USA)	Paclitaxel (3)	Urea	4–7	40, 60, 80, 120, 150
IN.PACT Pacific (Medtronic Inc, Minneapolis, MN, USA)	Paclitaxel (3)	Urea	4–7	40, 60, 80, 120

3. The excipient or carrier allows effective transfer of drug into the arterial wall, which can be contrast agent, urea, iopromide, or biodegradable polymer. Most of them are hydrophilic spacers that reduce the loss of hydrophobic paclitaxel microparticles in the systemic circulation.

DRUG-ELUTING BALLOONS IN FEMOROPOPLITEAL LESIONS

The successful performance of DEBs in FP arteries has been shown in several clinical studies.

THUNDER

THUNDER was double-blind, randomized trial in which154 patients with SFA lesions (stenosis and occlusions; mean length, 7.4 cm) were assigned to one of the following treatment groups: paclitaxel-coated balloon with an iopromide carrier (Paccocath, Medrad, PA) with standard nonionic contrast medium, standard PTA with uncoated balloon and nonionic contrast medium, or standard PTA with paclitaxel added to contrast medium. Despite a high procedural success rate in all groups, the need for bailout stenting was higher in patients treated with uncoated balloons. A significant reduction in 6-month late lumen loss and binary restenosis was observed in the DEB group. TLR was significantly lower in the paclitaxel-coated balloon group for up to 2 years of follow-up.[32]

FemPac

Eighty-seven patients (mean lesion length, 6 cm) with de novo FP lesions were randomly assigned to treatment with either uncoated or paclitaxel-coated balloon (Paccocath). At 6 months of follow-up, lumen loss and TLR were significantly lower in the DEB group, and this result was sustained up to 18 months.

Levant 1

Levant 1 was a prospective, randomized (1:1) trial comparing late lumen loss in FP lesions treated with the MOXY DEB (Lutonix, Murray Hill, NJ, USA) (with a low-dose 2 $\mu g/mm^2$ of paclitaxel and a coating containing a polysorbate/sorbitol carrier) versus an uncoated balloon. A total of 101 patients were enrolled. At 6 months, lumen loss (primary endpoint) was significantly lower in the Lutonix DEB group than in the uncoated balloon group (0.46 ± 1.13 mm vs 1.09 ± 1.07 mm, $P = .016$) with safety sustained up to 24 months.[33]

Pacifier

In the Pacifier study, 85 patients with FP lesions were randomly assigned to treatment with either the IN.PACT Pacific (paclitaxel-eluting with urea as carrier) (Medtronic, Inc, Santa Rosa, CA) or uncoated Pacific (Medtronic Inc). Lumen loss, restenosis, and re-interventions were significantly lower up to 1 year in the DEB group.[34]

Debellum

Fifty consecutive patients with FP or BTK lesions were randomly assigned to DEB or conventional balloon PTA. A lower rate of TLR was reported in the DEB group, and this translated into better clinical outcomes with significant improvements in ankle-brachial index and Fontaine stage.[35]

Biolux P-I

Biolux P-I was a first-in-man, prospective trial to evaluate the performance of the Passeo 18 LUX DEB (Biotronik, Berlin, Germany) versus standard PTA in 26 patients with FP lesions. Late lumen loss at 6 months was significantly lower in the DEB group as were TLR rates at 12 months.

DEBATE-SFA

DEBATE-SFA was a prospective, randomized trial that enrolled 104 patients to either predilation with DEB plus PTA with BMS or predilation with an uncoated balloon plus PTA with BMS. Binary restenosis at 1-year of follow-up was significantly inferior in the DEB treatment group. Moreover, a near-significant 1-year freedom from TLR advantage was observed.[36]

The preliminary results of the IN.PACT SFA clinical trial presented during CX 2014 by T. Zeller showed that the Admiral DEB (Medtronic, Inc) was superior to POBA for the treatment of SFA lesions.

DRUG-ELUTING BALLOONS IN BELOW-THE-KNEE LESIONS

Successful performance of DEBs in the treatment of BTK lesions has been shown in a registry that included patients treated with the IN.PACT Amphirion DEB (Medtronic Vascular) compared with historical controls who underwent conventional PTA. The restenosis rate at 3 months was lower for the DEB-treated patients (27% vs 69%).

The positive findings observed in the BTK arm of the DEBELLUM trial[35] were confirmed in the larger DEBATE-BTK study, which showed that binary restenosis was reduced from 74% with balloon angioplasty to 27% with a paclitaxel–urea DEB (IN.PACT Amphirion; *P*<.001).[37]

The preliminary results of the IN.PACT DEEP clinical trial presented during LINC 2014 by T. Zeller showed that the IN.PACT Amphirion DEB (Medtronic, Inc, Minneapolis, MN, USA) did not result in a differential treatment effect for patients with BTK lesions and CLI compared with use of a standard balloon PTA. Moreover, the study showed a safety potential risk in the DEB arm with a trend toward an increased rate of major amputation (above the ankle) compared with the PTA control.

Based on these findings, Medtronic voluntarily withdrew the IN.PACT Amphirion DEB from all markets worldwide in November 2013.

NEW DRUG-ELUTING BALLOONS

The introduction of innovative DEBs aims to overcome some of their potential drawbacks, such as the risk of distal embolization caused by dislodgment of paclitaxel particles, systemic toxic effects (in patients with long lesions), and local toxic effects (overlapping zones).

The Legflow DEB (Cardionovum Sp, Warsaw, Poland) has nanocrystalline paclitaxel formulation embedded underneath the surface and inside its shelloic acid (a natural resin) matrix. The stable coating minimizes drug wash out during catheter tracking. The RAPID trial (ISRCTN47846578) aims to recruit 176 patients with SFA lesions to be treated with the nitinol SUPERA stent (IDEV Technologies Inc, Webster, TX) or with the Legflow DEB. The primary endpoint is the absence of binary restenosis of the treated SFA segment. Secondary outcomes are TLR, clinical and hemodynamic outcome, amputation rate, mortality rate, adverse events, and device-specific adverse events.

The PRIMUS DEB (Cardionovum Sp) is similar to LegFlow (shelloic acid coating and nanoparticles of paclitaxel) and showed good performance in a first-in-man study involving 19 patients with coronary lesions.[38]

TIPS AND TRICKS FOR USE OF DRUG-ELUTING BALLOONS

To facilitate and ensure efficacy and uniform drug transfer to the vessel wall, pretreatment of the diseased vessel segment is recommended. Lesions can be prepared by the preliminary use of an uncoated balloon or a debulking device (atherectomy), particularly for heavily calcified lesions. Avoiding any "geographic miss" is also important; the length of the segment treated with the DEB must be the same as the segment predilated. In

the LEVANT 1 trial, accurate balloon apposition was associated with a better primary patency at 1 year (85.7% vs 44.4%) when misplacement of the balloon occurred. The use of landmarks or rules to guide the procedure should be encouraged. Accurate handling of devices and adequate insufflation times must be observed to avoid paclitaxel loss.

OTHER DRUG-ELUTING BALLOON APPLICATIONS
Dialysis Access

Percutaneous treatment of failing dialysis access with balloons or stents is associated with poor 1-year outcomes.[39,40] DEBs have been successfully used in 2 pivotal trials in the treatment of those lesions that occur at the venous anastomosis site of synthetic grafts or fistulas. The 6-month primary patency rates were significantly higher in the DEB group (IN.PACT Amphirion paclitaxel, coated) compared with the uncoated balloon group. Thus, the beneficial role of DEBs in the management of recurrent dialysis access failure needs to be further explored.[41,42]

No-Stenting Zone

The FP vasculature includes some relative no-stent zones in which the use of DEBs is beneficial. Included are:

- The common femoral artery, the function of which is essential for several reasons. It gives origin to the profunda femoral artery, which is the most important source of collateral branches in case of SFA occlusion. It is a site suitable for various types of bypasses.
- The ostial SFA. Stenting in this area can be challenging because of angles at the bifurcating ostia of the SFA and profunda femoral artery. Moreover, debulking devices can cause saddle embolization or perforation.
- Restenotic bypass grafts.

DRUG-ELUTING DEVICES AND IN-STENT RESTENOSIS

Mimicking the results reported in the treatment of coronary ISR, drug-eluting technologies have shown promising performance in the management of SFA ISR.[43] In a subcohort of 108 patients (119 lesions; mean lesion length, 133 mm) with ISR from the ZILVER-PTX trial, primary patency of 95.7% at 6 months and of 78.8% at 1 year were reported. Freedom from clinically driven TLR was 81% at 1 year and 60.8% at 2 years. Moreover, only 1.2% of the stents used in this study had detectable fractures at 12 months, and significant improvements in ankle-brachial index, walking and climbing distance, and Rutherford class were observed at 2 years.[44]

Promising data on the use of DEBs for the treatment of SFA-ISR come from a single center, prospective registry involving 39 patients (48.7% diabetics, 20.5% with CLI); all patients underwent conventional SFA PTA and postdilation with a paclitaxel-eluting balloon (IN.PACT). In 10% of patients, bailout stent placement was required to treat flow-limiting dissection. Technical and procedural success was achieved in all patients, and 1-year primary patency was 92.1%. This strategy has proven to be safe and effective at up

Table 3
Ongoing or planned randomized drug-eluting balloon trials

Trial	DEB	Comparator	Endpoint
Femoropopliteal *de novo* lesions			
RIVER	Paclitaxel coated	POBA	12 M patency (DUS)
ISAR-STATH (NCT00986752)	Paclitaxel-urea coated plus stent	Atherectomy or stent	6 M % diameter stenosis (DUS)
LEVANT 2 (NCT01412541)	Paclitaxel polysorbate/ sorbitol coated	Balloon angioplasty	12 M patency (DUS) 12 M freedom from index limb amputation, index limb re-intervention, and index-limb-related death
RAPID	Paclitaxel-shellac coated plus stent	Balloon angioplasty plus stent	12 M binary restenosis
IN.PACT SFA II (NCT01566461)	Paclitaxel-urea coated	Balloon angioplasty	12 M freedom from clinically driven TLR and from restenosis (DUS)
Advance 18 PTX Trial (NCT00776906)	Paclitaxel coated	Bare balloon	6 M late lumen loss
Freeride (NCT01960647)	Paclitaxel coated	Balloon angioplasty	6 M rate of clinically driven TLR
Femoropopliteal in-stent restenois			
COPA CABANA (NCT01594684)	Paclitaxel-iopromide coated	Balloon angioplasty	6 M late lumen loss
ISAR-PEBIS (NCT01083394)	Paclitaxel-urea coated	Balloon angioplasty	6 M % diameter stenosis (DUS)
PHOTOPAC (NCT01298947)	Paclitaxel coated	Laser atherectomy + DEB	12 M target lesion % stenosis
PACUBA I (NCT01247402)	Paclitaxel coated	Balloon angioplasty	6 M patency (DUS)
Below-the-knee de novo lesions			
ADCAT (NCT01763476)	Paclitaxel-urea coated	Atherectomy plus paclitaxel–urea-coated	6 M patency (DUS)
LUTONIX BTK (NCT01870401)	Paclitaxelpolysorbate/ sorbitol coated	Balloon angioplasty	1 M freedom from major adverse limb events and all-cause death
PICCOLO (NCT00696956)	Paclitaxel coated	Balloon angioplasty	6 M late lumen loss
EURO CANAL (NCT01260870)	Paclitaxel coated	Balloon angioplasty	1 M procedural safety
Below-the-knee in-stent restenosis			
BAIR (NCT01398033)	Paclitaxel-urea coated	Balloon angioplasty	3 M patency (angiography)

Abbreviations: DUS, Doppler UltraSound; M, months.

2 years' follow-up with a primary patency rate of 70.3%.[45,46]

In the Drug Eluting Balloon in Peripheral Intervention for the Superficial Femoral Artery (DEBATE) trial, treatment of ISR with DEB (44 patients, 64% with CLI) showed a significant reduction in restenosis recurrence when compared with conventional PTA. Primary patency and TLR at 12 months were 90.5% and 13.6%, respectively.[47]

Results of the multicenter, prospective Femoral Artery In-stent Restenosis Trial (FAIR) have been announced at Leipzig Interventional Course 2014. In 119 patients randomly assigned to DEB (IN.PACT Admiral; n = 62) or standard PTA (n = 57), the DEB strategy resulted in significantly decreased restenosis and clinically driven reinterventions through 6 and 12 months (15.4% vs 44.7% and 29.5% vs 62.5%, respectively); freedom from TLR was significantly lowered in the DEB group (90.8% vs 52.6%, P = .0001); clinical and functional benefit were similar in both groups at the price of significantly higher TLR in the PTA arm.

Ongoing randomized trials will address the unsolved issues about DEB performance in ISR lesions.

DRUG-ELUTING BIORESORBABLE SCAFFOLDS

Bioresorbable DES may have a dual role in overcoming limitations of both DES and DEBs in that they could avoid elastic recoil and flow-limiting dissection and could, at the same time, provide adequate drug transfer into the arterial wall with a temporary scaffold. The resorption that occurs after a predictable time allows the restoration of normal vessel function and eliminates the potential trigger for chronic inflammatory vessel reaction.

After the disappointing results obtained with the Igaki-Tamai device in the PERSEUS trial (primary patency decreased at 1 year from 90% to 40%–50%), novel expectations lie in the Absorb bioresorbable Vascular Scaffold, BVS (Abbott Vascular, Santa Clara, CA, USA). It releases everolimus while nonenzymatic hydrolysis of polymer and coating occurs. After 24 to 36 months, stent struts are completely replaced by SMCs.[48] The ESPRIT I trail is a single-arm, multicenter, prospective trial investigating the safety and performance of the Esprit BVS in patients (n = 35) with iliac or SFA lesions. At 30 days, preliminary results showed 100% technical success, no occurrence of clinical events or scaffold thrombosis, no binary restenosis on duplex evaluation, and a significant clinical improvement (percentage of severe claudicants decreased from 57% at baseline to 0% at 1 month).

OPEN QUESTIONS

More robust clinical evidence is needed to justify the role of drug-eluting devices as the new gold standard for the treatment of FP and BTK arteries. In particular, issues to be addressed include:

Drug-eluting Stents
- Can the permanent scaffold represent a problem for recrossing or future bypass grafting?
- How can the distribution of drug in the vessel wall be made more heterogeneous?
- Is there a sufficient economic benefit in their widespread use for the treatment of de novo lesions?

Drug-eluting Balloons
- How can they deal with the problem of acute vessel recoil?
- What about their performance after subintimal recanalization or heavily calcified lesions?

Table 3 provides an overview of ongoing trials that could address these concerns.

SUMMARY

The currently available body of evidence conveys that drug-eluting technology is a promising, safe, and efficient tool in the treatment of PAD. It seems important to underline that results from randomized trials cannot be easily generalized for several reasons: (1) they do not reflect a real world population; (2) many studies have been carried out by experienced and highly skilled interventionalists or have been funded by industry; and (3) the late lumen loss, frequently used as a primary study endpoint, is rather a surrogate marker of efficacy compared with binary restenosis or TLR.

To summarize current knowledge, however, it seems that a new paradigm must be formulated favoring the use of DES in FP and BTK arteries because DEBs represent useful tools in shorter lesions, ISR, and no-stenting zones. Their long-term performance in calcific lesions and occlusions could be improved by the additional use of debulking strategies.

REFERENCES

1. Adam DJ, Beard JD, Cleveland T, et al. Bypass versus angioplasty in severe ischaemia of the leg (BASIL): multicentre, randomised controlled trial. Lancet 2005;366(9501):1925–34.
2. Deloose K, Lauwers K, Callaert J, et al. Drug-eluting technologies in femoral artery lesions. J Cardiovasc Surg (Torino) 2013;54(2):217–24.

3. Schillinger M, Sabeti S, Loewe C, et al. Balloon angioplasty versus implantation of nitinol stents in the superficial femoral artery. N Engl J Med 2006; 354(18):1879–88.

4. Laird JR, Katzen BT, Scheinert D, et al. Nitinol stent implantation versus balloon angioplasty for lesions in the superficial femoral artery and proximal popliteal artery: twelve-month results from the RESILIENT randomized trial. Circ Cardiovasc Interv 2010;3(3):267–76.

5. Kasapis C, Henke PK, Chetcuti SJ, et al. Routine stent implantation vs. percutaneous transluminal angioplasty in femoropopliteal artery disease: a meta-analysis of randomized controlled trials. Eur Heart J 2009;30(1):44–55.

6. Schillinger M, Minar E. Percutaneous treatment of peripheral artery disease: novel techniques. Circulation 2012;126(20):2433–40.

7. Johnston KW. Femoral and popliteal arteries: reanalysis of results of balloon angioplasty. Radiology 1992;183(3):767–71.

8. Schillinger M, Sabeti S, Dick P, et al. Sustained benefit at 2 years of primary femoropopliteal stenting compared with balloon angioplasty with optional stenting. Circulation 2007;115(21):2745–9.

9. Krankenberg H, Schlüter M, Steinkamp HJ, et al. Nitinol stent implantation versus percutaneous transluminal angioplasty in superficial femoral artery lesions up to 10 cm in length: the femoral artery stenting trial (FAST). Circulation 2007;116(3):285–92.

10. Dick P, Wallner H, Sabeti S, et al. Balloon angioplasty versus stenting with nitinol stents in intermediate length superficial femoral artery lesions. Catheter Cardiovasc Interv 2009;74(7):1090–5.

11. Scheinert D, Grummt L, Piorkowski M, et al. A novel self-expanding interwoven nitinol stent for complex femoropopliteal lesions: 24-month results of the SUPERA SFA registry. J Endovasc Ther 2011; 18(6):745–52.

12. Sixt S, Scheinert D, Rastan A, et al. One-year outcome after percutaneous rotational and aspiration atherectomy in infrainguinal arteries in patient with and without type 2 diabetes mellitus. Ann Vasc Surg 2011;25(4):520–9.

13. Kedora J, Hohmann S, Garrett W, et al. Randomized comparison of percutaneous Viabahn stent grafts vs prosthetic femoral-popliteal bypass in the treatment of superficial femoral arterial occlusive disease. J Vasc Surg 2007;45(1):10–6 [discussion: 16].

14. Randon C, Jacobs B, De Ryck F, et al. Angioplasty or primary stenting for infrapopliteal lesions: results of a prospective randomized trial. Cardiovasc Intervent Radiol 2010;33(2):260–9.

15. Biondi-Zoccai GG, Sangiorgi G, Lotrionte M, et al. Infragenicular stent implantation for below-the-knee atherosclerotic disease: clinical evidence from an international collaborative meta-analysis on 640 patients. J Endovasc Ther 2009;16(3):251–60.

16. Byrne RA, Joner M, Alfonso F, et al. Drug-coated balloon therapy in coronary and peripheral artery disease. Nat Rev Cardiol 2014;11(1):13–23.

17. Seedial SM, Ghosh S, Saunders RS. Local drug delivery to prevent restenosis. J Vasc Surg 2013; 57(5):1403–14.

18. Stefanini GG, Holmes DR Jr. Drug-eluting coronary artery stents. N Engl J Med 2013;368(3):254–65.

19. Marx SO, Jayaraman T, Go LO, et al. Rapamycin FKBP inhibits cell cycle regulators of proliferation in vascular smooth muscle cells. Circ Res 1995; 76(3):412–7.

20. Duda SH, Bosiers M, Lammer J, et al. Sirolimus eluting versus bare nitinol stent for obstructive superficial femoral artery disease: the SIROCCO I trial. J Vasc Interv Radiol 2005;16(3):331–8.

21. Duda SH, Bosiers M, Lammer J, et al. Drug-eluting and bare nitinol stents for the treatment of atherosclerotic lesions in the superficial femoral artery long-term results from the SIROCCO trial J Endovasc Ther 2006;13(6):701–10.

22. Dake MD, Scheinert D, Tepe G, et al. Nitinol stents with polymer-free paclitaxel coating for lesions in the superficial femoral and popliteal arteries above the knee: twelve-month safety and effectiveness results from the Zilver PTX single-arm clinical study J Endovasc Ther 2011;18(5):613–23.

23. Dake MD, Ansel GM, Jaff MR, et al. Paclitaxel-eluting stents show superiority to balloon angioplasty and bare metal stents in femoropopliteal disease: twelve-month Zilver PTX randomized study results. Circ Cardiovasc Interv 2011;4(5): 495–504.

24. Dake MD, Ansel GM, Jaff MR, et al. Sustained safety and effectiveness of paclitaxel-eluting stents for femoropopliteal lesions: 2-year follow-up from the Zilver PTX randomized and single-arm clinical studies. J Am Coll Cardiol 2013;61(24):2417–27.

25. Lammer J, Bosiers M, Zeller T, et al. First clinical trial of nitinol self-expanding everolimus-eluting stent implantation for peripheral arterial occlusive disease. J Vasc Surg 2011;54(2):394–401.

26. Varcoe RL. Drug eluting stents in the treatment of below the knee arterial occlusive disease. J Cardiovasc Surg (Torino) 2013;54(3):313–25.

27. Rastan A, Brechtel K, Krankenberg H, et al. Sirolimus-eluting stents for treatment of infrapopliteal arteries reduce clinical event rate compared to bare-metal stents: long-term results from a randomized trial. J Am Coll Cardiol 2012;60(7):587–91.

28. Bosiers M, Scheinert D, Peeters P, et al. Randomized comparison of everolimus-eluting versus bare-metal stents in patients with critical limb ischemia and infrapopliteal arterial occlusive disease. J Vasc Surg 2012;55(2):390–8.

29. Scheinert D, Katsanos K, Zeller T, et al. A prospective randomized multicenter comparison of balloon

angioplasty and infrapopliteal stenting with the sirolimus-eluting stent in patients with ischemic peripheral arterial disease: 1-year results from the ACHILLES trial. J Am Coll Cardiol 2012;60(22): 2290–5.

30. Feiring AJ, Krahn M, Nelson L, et al. Preventing leg amputations in critical limb ischemia with below-the-knee drug-eluting stents: the PaRADISE (PReventing Amputations using Drug eluting StEnts) trial. J Am Coll Cardiol 2010;55(15):1580–9.

31. Fusaro M, Cassese S, Ndrepepa G, et al. Drug-eluting stents for revascularization of infrapopliteal arteries: updated meta-analysis of randomized trials. JACC Cardiovasc Interv 2013;6(12):1284–93.

32. Werk M, Langner S, Reinkensmeier B, et al. Inhibition of restenosis in femoropopliteal arteries: paclitaxel-coated versus uncoated balloon: femoral paclitaxel randomized pilot trial. Circulation 2008; 118(13):1358–65.

33. Scheinert D, Duda S, Zeller T, et al. The LEVANT I (Lutonix paclitaxel-coated balloon for the prevention of femoropopliteal restenosis) trial for femoropopliteal revascularization: first-in-human randomized trial of low-dose drug-coated balloon versus uncoated balloon angioplasty. JACC Cardiovasc Interv 2014;7(1):10–9.

34. Werk M, Albrecht T, Meyer DR, et al. Paclitaxel-coated balloons reduce restenosis after femoropopliteal angioplasty: evidence from the randomized PACIFIER trial. Circ Cardiovasc Interv 2012;5(6): 831–40.

35. Fanelli F, Cannavale A, Boatta E, et al. Lower limb multilevel treatment with drug-eluting balloons: 6-month results from the DEBELLUM randomized trial. J Endovasc Ther 2012;19(5):571–80.

36. Liistro F, Grotti S, Porto I, et al. Drug-eluting balloon in peripheral intervention for the superficial femoral artery: the DEBATE-SFA randomized trial (drug eluting balloon in peripheral intervention for the superficial femoral artery). JACC Cardiovasc Interv 2013,0(12).1295–302.

37. Liistro F, Porto I, Angioli P, et al. Drug-eluting balloon in peripheral intervention for below the knee angioplasty evaluation (DEBATE-BTK): a randomized trial in diabetic patients with critical limb ischemia. Circulation 2013;128(6):615–21.

38. Karimi A, de Boer SW, van den Heuvel DA, et al. Randomized trial of Legflow((R)) paclitaxel eluting balloon and stenting versus standard percutaneous transluminal angioplasty and stenting for the treatment of intermediate and long lesions of the superficial femoral artery (RAPID trial): study protocol for a randomized controlled trial. Trials 2013;14:87.

39. Bittl JA. Catheter interventions for hemodialysis fistulas and grafts. JACC Cardiovasc Interv 2010; 3(1):1–11.

40. Kanterman RY, Vesely TM, Pilgram TK, et al. Dialysis access grafts: anatomic location of venous stenosis and results of angioplasty. Radiology 1995;195(1): 135–9.

41. Haskal ZJ, Trerotola S, Dolmatch B. Stent graft versus balloon angioplasty for failing dialysis-access grafts. N Engl J Med 2010;362(6):494–503.

42. Kariya S, Tanigawa N, Kojima H, et al. Percutaneous transluminal cutting-balloon angioplasty for hemodialysis access stenoses resistant to conventional balloon angioplasty. Acta Radiol 2006;47(10):1017–21.

43. Franzone A, Stabile E, Carbone A, et al. Management of in-stent restenosis in peripheral arteries: are DEBs sufficient as stand-alone treatment for femoro-popliteal in-stent restenosis? J Cardiovasc Surg (Torino) 2014;55(3):335–8.

44. Zeller T, Dake MD, Tepe G, et al. Treatment of femoropopliteal in-stent restenosis with paclitaxel-eluting stents. JACC Cardiovasc Interv 2013;6(3): 274–81.

45. Stabile E, Virga V, Salemme L, et al. Drug-eluting balloon for treatment of superficial femoral artery in-stent restenosis. J Am Coll Cardiol 2012;60(18): 1739–42.

46. Virga V, Stabile E, Biamino G, et al. Drug-eluting balloons for the treatment of the superficial femoral artery in-stent restenosis: 2-year follow-up. JACC Cardiovasc Interv 2014;7(4):411–5.

47. Liistro F, Porto I, Grotti S, et al. Drug-eluting balloon angioplasty for carotid in-stent restenosis. J Endovasc Ther 2012;19(6):729–33.

48. Oberhauser JP, Hossainy S, Rapoza RJ. Design principles and performance of bioresorbable polymeric vascular scaffolds. EuroIntervention 2009; 5(Suppl F):F15–22.

49. Commeau P, Barragan P, Roquebert PO. Sirolimus for below the knee lesions: mid-term results of SiroBTK study. Catheter Cardiovasc Interv 2006; 68(5):793–8.

50. Scheinert D. Comparison of sirolimus-eluting vs bare-metal stents for the treatment of infrapopliteal obstructions. EuroIntervention 2006;2(2):169–74.

51. Bosiers M. Percutaneous transluminal angioplasty for treatment of 'below-the-knee' critical limb ischemia: early outcomes following the use of sirolimus-eluting stents. J Cardiovasc Surg (Torino) 2006; 47(2):171–6.

52. Feiring AJ, Wesolowski AA. Antegrade popliteal artery approach for the treatment of critical limb ischemia in patients with occluded superficial femoral arteries. Catheter Cardiovasc Interv 2007; 69(5):665–70.

53. Siablis D. Sirolimus-eluting versus bare stents after suboptimal infrapopliteal angioplasty for critical limb ischemia: enduring 1-year angiographic and clinical benefit. J Endovasc Ther 2007;14(2): 241–50.

54. Siablis D. Infrapopliteal application of paclitaxel-eluting stents for critical limb ischemia: midterm angiographic and clinical results. J Vasc Interv Radiol 2007;18(11):1351–61.
55. Grant AG. Infrapopliteal drug-eluting stents for chronic limb ischemia. Catheter Cardiovasc Interv 2008;71(1):108–11.
56. Rosales OR, Mathewkutty S, Gnaim C. Drug eluting stents for below the knee lesions in patients with critical limb ischemia: long-term follow-up. Catheter Cardiovasc Interv 2008;72(1):112–5.
57. Siablis D. Infrapopliteal application of sirolimus-eluting versus bare metal stents for critical limb ischemia: analysis of long-term angiographic and clinical outcome. J Vasc Interv Radiol 2009;20(9):1141–50.
58. Rastan A. Primary use of sirolimus-eluting stents in the infrapopliteal arteries. J Endovasc Ther 2010; 17(4):480–7.
59. Balzer JO. Percutaneous interventions below the knee in patients with critical limb ischemia using drug eluting stents. J Cardiovasc Surg (Torino) 2010;51(2):183–91.
60. Karnabatidis D. Primary everolimus-eluting stenting versus balloon angioplasty with bailout bare metal stenting of long infrapopliteal lesions for treatment of critical limb ischemia. J Endovasc Ther 2011; 18(1):1–12.
61. Werner M. Sirolimus-eluting stents for the treatment of infrapopliteal arteries in chronic limb ischemia: long-term clinical and angiographic follow-up. J Endovasc Ther 2012;19(1):12–9.

Index

Note: Page numbers of article titles are in **boldface** type.

0733-8651/15/$ – see front matter © 2015 Elsevier Inc. All rights reserved.

Moving?

Make sure your subscription moves with you!

To notify us of your new address, find your **Clinics Account Number** (located on your mailing label above your name), and contact customer service at:

Email: journalscustomerservice-usa@elsevier.com

800-654-2452 (subscribers in the U.S. & Canada)
314-447-8871 (subscribers outside of the U.S. & Canada)

Fax number: 314-447-8029

Elsevier Health Sciences Division
Subscription Customer Service
3251 Riverport Lane
Maryland Heights, MO 63043

*To ensure uninterrupted delivery of your subscription,
please notify us at least 4 weeks in advance of move.

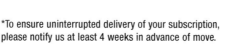